Mental Health in Historical Perspective

Series Editors

Catharine Coleborne, School of Humanities and Social Science,
University of Newcastle, Callaghan, NSW, Australia
Matthew Smith, Centre for the Social History of Health and Healthcare,
University of Strathclyde, Glasgow, UK

Covering all historical periods and geographical contexts, the series explores how mental illness has been understood, experienced, diagnosed, treated and contested. It will publish works that engage actively with contemporary debates related to mental health and, as such, will be of interest not only to historians, but also mental health professionals, patients and policy makers. With its focus on mental health, rather than just psychiatry, the series will endeavour to provide more patient-centred histories. Although this has long been an aim of health historians, it has not been realised, and this series aims to change that.

The scope of the series is kept as broad as possible to attract good quality proposals about all aspects of the history of mental health from all periods. The series emphasises interdisciplinary approaches to the field of study, and encourages short titles, longer works, collections, and titles which stretch the boundaries of academic publishing in new ways.

Kevin Matthew Jones

Psychological Classification and Diagnosis in Asylum Statistics, 1800–1948

The British Table of the Forms of Insanity

palgrave
macmillan

Kevin Matthew Jones
Department of History
University of Nottingham
Nottingham, UK

ISSN 2634-6036 ISSN 2634-6044 (electronic)
Mental Health in Historical Perspective
ISBN 978-3-031-46156-9 ISBN 978-3-031-46154-5 (eBook)
https://doi.org/10.1007/978-3-031-46154-5

This Palgrave Macmillan imprint is published by the registered company Springer Nature Switzerland AG
The registered company address is: Gewerbestrasse 11, 6330 Cham, Switzerland

After initial publication of the book, minor corrections to the text were made. These do not constitute a substantive change to the book's contents.

For Judith, Leonard, Maurice and Philip.

Acknowledgements

Many people have generously given their time, knowledge and expertise to help complete this volume. Firstly, the study would not have been possible without the continued support of the Centre for the History and Philosophy of Science at the University of Leeds. Aside from the financial support granted to help complete the study during my doctorate, I am grateful to have been based in a unique and eclectic research environment during my postdoctoral years. I would like to thank fellow Ph.D. students who were a source of support and encouragement during my time completing the thesis on which this volume is based, and Dr. Michael Finn and Dr. Adrian Wilson for their sagacity as dissertation supervisors, and their continued support as colleagues in Leeds. I would like to thank Professor Jonathan Topham for offering his encyclopaedic knowledge of Victorian periodicals and the finer details of scientific publications; this was indispensable for helping to develop the work presented in the first two chapters of this volume. I would like to thank Professor Gregory Radick for his tips on investigations into insanity conducted by the Galton Laboratories during the first years of the twentieth century, and the broader links between psychiatry and genetics. I am grateful to the organisers of the many conferences who have provided me with the opportunity to present the research included in this volume in some form or another. In particular, I would like to thank the British Society for the History of Science; the Committee for the Integrated History and Philosophy of Science; the History, Science, Technology and Medicine

Network of Ireland; the Northern Network for Medical Humanities; and the International Society for the History, Philosophy, and Social Studies of Biology (ISHPSSB). The Philosophy of Psychiatry workshop at Lancaster University also deserves special mention for helping to develop this work during its early stages, as does the Foundlaw Project's Conceptual Change in History Conference at the University of Helsinki in 2016. During the final stages of the project, I was lucky enough to spend eighteen months at the National Archives, where I could appreciate first-hand the hard work and skill of librarians and archivists. I would like to thank Dr. Jenny Bunn for her patient guidance during my time there, the rest of the Research and Academic Engagement team, and Barbara Packard and Jo Pugh for their insights into the archives sector. I would also like to acknowledge the efforts of archivists at the Wellcome Institute, the Royal College of Psychiatrists, UCL Special Collections and the West Yorkshire Archive Services.

Many have generously given their time over the years to look through material that has found its way into this volume. In particular, I would like to thank Mike and Adrian again for having read the work at an early stage. I would like to thank Sean Dyde for looking over a great deal of the material from the first section, and having the gumption to tear into the early drafts of the work. Åsa Jansson's helpful insights on an early version of the third chapter 3 gave me the conviction that I was on to something with the history of the Table of the Forms. Thanks also to Jennifer Wallis and Chris Millard for having taken the time to critically assess chapters from this volume in various embryonic forms. I would like to thank Rhodri Hayward for acting as an external examiner as this work monograph builds upon the discussion conducted during the viva voce examination. Thanks to Dr. Chris Renwick and Dr. Amanda Rees for their help in developing the research during my postdoc period, especially the material related to the International Classification of Diseases and the National Health Service presented in the final chapter. I would also like to thank Professor Rachel Cooper and Professor David Healy for providing useful pointers that have enriched the research. I would like to acknowledge Professor Joe Cain's recent guide to the research publications of the Galton Laboratory was incredibly helpful.[1] Finally, I would

[1] Joe Cain, 'Publications produced by the Francis Galton Laboratory for National Eugenics' in *The Library*, vol.22, no.4, pp.523-548.

like to thank Dr. Andrew Edgar for being a source of continuing scholarly inspiration over the years: our conversations, whether on the history of magic or Frankfurt School philosophy have found their way into this book in some form or another.

Praise for *Psychological Classification and Diagnosis in Asylum Statistics, 1800–1948*

"Kevin Jones's book provides the first detailed reconstruction of the nineteenth and twentieth-century debates about psychiatric classification. These classifications are now foundational to the ways we see ourselves and our relationships with others, so much so that it is difficult to imagine life without them. Problems in the workplace, classroom or family home are often framed through reference to putative psychiatric diagnoses or psychological conditions. This transformation has been widely commented upon, but an overarching historical analysis of these categories has been absent. Moving from the Victorian statistical Tables of Insanity through to the World Health Organisation's International Classification of Diseases, Jones presents a thoughtful and intelligent analysis of the medical debates that ground the identities we live with in Britain today."

—Rhodri Hayward, *Reader, Queen Mary University London*

"The media give supposed psychiatric classifications, like the American Diagnostic and Statistics Manual (DSM), extensive coverage in debates about mental illness. DSM looks like a classification system that makes mental illness a part of medicine but it's not. It's a dictionary of symptoms or collections of symptoms. For nearly two centuries there has been a confusing divide between dictionaries and classifications, beginning with the Table of Forms put in place to track outcomes and value for money in British asylums. Kevin Jones' fascinating account of a century of debate on how to do this sheds light on problems that endure today."

—David Healy, *Professor of Psychiatry, Bangor University*

Terminology

Although I have made attempts to clarify terminology throughout the book, I thought it wise to include the following notes of clarification and explanation of key terms.

The Table of the Forms of Insanity/Mental Disorder: The document was known for much of its life as the Table of the Forms of Insanity until the final round of revisions were undertaken by the MPA in 1934. This is when it became known as the 'Table of the Forms of Mental Disorder'. For brevity's sake, I refer to it generally as the 'Table of the Forms', but when I am specifically referring to the document that was used from 1845 until the beginning of the twentieth century, I refer to it as the 'Table of the Forms of Insanity'. In the fourth chapter onwards, which covers the period between 1932 and 1948, I refer to the document as 'the Table of the Forms of Mental Disorder'. There are parts of the work when the Table of the Forms reads awkwardly and saying 'classification' would make it read more elegantly, but I have decided to continue using 'Table of the Forms' because it expresses the ambiguous function of the document, with some believing that it described different manifestations of one disease, and others regarding it as classifying different species or natural kinds.

The Medico-Psychological Association of Great Britain and Ireland (MPA): The Medico-Psychological Association has existed under four different guises since its establishment: the Association of Medical Officers of Asylums and Hospitals for the Insane between 1841 and 1865, the Medico-Psychological Association from then until it received its Royal Charter in 1926 from whence it became the Royal Medico-Psychological Association until 1971 when it became the Royal College of Psychiatrists. I attempt to use the historically correct moniker where appropriate, but the Medico-Psychological Association, or simply 'the Association' has been used as the defaults when discussing a period that straddles change in name.

The Commissioners in Lunacy for England and Wales: I have referred to this as the Lunacy Commission for a great deal of this study for simplicity's sake, and have specified when I am talking about similar bodies in Scotland and Ireland.

1882 Revision: This refers to the Table of the Forms that was published after the first series of revisions taking place between 1869 and 1881. For simplicity's sake, I have, as with the other revisions to the document, referred to them by the date they were published.

1907 Revision: As above, this refers to the second set of revisions that took place between 1902 and 1906, and which was formally published in 1907.

1934 Revision: This refers to the final set of revisions to the Table, which took place between 1929 and 1932 and was published in 1934.

1845 Lunacy Act: For much of the text, I use the term 1845 Lunacy Act to refer to both the Lunacy Act and the County Asylums Act of 1845. The two acts were passed simultaneously and were designed to work in conjunction. Until the next piece of landmark legislation was passed with the 1890 Lunacy Act, both acts were repealed and replaced by amendment acts during the intervening years. It would be technically correct to refer to them by name, but I fear this would be unnecessarily confusing and detract from the purposes of this study, so I have followed a convention in the history of medicine to refer to the acts as the 1845 Lunacy Act.

International Statistical Classification of Diseases, Injuries and Causes of Death (ICD): This study ends with the adoption of the World Health Organisation's first formal classification of diseases, the International Statistical Classification of Diseases, Injuries and Causes of Death. This has come to be known as the ICD-6, or sixth edition, since it was based on the International List of Causes of Death that had been developed by a number of organisations, but most prominently, the Statistical Services of Paris under the chairmanship of Jacques Bertillon, and the International Statistical Institute. The convention is to call it the sixth edition since five International Conferences for the Revision of the International List of Causes of Death had sat. Labelling the World Health Organisation's classification the sixth edition is of questionable accuracy since it was the first to not be limited to causes of death by including diseases and mental health conditions. It therefore stands as the first international classification of diseases. Since this study only considers the 1948 ICD, I have decided to refer to it simply as the ICD and not include the '6'.

Contents

About the Author

Kevin Matthew Jones is a Lecturer in History at the University of Nottingham.

List of Figures

List of Tables

CHAPTER 1

Introduction

> Why do you keep me here?
> Because you are ill.
> Yes, I am ill. But surely there are scores of madmen, hundreds, walking about unmolested, simply because in your ignorance you're incapable of distinguishing them from healthy people! Why then should I and these unhappy wretches be kept here, like so many scapegoats for the others? You, your assistant, the superintendent, and the rest for the scoundrels employed in the hospital - you're morally infinitely lower than any of us! Why then must we be kept here and not you? Where's the logic?
> I'm afraid morality and logic have nothing to do with it. It's all a matter of chance. Those who are put here stay here, and those who are not here are free to live as they like. That's all. There's neither morality nor logic in the fact that I am a doctor and you are a mental patient. It's just mere *chance*.
> 'I don't understand this nonsense,' Gromov said in a dull voice, sitting down on his bed.
> Anton Pavlovich Chekhov, *Ward no.6*, 1892.

This book explores the development of the terminology used to diagnose psychological conditions and their use in mental health statistics collected by lunacy administration and public health authorities. It does so through the presentation of the story of the Table of the Forms, a list of

K. M. Jones, *Psychological Classification and Diagnosis in Asylum Statistics, 1800–1948*, Mental Health in Historical Perspective,
https://doi.org/10.1007/978-3-031-46154-5_1

diagnostic categories used in Britain between 1845 and 1948. The Table of the Forms' principal use was in statistical paperwork used to collect patient data returned from asylums. The story presented in this volume begins with large-scale expansion of the asylum system that commenced with the passing of the 1845 Lunacy Act and ends with changes to health services included under the terms of the 1946 National Health Service Act. As we will see, the history of psychological diagnosis cannot be told without charting concurrent developments in asylum administration that shaped mental health statistics. Although statistics were initially considered a matter for bureaucracy and asylum administration, interest in the scientific potentials for statistical enquiry increased throughout the second half of the nineteenth century and peaked at the beginning of the twentieth century. The discussions over classification used in asylum statistics that are assessed in this volume involved not only medical staff, but also statisticians, lunacy administration and public health officials. The efforts to standardise psychological diagnosis caused disagreement and controversy, leading to drawn out debates that hampered measures to develop national statistics on psychological diagnosis. As interest grew in the scientific potential of asylum medical statistics on classification, the debates surrounding the Table of the Forms intensified. This is within the context of an increased interest in vital statistics during the Victorian period that ran alongside the expansion of the asylum system during the second half of the nineteenth century.[1]

The diagnostic terms included in The Table of the Forms are the closest to being a set of standard terms used in British asylums during the heyday of the Victorian Asylum, and for much of the first half of the twentieth century. The requirement to collect and submit patient information marked the beginning of an age of mass mental health data collection that continues today. The document's use as a table in statistical paperwork made it tantamount to being the standard classification of psychological diagnosis between 1845 and the implementation of the NHS in 1948. It stood at the centre of debates over the standardisation of terms used in diagnosis to enable the compilation of statistics on psychological diagnosis. It came into existence as a result of legal changes introduced under the terms of the 1845 Lunacy and the County

[1] Eileen Magnello, 'The Introduction of Mathematical Statistics into Medical Research: The Roles of Karl Pearson, Major Greenwood and Austin Bradford Hill' in *The Road to Medical Statistics*, edited by Eileen Magnello and Ann Hardy, Rodopi, 2002, pp. 95–123.

Asylums Acts. This legislation led to the massive expansion of the asylum system and made doctors running these institutions legally responsible for recording information about any person admitted. From this point on, asylums were legally obliged to collect and record information on all who passed through the doors of the institution, and this included the psychological diagnosis they had received. The submission of patient data to authorities through annual statistical returns to the Lunacy Commission, the body established to oversee and regulate asylums, was also made a legal responsibility. These developments created large-scale mental health statistics in the form of asylum medical data, which would be published in annual reports of the Lunacy Commission. Although these developments did not lead immediately to national statistics on psychological diagnosis, they allowed the possibility for data on diagnosis from a large number of institutions to be compiled and analysed. Once the conditions for the collection of this data had been established, attention turned towards standardising the terms used in psychological diagnosis to make the data useful. This led to the Table of the Forms becoming the focus of an increasingly intense series of debates over the most appropriate means of standardising terms of psychological diagnosis.

The discussions would frequently emerge from revisions to bureaucratic procedures associated with the aforementioned legal obligations on patient record-keeping. Although the completion of statistical returns was usually the initial focus of attempts to revise the table, these attempts at standardisation frequently developed into broader philosophical disputes: these included what exactly was the nature of insanity, how should madness be understood by medical science and how should its different forms be classified. Revisions to administrative tables used for record-keeping purposes would at times escalate into all-out warfare between camps promoting fundamentally differing approaches to psychological diagnosis. The Table of the Forms would subsequently become subject to three sets of revisions undertaken by the principal representative body of alienists, the Medico-Psychological Association (MPA). The debates surrounding each of the revisions to the Table of the Forms constitute the focus of this study. The first of these revisions was published in 1882 after nearly two decades of debate over asylum medical statistics. These commenced in 1863 in reaction to a lecture that proposed a classification of insanity that would replace the forms of insanity then in use asylum medical statistics. The second revision was published in 1907 after an intense five-year long set of debates over psychological classification that were triggered by calls to change asylum admissions procedures. The final set of revisions were published in 1934 and were the last set of changes to the Table of the Forms as the document was replaced by the *International Classification of Diseases (ICD)* issued by the World Health Organisation in 1948. This was due to reforms to data collection processes and record-keeping protocols that were developed in anticipation of a new health service and were implemented under the terms of the 1946 National Health Service Act.

In its assessment of these developments, this volume argues that the interconnected history of the terms used in psychological diagnosis and their application in asylum statistics makes considerations of bureaucratic procedures an inexplicable part of understanding the history and philosophy of psychiatric classification.[2] In other words, the research presented in this volume shows that any account of what constitutes a mental disorder must incorporate the social and administrative factors that have shaped clinical diagnosis.

The Table of the Forms was a central feature of asylum medical statistics on psychological diagnosis, and it bears some resemblances to the classifications currently used in psychiatric epidemiology. Saying this, the Table defies many of the expectations we may have come to expect from a medical classification in the age of global epidemiology that developed since the Second World War. Psychiatric epidemiology is currently structured around the categories included in the WHO's *ICD* and the APA's *Diagnostic and Statistical Manual of Mental Disorders* (DSM).[3] Given the controversy surrounding it, the Table may appear to be a 'Victorian DSM' of sorts to those already acquainted with the recent history of psychiatric classification, and the division caused by the APA's diagnostic labels. This characterisation is in some ways helpful to make sense of the chequered history of the table, with the most apparent similarities being the role

[2] Charles Rosenberg, 'The Tyranny of Diagnosis: Specific Entities and Individual Experience' in *the Milbank Quarterly*, vol. 80, no. 2, June 2002, pp. 237–260.

[3] In his discussion of the origins of psychiatric epidemiology, Steeves Damazeux places many of the major developments in modern psychiatric epidemiology within the post-World War II era: Steeves Demazeux, 'Psychiatric Epidemiology, or the Story of a Divided Discipline' in *International Journal of Epidemiology*, vol. 43, 2014, pp. 53–66. See also: Harry Yi Jui-Wu, *Mad by the Millions, Mental Disorders and the Early Years of the World Health Organization*, MIT Press, 2021; Ana Antic, 'Transcultural Psychiatry: Cultural Difference, Universalism and Social Psychiatry in the Age of Decolonisation' in *Culture, Medicine, and Psychiatry*, vol. 45, 2021, pp. 359–384.

both have played in standardising diagnosis within mental health statistics. Similar controversies have surrounded both the Table of the Forms and the *DSM*, with quibbles over terminology often being based on broader philosophical considerations on what constitutes a mental health disorder, and what a psychiatric classification ought to achieve. Similarly, the historical actors engaged in debates over the Table of the Forms believed terms of psychological diagnosis should do nothing less than scientifically map natural kinds, whereas others did not think scientific classification equates to clinical or therapeutic effectiveness, which should be the priority over anything else.[4] Debates between these broad schools in the case of the Table were based on a conception of mental health that resembles what we now call the medical model, with the debates surrounding the Table of the Forms resting on similar assumptions that insanity was a biological, psychological or behavioural dysfunction.[5] Like the *DSM*, the Table of the Forms is also the product of a psychiatric association, and was a rival to the mental health classification drawn up by the Royal College of Physicians (RCP). As we will see, the mental health section of the *ICD*, which replaced the Table of the Forms for use in mental health statistics in the United Kingdom, was partly based upon the classification of the RCP and not the Table of the Forms.

There are however important differences that complicate a simple comparison between the Table of the Forms and the *DSM*. The scope and function of each of these psychiatric classifications are shaped by their differing historical contexts. The Table of the Forms came into existence at an embryonic point in the development of formal psychiatric diagnosis, medical bureaucracy and mental health statistics. Accordingly, its status as a classification is somewhat unstable, since it was originally conceived as a

[4] It is important to note that the arguments between these schools are not drawn along professional interests or boundaries, with many clinicians offering classifications they wanted to be regarded as scientific, and others thinking a science of diagnosis was not possible. Steve Sturdy cautions against overestimating tensions in scientific and clinical practice, claiming that an over-eagerness on the part of historians to write about conflict between the two has translated itself into a historiography that has provided a distorted view of an antagonistic relationship between science and the clinic; Steve Sturdy, 'Looking for Trouble: Medical Science and Clinical Practice in the Historiography of Modern Medicine' in *Social History of Medicine*, vol. 24, no. 3, pp. 739–757.

[5] Dan J. Stein, Katharine A. Phillips, Derek Bolton, K.W.M Fulford, John Z. Sadler, and Kenneth S. Kendler, 'What Is a Mental/Psychiatric Disorder? From DSM-IV to DSM-V' in *Psychological Medicine*, vol. 40, no. 11, November 2010, pp. 1759–1765.

set of recommended terms for use in record-keeping and the completion of asylum statistical returns. The document only came to be referred to as a 'classification' quite late on, around the time revisions were made to the document at the beginning of the twentieth century. In contrast, by the time of the *DSM*'s first edition in 1951, psychiatry was a well-established medical discipline, with the foundations of mental health epidemiology being established through a sprawling American asylum system that was accompanied by a well-developed national framework for the collection of asylum medical statistics. One of the key differences that reflects these differing historical contexts is that from the outset, the *DSM* included descriptions of the conditions it listed, whereas the Table of the Forms only included definitions very late on and not until the final 1934 Revision to the document. In addition, those revising the Table of the Forms did not make any attempt to provide a definition of terms like insanity, lunacy or mental disorder, whereas from the *DSM-III*, broad definitions of 'mental disorder' were added to serve as a foundation to the classification. These definitions of mental disorder have become as much a target of debate surrounding the *DSM* as the specific conditions included in the document.[6] Criticisms have come from a variety of perspectives, including those who do not think definitions of mental disorder have properly captured their status as natural kinds, and those who think that they do not capture their social or cultural character.

As we will see, although there are echoes of these debates present in the history of the Table of the Forms, it did not receive the same sort of criticisms since little attempt was made to provide the kinds of definitions that are present in more recent classifications of mental health conditions. Instead, operational terms like 'lunacy' and 'idiocy' relied on legal definitions included in the 1845 and 1890 Lunacy Acts, as well as the 1886 Idiot's Act. Responding to changes in legal definitions, from the 1907 Revision onwards, the Table came to be split into two sections to reflect legal distinctions between 'idiots', 'deficients', 'imbeciles' and 'lunatics'. Victorian legislation on lunacy provided definitions for 'lunatics' that differentiated this class of patients from other medico-legal categories. In following legal definitions of insanity, the committees revising the Table of the Forms relied on operational definitions that informed bureaucratic mechanisms set out by law and which enabled the collection of mental

[6] Allan V. Horwitz, *DSM: A History of Psychiatry's Bible*, John Hopkin University Press, 2021.

health statistics in the form of asylum medical data. When it came to the definitions for each of the disorders included in the Table, revisions committees rarely offered definitions of their own and instead relied upon the accumulated knowledge of medical publications. In doing so, the aim was to make a classification suitable for the overworked asylum doctor, whose practice lay between specialisms and before the advent of psychiatry as an established branch of medicine. In contrast, the American Psychiatric Association, as devisors of the *DSM*, proposed definitions of mental disorder and thereby could assert clinical definitions independently from law.

This study does not frame the development of the concepts of psychopathology included in the Table of the Forms in relation to those employed today. Whilst many of the problems over definition and classification encountered during these discussions are still being played out, I have emphasised the role they played in the communication and formulation of statistical knowledge on mental health between 1800 and 1948. This is an important historiographical point that the historian of medicine Adrian Wilsons explores in his analysis of past disease concepts; Wilson outlines a dialogue of sorts that has taken place between historians who have emphasised scientific discoveries and clinical breakthroughs in medical research, and those who argue that the formulation of clinical knowledge is a social process.[7] He warns of the danger of writing the history of disease concepts from the perspective of their role in the constitution of current knowledge, and that this can open 'a conceptual space in which the historicity of all disease-concepts, whether past or present, has been obliterated'.[8] Wilson views this as a problem specific to the history of science and medicine, with triumphant celebration of the discoveries of clinical science serving to bury the ideas of those who were ultimately proven to have held ideas not in line with the progression of knowledge.[9] Partly in response to Wilson, Andrew Cunningham suggests that to recover the historicity and contingent development of disease concepts, we must look at diagnostic procedures and labels.[10] When practitioners

[7] Adrian Wilson, 'On the History of Disease Concepts: The Case of Pleurisy' in *History of Science*, vol. 38, no. 3, 2000, pp. 271–319.

[8] Ibid., p. 273.

[9] Ibid.

[10] Andrew Cunningham, 'Identifying Disease in the Past: Cutting the Gordian Knot' in *Asclepio*, vol. 54, 2002, pp. 13–34.

diagnose, Cunningham claims they select from what he terms an 'array of available diseases' in any given period's clinical knowledge.[11] To highlight his point, Cunningham discusses and analyses statistical records which list the array of diseases available to coroners making diagnoses on causes of death during the seventeenth, nineteenth and the late twentieth centuries.[12] Causes of death are a particularly important resource for historians because the concept 'disease' was typically construed as causal by coroners when making post-mortem judgements. Historians should exercise caution and not take a listed cause of death at face value as a biological cause since the biological element of disease is just one component that a historian needs to pay attention to. To highlight his point, Cunningham uses the example of cancer to describe the social stigma that surrounds a disease.[13] The identity of a disease is made up 'of a compound of elements' according to Cunningham, and the biological and medical are just two of them.[14] Indeed, within historical research, these are not always the most important elements to consider, since a person's death may be *caused* by the disease to which the concept refers, but the disease concept cannot be reduced to the biomedical element and needs to be viewed in terms of the limitations of knowledge that shaped communication. Considerations on the social and cultural influences on the naming of diseases echo Ian Hacking's understanding of the looping effects of humankinds used by the social sciences and industrial bureaucracies to 'sort people, their actions and their behaviour' into discreet categories.[15] There is however a key difference, since Cunningham and Wilson do not seek to find the fact of the matter, and merely seek to chart the concept of disease through history whereas Hacking seeks to offer a positive and ontological thesis about the constitution of disease concepts,

[11] Ibid., p. 21.

[12] Ibid., p. 30.

[13] Cunningham describes how the social stigma surrounding cancer led to it being known as the 'disease which dare not speak its name' since cancer comes with 'overtones of dirt and shame, and of blame and punishment, which few other diseases have', and that since it attacks individuals one at a time, there is viewed to be some sort of responsibility the person feels for having brought it upon themselves. Ibid., pp. 18–20.

[14] Ibid.

[15] He contrasts these to the natural kinds of the natural sciences that are said to carve nature at the joints; Ian Hacking, 'The Looping Effects of Human Kinds' in *Causal Cognition: A Multidisciplinary Debate*, Oxford, 1996, pp. 352–382.

which for him is historical and cultural as much as it is a formal clinical exercise.[16] Similarly, Bowker and Star's discussion of the *ICD* addresses the extent to which social and cultural factors shaping medical conditions listed in the classification have been stripped away in favour of the biomedical.[17]

This study follows Cunningham and Wilson in its concern with the historiography of disease concepts, placing its emphasis on the bureaucratic context in which concepts of psychopathology have been developed. The history of the Table of the Forms is, then, the story of the development, within an administrative context, of a classification designed to standardise terms used in psychological diagnosis for the purposes of developing mental health statistics.[18] By providing a case study that looks at the early history of attempts to standardise concepts of psychological diagnosis for the purposes of asylum statistics, this work seeks to question distinctions that inform the history of medicine between clinical and administrative concerns. The discussions outlined in this volume provide new contributions to recent scholarship that assesses the significance of public health records and bureaucratic procedures to the history of science, technology and medicine.[19] Through these interconnected stories, this study provides a long durée view of the way psychiatric classification is embedded within practices of clinical diagnosis and public health administration. Accordingly, this volume explores the links between governance and the development of clinical classifications of mental disorder, its diagnosis and the way it shaped early mental

[16] Chris Millard provides a historical meta-critique of the use of Hacking's *looping kinds* that asks if it is legitimate to apply concepts formed by current scholarship, such as Hacking's, to historical works on disease identity: Chris Millard, 'Concepts, Diagnosis and the History of Medicine: Historicising Ian Hacking and Munchausen Syndrome' in *Social History of Medicine*, vol. 30, no. 3, August 2017, pp. 567–589.

[17] Geoffrey Bowker and Susan Leigh Star, *Sorting Things Out: Classification and Its Consequences*, MIT Press, Cambridge, MA, 1999.

[18] Gerald Grob, 'Origins of DSM-I: A Study in Appearance and Reality' in *the American Journal of Psychiatry*, vol. 148, no. 4, pp. 421–431.

[19] For instance, Timmermann et al. present the argument that developments in admissions records were a vital factor behind making mental health biomedical, and Filippo Maria Sposini assess the implications of certification for global mental health: Handerer, Kinderman, C Timmermann, Tai, 'How Did Mental Health Become So Biomedical? The Progressive Erosion of Social Determinants in Historical Psychiatric Admission Registers' in *History of Psychiatry*, vol. 32, no. 1, 2021, pp. 37–51; Fillipo Maria Sposini, *The Certification of Insanity: Local Origins and Imperial Consequences*, Palgrave, 2023.

health data in the form of asylum medical statistics on psychological diagnosis.[20] This study also seeks to contribute to recent work that explores the role of institutional, social and technological changes in yielding data used to formulate scientific knowledge.[21] The history of the MPA's classification entails an exploration of public records that collected patient information, and demonstrates that governance played a pivotal role in attempts to standardise psychological diagnosis since considerations on asylum management had instigated discussions over classification on a number of occasions.[22] The history presented in this volume attempts to show how bureaucratic processes have therefore not only influenced the development of clinical concepts, but have proven to act as the foundation and catalyst for the standardisation of concepts of diagnosis. This is no more clearly seen in the way debates over the Table were driven by divisions over asylum governance, with theoretical considerations on what mental disorders were and how they ought to be classified often arising during discussions over standardisation.

The research presented in this case study draws upon the records of these debates which were published in the MPA's *Journal of Mental*

[20] The links between governance, statistics and psychological medicine have been explored by academic scholarship informed by Foucauldian critiques of psychiatric practice. Nikolas Rose and Alain Desrosières, for instance, argue that quantification is linked to measures undertaken by states to govern social and economic life. More recent work from Nima Bassiri has built on this work to provide a picture of the ways that psychiatry from the late nineteen and early twentieth centuries increasingly paid attention to an individual's fitness to participate in the economy. See: Nikolas Rose, 'Calculable Minds and Manageable Individuals' in *History of the Human Sciences,* vol. 1, no. 2, October 1988, pp. 179–200; Alain Desrosières, *The Politics of Large Numbers: A History of Statistical Reasoning*, Harvard University Press, 1998.; Nima Bassiri, *Madness and Enterprise: Psychiatry, Economic Reason, and the Emergence of Pathological Value*, Chicago University Press, 2024.

[21] Steffan Müller-Wille, 'Names and Numbers: "Data" in Classical Natural History, 1758–1859' in *Osiris*, vol. 32, no. 1, 2017, pp. 109–128; David Sepkoski and Marco Tamborini, '"An Image of Science" Cameralism, Statistics, and the Visual Language of Natural History in the Nineteenth Century' in *Historical Studies in the Natural Sciences*, vol. 48, no. 1, 2018, pp. 56–109; Marco Tamborini, 'Series of Forms, Visual Techniques, and Quantitative Devices: Ordering the World Between the End of the Nineteenth and Early Twentieth Centuries' in *History and Philosophy of the life Sciences*, vol. 41, 2019, pp. 1–20.

[22] G.E. Berrios's conceptual history of classification, for instance, makes no mention of mental health statistics or the use of diagnostic terms in clinical records: see G.E. Berrios, 'Classifications in Psychiatry: A Conceptual History' in *Australian and New Zealand Journal of Psychiatry,* vol. 33, 1999, pp. 145–160.

Science. In doing so, I hope to offer an alternative view to histories of diagnostic concepts and psychiatric classification that have for the most part have for the most part used textbooks and medical journals as primary sources.[23] Whilst acknowledging the important contribution made by these works, this study takes an alternative approach through its attempts to broaden our understanding of the use of diagnostic categories in public records and public health reports. In doing so, the implications of record-keeping procedures are explored for the way they shaped psychological diagnosis, as is the relationship between the development of clinical concepts and record-keeping practices. By focusing on data and statistics relating to psychological diagnosis, this study challenges the prevailing view that the means to understand the history of diagnostic categories is primarily through the analysis of medical textbooks and scientific research papers. In turn, the discussions on classification can provide insights into the language used to diagnose patients, and how these diagnoses were recorded in asylum casebooks that eventually were published as statistical data on psychological diagnosis in reports issued by bodies involved in public health governance such as the Lunacy Commission. A distinction between matters of governance and clinical science has informed a historiography of psychiatric classification that is largely responsible for the lack of a comprehensive treatment of the Table of the Forms. This has led to the view amongst historians of medicine that the Table of the Forms was an administrative classification worthy only of a passing mention.[24] An emphasis on published clinical documents has formulated a historiography that has until only relatively recently given attention to administrative procedures in the development of clinical ideas.[25] To some extent, the distinction between clinical discoveries

[23] Edward Shorter, 'The History of Nosology and the Rise of the Diagnostic and Statistical Manual of Mental Disorder' in *Dialogues in Clinical Neuroscience*, vol. 17, no. 1, pp. 59–67; *A History of Clinical Psychiatry: The Origin and History of Psychiatric Disorders*, edited by German Berrios and Roy Porter, London, 1995.

[24] William Bynum, for instance, makes a small reference to the classification used in asylum statistics in his authoritative treatment of Bucknill and Tuke's *Dictionary of Psychological Medicine*. See: W.F. Bynum 'Tuke's Dictionary and Psychiatry at the Turn of the Century' in *150 Years of British Psychiatry: 1841–1991*, edited by Berrios and Freeman, Gaskell, 1991, pp. 163–179.

[25] Much scholarship has been devoted to the internal processes and deliberations that have developed categories of mental disorder included in the ICD and DSM: see Hannah Decker, 'How Kraepelinian Was Kraepelin? How Kraepelinian Are the Neo-Kraepelinians?

and bureaucratic procedures has been reflected in wider philosophical disputes over mental health classification that overlook their administrative bureaucratic function.[26] This study attempts to show that matters of medical governance are necessary to tell a meaningful history of psychiatric classification. A full historical account requires an understanding of the ways institutional, social and technological changes have shaped the fundamental terms used in psychological diagnosis and mental health statistics. Therefore, a realist account of mental disorder must examine the ways that bureaucratic processes have contributed to the development of classification used for the purposes of diagnosis. It is therefore hoped that the account of the social institutions and practices that shaped a document like the Table of the Forms will enrich an understanding of mental disorders as real entities, understandings of which are shaped by their social context and social history.

Linked to this aim is the goal of this study to provide an account of the procedures that shaped statistical data on diagnosis emerging from asylums. The Table of the Forms was used to structure data on diagnosis amongst asylum admissions published in reports of the Lunacy Commission from its establishment in 1845, until its responsibilities were transferred to the Board of Control for Lunacy and Mental Deficiency under the terms of the Mental Deficiency Act 1913. Although existing until the passing of the Mental Health Act 1959, the Board of Control had ceased to publish medical statistics after the implementation of the National Health Service Act in 1948, when these responsibilities were transferred to the Ministry of Health and the General Records Office. The reports issued from 1845 to 1948 remain an important source of information to historical scholarship, and although historians have frequently drawn upon asylum medical statistics, study of the processes

From Emil Kraepelin to DSM-III' in *History of Psychiatry*. vol. 18, no. 3, 2007, pp. 337–360; J.R.M. Copeland, 'Classification and the British Glossary of Mental Disorders' in *British Journal of Psychiatry*, vol. 119, no. 551, October 1971, pp. 413–418; R.E. Kendell et al., 'Diagnostic Criteria of American and British Psychiatrists' in *Archives of General Psychiatry*, vol. 5, 1971, pp. 123–130; Edward Shorter, 'The History of Nosology and the Rise of the *Diagnostic and Statistical Manual of Mental Disorder*' in *Dialogues in Clinical Neuroscience*, vol. 17, no. 1, pp. 59–67.

[26] Jonathan Tsou, *Philosophy of Psychiatry*, Cambridge University Press, 2021.

that shaped asylum statistics has been lacking.[27] Although it is out of the scope of this study to provide a full history of asylum medical statistics since the primary focus is charting the development of the Table of the Forms, I only discuss other tables included in statistical returns only inasmuch as they assist in furthering the story of the Table. In undertaking this task, I hope this study can begin to shed some light on the historical significance of the table and the debates that surrounded each of the revisions made to it. It is also important to note that this study is not a work of cliometrics, so does not employ historical statistics on psychological diagnosis to arrive at any conclusions over the rate or prevalence of insanity during these years; indeed, given the concerns aired during the debates about the replicability of psychological diagnosis and frequent misdiagnosis occurring within asylums, it is unclear whether the data on diagnosis included in the reports of bodies like the Board of Control are reliable enough to provide a firm ground for any assessment of this sort. Nevertheless, I do outline some of the ways psychiatrists, statisticians and public health bodies interpreted data which appeared to show that there was an increase in certain forms of insanity during the second half nineteenth century and the first half of the twentieth. Furthermore, the interrogation of the categories developed for statistics on diagnosis reveals the attitudes that informed the early years of mental health statistics, even if the data provided by these procedures does not fulfil the standards demanded by contemporary data science.

The development of nationwide statistics on psychological diagnosis in admissions was slow and chequered. As we will see, nationwide statistics on diagnosis were not published in asylum reports immediately following the passing of the 1845 Lunacy Act, and statistics are not available for periods during the years covered by this study. The first table that collated national statistics on diagnosis did not appear in reports of the Lunacy Commission until 1866, and it would not be until 1878 that tables on admissions diagnosis would regularly appear. Many larger institutions, such as the Manchester Royal Lunatic Asylum and the West Riding Pauper Lunatic Asylum, published their information on diagnosis in their own annual reports, but the terms of diagnosis used in the tables often did not follow those recommended by the Lunacy Commission in their

[27] Peter Bartlett, 'The Asylum, the Workhouse, and the Voice of the Insane Poor in 19th-Century England' in the *International Journal of Law and Psychiatry*, vol. 21, no. 4, 1998, pp. 421–432.

first report of 1845. As a result, it was difficult and time-consuming for the Lunacy Commission to compile data on diagnosis for publication in annual reports. Gradual standardisation made compiling the data simpler, and towards the end of the nineteenth century, the Lunacy Commission began to publish national statistics on psychological diagnosis. These were frequently accompanied by lengthy analyses of the prevalence of certain forms of insanity by gender, locale and occupation. After the report for the year 1913, the links between lunacy administration and the publication of medical data began to break down, and only basic information on admissions, discharges and deaths would be published until reforms were made to the procedures that collected mental health statistics from the early 1940s and as preparations were underway for a future national health service.

Through an investigation into the terms of psychological diagnosis used in medical statistics, the study aims to traverse a cleft in the historiography between studies of the Victorian asylum and the twentieth-century history of psychiatry.[28] Diagnosis during the age of the asylum primarily operated according to what is conventionally viewed as the classical division of insanity into forms of mania, idiocy, melancholia and dementia, with additional diagnostic terms such as moral insanity and general paralysis of the insane becoming firmly established by the 1860s onwards.[29] Textbooks offered various sub-types and modifications of these disease concepts, with many influential classifications of the nineteenth century employing the terms mania, melancholia and dementia in some form or another.[30] The dominant view of twentieth-century psychiatry is that

[28] John Turner et al., 'The History of Mental Health Services in Modern England: Practitioner Memories and the Direction of Future Research' in *Medical History*, vol. 59, no. 4, 2015, pp. 599–624.

[29] German Berrios, *The History of Mental Symptoms: Descriptive Psychopathology Since the Nineteenth Century*, Cambridge University Press, 1996.

[30] These included the work of Philippe Pinel, Wilhelm Griesinger and many of the diagnostic concepts within John Charles Bucknill and Daniel Hack Tuke's *Dictionary of Psychological Medicine*. The most comprehensive treatment of notions of psychopathology within the British context during the latter half of the nineteenth century comes in the form of William Bynum's analysis of Tuke and Bucknill's *A Dictionary of Psychological Medicine*. The dictionary was a compendium of research from neurologists, psychiatrists, psychologists, surgeons, pathologists, physicians and obstetricians, and was designed to provide a snapshot of the cutting-edge of research into the mental sciences. Bynum focused upon this seminal work because it was, like the Table of the Forms, a consensus-based classification of insanity: the ideas in it were formulated by contributions from

it saw a conflict between Kraepelinian diagnostic concepts and psychoanalysis.[31] Dementia praecox and manic-depressive insanity, historically linked to schizophrenia and manic depression that are still used today, became widespread terms of diagnosis in an astonishingly brief period during the first quarter of the century, at least in the British context.[32] Mindful of these strands in the historiography, this study attempts to draw continuities between asylum classifications and the early years of psychological concepts that are still in use in some form during the current Neo-Kraepelinian era of diagnosis. The debates surrounding the Table of the Forms provide an opportunity to chart the rise of Kraepelinian psychology within debates over classification from era of the asylum to those taking place up until the end of the Second World War. Chapter 5 argues the 1907 Revisions to the Table of the Forms played a role in this rise because of the introduction of diagnostic concepts that attempted to provide greater reliability to prognosis. It argues that the 1907 Revision was a Kraepelinian document because those involved in discussions to revise the Table of the Forms had sought to realise what Kraepelin was hailed to have achieved: the collection and management of large amounts of patient data that linked symptoms and diagnosis to prognosis. At the beginning of the twentieth century, asylum superintendents hoped that statistical methods could eventually provide diagnostic concepts that would go on to provide a reliable indication of the outlook of a patient. This emphasis on prognosis was linked to a broader loss

asylum superintendents working in larger institutions in the British Isles, like James Crichton-Browne, who established his own research centre at the West Yorkshire Lunatic Asylum. The key difference between these histories and the history of the Table of the Forms which is presented in this study is that the emphasis is on the discussions that led to the formulation of an array, to borrow Cunningham's term, of diagnosis concepts. William F. Bynum, 'Tuke's *Dictionary* and Psychiatry at the Turn of the Century' in *150 Years of British Psychiatry: 1841–1991*, edited by Berrios and Freeman, Gaskell, 1991, pp. 163–179.

[31] Edward Shorter, 'The History of Nosology and the Rise of the Diagnostic and Statistical Manual of Mental Disorder' in *Dialogues in Clinical Neuroscience*, vol. 17, no. 1, pp. 59–67.

[32] In the British Isles at least, they were routinely used by psychiatrists during and after the Great War, only twenty years after they had first been introduced in the first editions of Emil Kraepelin's textbooks. See for instance Edgar Jones, 'An Atmosphere of Cure: Frederick Mott, Shell Shock and the Maudsley' in *History of Psychology*, vol. 25, 2014, pp. 412–421 (p. 415).

of faith in the power of asylum treatment towards the end of the nineteenth century, with many hoping that an accurate prediction on the outlook of a form of insanity either preventing unnecessary admission to increasingly over-crowded asylums, or heightening the chances for a speedy discharge through administering treatment specific to the form of insanity encountered during an admission inspection.

Law, Medicine and Mental Science

In its critical assessment of the development of the Table of the Forms, this book aims to provide insights into the history of public health data on psychological diagnosis. It aims to makes sense of public health data on psychological diagnosis contained within lunacy reports by presenting considerations on the factors that shaped the fundamental categories of diagnosis. Accordingly, the discussions on psychological classification undertaken by the MPA constitute the central focus of this volume.[33] I have also consulted lunacy administration reports to understand the application of the classifications developed in these debates. I have at times drawn upon publications with mass readerships to demonstrate how the statistics generated by asylums admissions procedures attracted public interest; far from being merely the reserve of asylum management and lunacy administration, statistics on psychological diagnosis were debated in newspapers and periodicals with large, non-specialist audiences. At the same time, a few omissions have been required. Running almost concurrently to the story of the Table of the Forms was the development of the Mental Diseases section of the College of Physicians' Nomenclature of Diseases. This is another fascinating story and where possible I have tried to interweave important moments that cross over with the MPA's Table, but a full scholarly study of the relationship between it and the Table of the Forms is outside the scope of this enquiry. The study is ordered chronologically for ease of navigation; whilst intended to be read as one

[33] For some details on the history of the Association, see the official history of the Royal College of Psychiatrists, though as Gerald Grob notes, this is by no means an authoritative history: Thomas Bewley, *From Madness to Mental Disorder: A History of the Royal College of Psychiatrists*, RCPsych Publications, 2008; and Gerald N. Grob, 'Review: *Madness to Mental Illness: A History of the Royal College of Psychiatrists*' in *Journal of the History of Medicine and Allied Sciences*, vol. 67, no. 3, July 2012, pp. 509–510.

story, the chapters in this book have been designed to allow the reader to jump to a period of particular interest.

Although there have been recent turns towards looking at the bureaucratic procedures that have shaped psychiatric classification, the distinction between scientific and administrative considerations is firmly lodged in the historiography. As mentioned, this is one of the reasons why, until now, the full history of the Table of the Forms has not been considered worthy of scholarly attention. It is also a result of a distinction long informing the social history of psychiatry between legalism and medicalism to understand the relationship between clinical practice and the legal obligations placed upon medicine that are outlined in legislation.[34] The legalism/medicalism distinction is typically deployed to make sense of mental health legislation and its relationship to clinical practice, specifically, the powers medical staff and institutions are granted by law to detain patients. On the one hand, legalism understands the lunacy laws from 1845 to have placed increasingly greater legal constraints and restrictions on medical practice. On the other hand, medicalism refers to laws, most notably the 1959 Mental Health Act, that grant greater powers to clinicians and fewer oversights from regulatory bodies. Building on Roger Smith's observation that it is not possible to neatly disentangle clinical practice and the law in order to make judgements on where the law begins and psychiatry ends, this study aims to show how the standardisation of the fundamental categories of diagnosis were shaped by debates frequently triggered by legal and administrative considerations.[35] In particular, the 1845 Lunacy Act played a central role in formalising psychological diagnosis, and establishing the bureaucratic frameworks that enabled mental health data to be collected from asylums. Therefore, whilst Smith argues that mental health legislation is in many ways central and indistinguishable from psychiatric practice, this study makes the argument that mental health law has shaped

[34] For instance, Kathleen Jones famously considers the 1890 Lunacy Act to be a triumph of legalism since it placed greater restrictions on psychiatry's powers of detention, and oversight on medical practice in response to widespread fear of wrongful confinement. On the other hand, Jones considers the 1959 Mental Health Act to be a triumph of medicalism due to the powers it gave doctors. See Kathleen Jones, 'Law and Mental Health: Sticks or Carrots' in *150 Years of British Psychiatry*, edited by Berrios and Freeman, Gaskell, 1991, pp. 89–102.

[35] Roger Smith, 'Legal Frameworks for Psychiatry' in *150 Years of British Psychiatry 1841–1991*, edited by German Berrios and Hugh Freeman, London, Gaskell, 1991.

the epistemic frameworks of psychiatry by providing a catalyst to standardise the categories used in statistical data on psychological diagnosis. In turn, this developed medical science by allowing diagnosis to be better communicated amongst the emerging psychiatric profession, and the data on diagnosis to be compiled into use in mental health statistics.

A brief version of the century-long history of the Table of the Forms can be told in relation to the mental health legislation passed during the document's existence. Due to its connections to medico-legal definitions of mental disorder, the Table of the Forms was first published in response to the passing of mental health legislation outlining changes to asylum administration in 1845. It was a product of the mass expansion of the asylum system in the British Isles under the terms of the 1845 Lunacy Acts, and the requirements it outlined to hold records on so-called pauper or rate-aided patients.[36] The supply of information through annual statistical returns to the Lunacy Commission was designed to keep track of patients in the growing network of county asylums, and avoid the possibility of an individual becoming lost in the system.[37] As admissions data came to be published in annual reports of the Lunacy Commission, alienists increasingly regarded administrative data as a possible knowledge-resource that could provide alternatives to the investigations into the body that characterised much of the research undertaken in Victorian asylums.[38] Although the terms of psychological diagnosis used for statistical purposes were a source of interest from the early years of the MPA in the 1840s, they had faded from sight during the 1850s before a resurgence of interest in the forms of insanity used in asylum administrative data occurred around the 1860s. The debates that followed, which

[36] Peter Bartlett states that the technical meaning of a pauper lunatic was 'a person whose maintenance was paid for by their local parish or union', but cautions against understanding the term too literally because the families of many pauper lunatics reimbursed the poor law authorities for the cost of their care: see Peter Bartlett, The Poor Law of Lunacy: The Administration of Pauper Lunatics in Mid-Nineteenth Century England (with special Emphasis on Leicestershire and Rutland), PhD Thesis, UCL, 1993, pp. 221–222 (p. 57).

[37] William Llewelyn Parry-Jones, *The Trade in Lunacy: A Study of Private Madhouses in England in the Eighteenth and Nineteenth Centuries*, Routledge, 1972.

[38] Jennifer Wallis, *Investigating the Body in the Victorian Asylum Doctors, Patients, and Practices*, Palgrave Macmillan, 2017; Michael J. Clarke, 'The Rejection of Psychological Approaches to Mental Disorder in Late Nineteenth Century British Psychiatry' in *Mad Houses, Mad Doctors and Madmen: The Social History of Psychiatry in the Victorian Era*, edited by Andrew Scull, Athlone, 1981.

would wage on until the 1882 Revision was published, were triggered by the offering of an alternative classification in 1864 from David Skae (1814–1873) that catered to a growing demand for a scientific classification of the insanities. The passing of the 1886 Idiot's Act would have important implications for subsequent revisions to the Table of the Forms, with the legal distinction between congenital insanity and insanity occurring later in life articulated in the 1907 and 1934 Revisions.[39] The 1907 Revisions were partly conducted in response to changes introduced through the 1890 Lunacy Act, which are conventionally regarded by historians as having placed greater legal restrictions upon the asylum, and which extended the requirement to include information on voluntary patients within statistical returns.[40] The 1913 Mental Deficiency Act would include a definition of 'feeble-mindedness' that was included in the 1907 revisions under the guise of congenital forms of insanity, with the classification making a distinction between mental illnesses that had occurred later in life and those that were thought to be hereditary. The subsequent 1934 Revision to the Table of the Forms would anticipate the use of psychopathy as a legal category under the terms of the 1959 Mental Health Act.[41] The reforms to admissions procedures which were conducted during the early 1940s as planning was taking place for a health service—an account of which ends this study—led to the Table of the Forms being replaced by the mental health section of the World Health Organisation's (WHO) *Manual of the International Statistical Classification of Diseases, Injuries and Causes of Death* (ICD) .[42] The 1946 National Health Service Act would formalise these changes before it came into effect in July 1948.

Participants in the debates conducted from the 1860s onwards aired hopes that the standardisation of diagnostic terms used in statistical returns would further the development of mental science by improving

[39] Peter Bartlett, The Poor Law of Lunacy: The Administration of Pauper Lunatics in Mid-Nineteenth Century England (with special Emphasis on Leicestershire and Rutland), PhD Thesis, UCL, 1993, pp. 221–222.

[40] Kathleen Jones, *Mental Health and Social Policy, 1845–1959*, Routledge, 1960.

[41] Matthew Thomson, *The Problem of Mental Deficiency: Eugenics, Democracy and Social Policy in Britain, 1870–1959*, Oxford University Press, 1998.

[42] Charles Webster, 'Psychiatry and the Early National Health Service: the role of the Mental Health Standing Advisory Committee' in *150 Years of British Psychiatry*, edited by G. Berrios and H. Freeman, Gaskell, 1991, pp. 103–106.

the quality of data on psychological diagnosis returned from asylums. Greater standardisation would make it simpler to compile the data into a format that could allow the data to be fruitfully analysed, yielding findings that could improve the state of the art. The Holy Grail for members of the MPA was to find correlations between data recorded on psychological diagnosis, and data recorded on the physical condition of patients admitted to an asylum. As is apparent from the discussions covered in Chapter 3, this is down to the widespread assumption held during the second half of the nineteenth century that psychological symptoms were dependent upon physical states.[43] Data on the social background of a patient was also recorded in asylum records, including information on their occupation and marital status prior to their admittance. The family background of a patient was also captured in these statistics, with any information that could be gleaned from patients or their family members on attacks of insanity amongst immediate family members being recorded, however valid it may be. Despite a prevailing preoccupation with physical aetiology, there were attempts to incorporate data like this on the social background of a patient into asylum medical statistics, although it was viewed as unreliable due to it having come from the personal testimony of patients and their families. This data also fuelled the interest in heredity during the second half of the nineteenth century and the first part of the twentieth, but, as we will see, this was not at the complete exclusion of attempts to understand what can be termed environmental and social causes of mental disorder.[44] The advent of therapeutic despair towards

[43] Tom Quick, 'From Phrenology to the Laboratory: Physiological psychology and the Institution of Science in Britain' in *History of the Human Sciences*, vol. 27, no. 5, 2014.

[44] Porter looks at the statistics collected by asylum medical superintendents before statisticians and eugenicists became interested in the role of heredity in the causation of mental disorders during the last quarter of the nineteenth century. He claims that in collecting and ordering data about those admitted to the asylum, doctors were proto-geneticists who sought to explain the inheritance of mental disorders in their patients. Porter's book focuses on the work of individual doctors such as John Thurnam—who worked at the Retreat in York and whom we encounter in this book—and how his practice of collecting exhaustive lists of data relating to the conditions of the patients admitted to the institution. Porter's account looks in depth at the paper technologies that allowed statistical data to be recorded in asylums. These take the form of tables like that of the Forms of Mental Disorder that were either devised by individual asylum superintendents like Thurnam, or issued by central authorities including medical associations and administrative bodies. Missing from Porter's account though is an analysis of the concepts of psychopathology that were used within data collection, and in particular, the tables that were published by

the end of the nineteenth century, the influence of degeneration and the rise of the eugenics movement shaped views on the purposes of asylum medical statistics, with the heredity of insanity becoming the dominant view and eclipsing social considerations during discussions over the Table of the Forms during the first half of the twentieth century.

Statistical returns were arteries in a national bureaucracy that collected and transmitted patient information recorded in asylum logbooks. Paper technologies including logbooks and the returns themselves were a crucial factor in the establishment of asylum administration from the beginning of the nineteenth century, and which saw wholesale expansion under the 1845 Lunacy Acts.[45] Legal changes to admissions procedures under the act shaped diagnosis, making it a formal legal requirement at the point of entry to an asylum. These legal procedures gave rise to increasingly more sophisticated efforts to collate and count the diagnoses of psychological disorders. During the first set of revisions to the statistical table, the MPA devised a 'Schedule of Aetiologies' that was commonly known as the Table of the Causes of Insanity. As per its title, this was a list of the suspected physical cause of a disorder in the hope that data from it and the Table of the Forms could be compared and collated. Although the hope to use paper technologies to assemble mass patient data on psychological diagnosis was frequently expressed by Lunacy Commissioners and alienists alike, the promise never reached its full potential, and there is little evidence to suggest that anything beyond the crudest comparisons of these data sets ever occurred. This can be explained partly by the slow speed of reforms to the large bureaucratic frameworks that accompanied asylum statistics. The systems that would allow the flows of information to come anywhere near to the ideal imagined by Lunacy Commissioners and alienists alike were obstructed by the quotidian demands of medical practice. As we will see, the slow uptake of mechanical counting technologies that would allow the rapid collation of the statistical returns came to be rued by those in charge of reforming the data collection

the Medico-Psychological Association. We will also see within these discussions that whilst heredity was an interest held by some involved in the discussions, it was by no means the only one, with many considering certain forms of insanity to have predominantly environmental or social causes. See Ted Porter, *Genetics in the Madhouse: The Unknown History of Human Heredity*, Princeton University Press, 2018.

[45] Volker Hess and J. Andrew Mendelsohn, 'Case and Series: Medical Knowledge and Paper Technology, 1600–1900' in *History of Science*, vol. 48, no. 3, 2010, pp. 287–314.

practices that produced mental health statistics during the Second World War. There was also a degree of resistance from within medicine to procedures designed to collect statistical data, as certain asylum medical superintendents frequently complained about the effort it took to fill in statistical returns, and could not see the worth of this time-consuming task. Statistical returns were viewed by some as a burden imposed by lunacy regulation, and only served to interfere with medical practice. Despite objections from some, hopes for an industrial collection and collation of national asylum medical statistics on psychological diagnosis came to be realised by the end of the 1870s. Despite this achievement, these were nowhere near the aspirations of advocates, who had hoped that collected patient histories could provide a stable foundation to medical knowledge, especially in the absence of breakthroughs in pathology and anatomy.[46]

Transnational Mental Health Epidemiology and Global Classification

Although international mental health epidemiology is usually considered to have commenced as a project with the establishment of the WHO, psychological classification used in early mental health statistics was a transnational project from its very beginnings.[47] In their assessment of the origins of psychiatric epidemiology, Anne M Lovell and Ezra Susser note that historians of psychiatry such as Gerald Grob have labelled developments before the post-World War II era, including asylum

[46] Åsa Jansson, for instance, shows how statistics came to associate suicidal tendencies with melancholia during the second half of the nineteenth century chiefly through the diagnoses that were recorded in asylum admissions books from 1845 onwards, but the studies that made this association were largely limited to individual asylums and not figures collated from across England and Wales: Åsa Jansson, 'From Statistics to Diagnostics: Medical Certificates, Melancholia, and "Suicidal Propensities" in Victorian Psychiatry' in *Journal of Social History*, vol. 43, no. 3, Spring 2013, pp. 716–731; 'Mood Disorders and the Brain: Depression, Melancholia, and the Historiography of Psychiatry' in *Medical History*, vol. 55, no. 3, July 2011, pp. 393–399.

[47] Anne M. Lovell, 'The World Health Organization and the Contested Beginnings of Psychiatric Epidemiology as an International Discipline: One Rope, Many Strands' in *International Journal of Epidemiology*, vol. 43, 2014, pp. 6–18.

statistics, as being a part of the pre-history of modern psychiatric epidemiology.[48] Accordingly, documents used in early mental health statistics like the Table of the Forms are described as 'proto-epidemiological texts'.[49] Whilst this volume is focused on the British context prior to the age of international psychiatric epidemiology, the Table of the Forms was in many ways a global construct, with it bearing influences from across Europe. Britain's predominant role as a synthesiser of breakthroughs emerging from other parts of the world is perhaps why Edward Shorter claims the British made fewer contributions to the development of psychological diagnosis and classification than France or Germany.[50] Whilst it is certainly the case that asylums in the British Isles were not as well-established as in the French system, and lacked the sophistication of the clinics associated with psychiatric hospitals of Imperial Germany, the view that there were no original contributions does not take into account many of the ideas that were distinctive to British psychiatry.[51] Sophisticated research was undertaken in larger asylums that had laboratories, such as the West Riding Lunatic Asylum, with those conducting it often having to balance their investigations into the nature of insanity with the everyday demands of asylum management and medical practice.[52] Despite these pressures, we will encounter characters from British asylums who offered their own terms of diagnosis and classification systems which were original and innovative despite them not having stood the test of time. The same can be said for the Table of the Forms, whose historical importance is easily overlooked if assessed solely in terms of its contribution to current knowledge. At first glance, the Table amalgamated and adapted ideas that were developed in other countries, and appears to be a derivative classification merely used to fulfil a legally required administrative

[48] Anne M. Lovell and Esra Susser, 'What Might Be a History of Psychiatric Epidemiology? Towards a Social History and Conceptual Account' in *International Journal of Epidemiology*, vol. 43, 2014, pp. 1–5.

[49] Ibid., p. 2.

[50] Edward Shorter, *A History of Psychiatry: From the Age of the Asylum to the Age of Prozac*, Wiley and Sons, 1997.

[51] Eric J. Engstrom, *Clinical Psychiatry in Imperial Germany*, Cornell University Press, 2003.

[52] Michael Anthony Finn, The West Riding Lunatic Asylum and the Making of the Modern Brain Sciences in the Nineteenth Century, PhD Thesis, University of Leeds, 2012.

task. However, if it is appraised in terms which acknowledge its role in the communication and development of scientific knowledge, then the classification and the debates surrounding it take on a new significance. The Table of the Forms and asylum medical statistics stimulated communication about mental health and the kinds of diagnosis people were receiving when admitted to an asylum. Communication of course is conducted in many different ways with different audiences and for different purposes. Accordingly, I have drawn upon medical journals, textbooks and public health reports, but also transactions, speeches, newspaper articles and correspondence as primary sources. In doing so, I hope to add to the literature within the history of science that shows how the borders between public science and specialist science are increasingly porous when we pay attention to the role that communication plays in the development of clinical knowledge.[53]

The existence of large state-run asylums and a post-Revolutionary materialist turn has been credited by Jan Goldstein as a main cause of diagnostic categories that emerged from the French Republic during the first half of the nineteenth century.[54] For the purposes of this study, the work of Philippe Pinel (1745–1826) is particularly important because the debates on classification outlined in this volume were in many ways responses to his nosography of mental disorder. As we will see in the next chapter, Pinel's nosography built on the work of English medical nosologists and made a lasting mark across Europe from its first publication in 1800, with his concepts providing the basis for the terms used in the Table of the Forms published in 1845. The terms Pinel adopted to classify symptoms—*melancholia, mania, mania without delusions, dementia* and *idiocy*—became a standard means of classifying mental disorders for much

[53] At the time of writing, it is three decades since Roger Cooter and Stephen Pumfrey called for an understanding of the gap between histories of scientific ideas and collective public behaviour through an attention to science popularisation. Much work has been conducted to understand how communication operates across these spheres in the formulation of scientific knowledge. Susanne Schmidt interrogates the age-old prioritisation of specialist science over public science by showing how in the case of the midlife crisis, it was the work of a journalist and academic outsider Gail Sheehy who had been pivotal in providing the concept its meaning. See Roger Cooter and Stephen Pumfrey, 'Separate Spheres and Public Places: Reflections on the History of Science Popularisation and Science in Popular Culture' in *History of Science*, no. 33, 1994; Susanne Schmidt, *Midlife Crisis: The Feminist Origins of a Chauvinist Cliché*, Chicago University Press, 2020.

[54] Jan Goldstein, *Console and Classify: The French Psychiatric Profession in the Nineteenth Century*, Cambridge University Press, 1988.

of the nineteenth century.[55] They would in some form appear in every version of the Table of the Forms published between 1845 and 1948. In the wake of Pinel came the work of his students, principally Jean Étienne Dominique Esquirol (1772–1840) and Jean-Pierre Falret (1794–1870), who would further develop and refine Pinel's nosography. These developments included coining the terms monomania and circular insanity, both of which would be included in versions of the Table of the Forms published in the nineteenth and twentieth centuries. Diagnostic concepts emerging from France during the first half of the nineteenth century were based upon descriptions of sets of symptoms, which were grouped into clusters to create concepts of psychological diagnosis. This approach, sometimes described as a symptomology by historians, was developed by Pinel and stood in contrast to the nosologists that came before him since it provided little in the way of a physical explanation for the disorders it listed.[56] As we will see in this volume, Pinel's nosography was hugely influential, if not without its critics, and it enjoyed longevity precisely because of the lack of a physical aetiology that could be disproven by empirical research. This was by design, and although he did not seek to provide a speculative theory of causation to explain observations gathered from the cases he observed at the Salpêtrière hospital in Paris, he did not discount the possibility that future discoveries may be made which could explain psychological conditions through physical states and causes. In addition to providing the foundations of symptomology, the French School established in the wake of Pinel was responsible for the rise of the language of *forms* to describe mental health conditions, at least during modern history.[57] Descriptions of forms of insanity point towards key

[55] David Wright notes in his analysis of admissions to the Buckinghamshire County Asylum that the concepts of Pinel and Esquirol were the 'standard classifications in the mid-Victorian period', as does Michael J. Clarke in his assessment of intellectual cultures in Victorian psychiatry: David Wright, 'Delusions of Gender?: Lay Identifications and Clinical Diagnosis of Insanity in Victorian England' in *Sex and Seclusion, Class and Custody: Perspectives on Class and Gender in the History of British and Irish Psychiatry*, edited by Jonathan Andrews and Anne Digby, Rodopoi, 2004, pp. 149–171; and Michael J. Clarke, 'The Rejection of Psychological Approaches to Mental Disorder in Late Nineteenth Century British Psychiatry' in *Mad Houses, Mad Doctors and Madmen: The Social History of Psychiatry in the Victorian Era*, edited by Andrew Scull, Athlone, 1981.

[56] German Berrios, *The History of Mental Symptoms: Descriptive Psychopathology Since the Nineteenth Century*, Cambridge University Press, 2008.

[57] The term 'forms' will be used throughout this study as it was the prevailing terminology employed by those who attempted to classify insanity for a great deal of the

ambiguities over whether different forms were different stages or manifestations of one illness, or whether they were separate kinds of disorder that each had different physical causes. Pinel's work itself was based on abstractions from a pool of cases, drawing together common features from different instances to arrive at disease categories that captured the essentials of the different forms. Bénédict Morel's (1809–1873) degeneration theory followed in the French tradition, but took a departure from Pinel's ambivalence on the physical causes of the different forms of insanity. He offered a theory of causation that relied on heredity to explain psychological disorder, and placed it at the centre of a clinical picture of social degeneration that would find articulation in the fiction of Emile Zola and the social-psychology of Gustave Le Bon.[58] Morel believed that the root cause of all forms of insanity were constitutional weaknesses in the body, and these could be detected through physical characteristics such as hairline and facial structure.[59] Morel's degeneration theory, the influence of Darwinian evolutionary theory and Spencerian social theory, had influenced notable British alienists like Skae and Henry Maudsley (1835–1918).[60] As Theodor Porter notes, heredity as a causing factor of mental disorders was a preoccupation of alienists before the eugenics movement had become fully established at the beginning of the twentieth

nineteenth century. It is possible that the distinction made between the form of madness, structured by observed trends in the course of an illness, and the psychological contents of particular cases, dates back further. Berrios, for instance, claims that the distinction between the 'form' and 'content' of insanity informed knowledge of mental disorders since antiquity, at least in Western thought, and links this to the application to the mental sciences of the Aristotelian idea that a common essence, character or 'eidos' bound together objects of a similar nature. See German Berrios, *The History of Mental Symptoms: Descriptive Psychopathology Since the Nineteenth Century*, Cambridge University Press, 2008.

[58] Daniel Pick, *Faces of Degeneration: A European Disorder c.1848–1918*, Cambridge University Press, 1993.

[59] Ian Dowbiggin, *Inheriting Madness: Professionalisation and Psychiatric Knowledge in Nineteenth Century France*, University of California Press, 1991.

[60] In the estimation of Trevor Turner, 'the scepticism that [Maudsley] was to ally to the degenerationist theories of Morel accompanied a dreadful paralysis in the profession as a whole' by the end of the nineteenth century'. See Trevor Turner, 'Henry Maudsley: Psychiatrist, philosopher and entrepreneur' in *Psychological Medicine*, vol. 18, no. 3, August 1988, pp. 551–574; Charlotte MacKenzie argues that Skae's classification was a degenerationist document, see Charlotte Mackenzie, *Psychiatry for the Rich, A History of Ticehurst Private Asylum, 1792–1917,* Routledge, 1993. (p. 177).

century, with some forms of insanity being more firmly linked to inheritance than others.[61] Stagnation in British psychiatry towards the end of the nineteenth century, and the lack of a breakthrough in the mental sciences fuelled the popularity of degeneration that later coalesced around eugenics, with concerns over burgeoning asylum populations frequently aired during the revisions to the Table of the Forms that took place between 1902 and 1907. Morel's degeneration theory had a lasting legacy in Britain, with vestiges of it remaining until at least the time of the 1934 Revision.

Despite Morel's legacy lasting well into the twentieth century, medical psychology was starting to turn its attention away from France during the mid-late nineteenth century and increasingly towards the ideas emerging from German research institutes. This was largely because of the relative sophistication of the clinical system within Imperial Germany.[62] British psychiatrists admired the research being published by figures like Karl Ludwig Kahlbaum (1828–1899), Ewald Hecker (1843–1909) and Wilhelm Griesinger (1817–1868), who would all make attempts to connect physiology and symptomology within expansive and highly technical clinical classifications.[63] Although these were respected by certain members of the MPA, others would criticise the work of Griesinger in particular for being too complicated and detail-laden for effective practical use. The work of Emil Kraepelin (1856–1926) however attracted nearly universal acclaim from all corners of British medical psychology from the end of the nineteenth century onwards partly because it was viewed as having made a division of the insanities that provided reliable indications of prognosis since it was based upon data that tracked the

[61] Theodor Porter, *Genetics in the Madhouse: The Unknown History of Human Heredity*, Princeton University Press, 2018.

[62] Eric Engstrom, *Clinical Psychiatry in Imperial Germany*, Cornell University Press, 2003.

[63] Ewald Hecker, 'Classic Text no. 55: Cyclothymia, a Circular Mood Disorder [originally published 1882]' in *History of Psychiatry*, vol. 14, no. 3, 2003, pp. 377–399; Karl Wilmanns, 'Ewald Hecker (1843–1909)' in *History of Psychiatry*, vol. 13, no. 52, 2002, pp. 377–399; Juan Goldar et al., 'Karl Ludwig Kahlbaum's Concept of Catatonia' in *History of Psychiatry*, vol. 6, no. 22, 1995, pp. 201–207; Otto Marx, 'Wilhelm Griesinger and the History of Psychiatry: A Reassessment' in *Bulletin for the History of Medicine*, vol. 46, no. 5, 1972, pp. 519–544.

outcome of diseases amongst many patients admitted to his asylum.[64] Kraepelin's work held huge appeal because of its simplicity in predicting the outlook of those diagnosed with dementia praecox, and those diagnosed with manic-depressive insanity. His work was therefore viewed by many as having incorporated a reasonably accurate prognosis within diagnostic concepts. The fact that he had done this through the collection and analysis of statistical evidence on asylum inmates added to its appeal. Kraepelin was viewed as having to some extent successfully realised the potential of mental health statistics, and their potential to inform clinical classifications that could provide some indication of the outlook of a patient. Kraepelin's work on prognosis was interwoven with his concerns of the degeneration of the German Volk, which along with the Neo-Lamarckian views he held, had motivated his epidemiological research.[65] Eugen Blueler's (1857–1939) term schizophrenia would replace Kraepelin's dementia praecox in much clinical literature, and his combination of Kraepelinian ideas with those of psychoanalysis would become popular in the US, but less so in the UK.[66] During the interwar period, the new science of phenomenology developed by Edmund Husserl (1859–1938) would have an influence on German ideas of psychopathology, most notably through the work of Karl Jaspers (1883–1969). The influence of German clinics started to wane as the Nazi regime began to use medicine to pursue euthanasia policies that shocked even committed members of the eugenics movement, with antisemitic policies seeing prominent German psychiatrists emigrate to the United Kingdom and the US. They brought with them a working understanding of the diagnostic concepts of German psychiatry, which had an impact upon the intellectual landscape of interwar British psychiatry.[67]

[64] Ian Dowbiggin tells the story of Valentin Magnan to explore the nationalist reaction to German psychiatry that penalised French Kraepelinians: 'Back to the Future: Valentin Magnan, French Psychiatry, and the Classification of Mental Diseases, 1885–1925' in *Social History of Medicine*, vol. 9, no. 3, December 1996, pp. 383–408.

[65] Eric J. Engstrom discusses whether it is possible to separate his work on nosology and his Neo-Lamarckian informed epidemiology in his introduction to: Emil, Kraepelin, 'On the Question of Degeneration' in *History of Psychiatry*, vol. 19, no. 3, 2007, pp. 399–404.

[66] Richard Noll, *American Madness: The Rise and Fall of Dementia Praecox*, Harvard University Press, 2011.

[67] These would include figures who would have a dramatic impact on psychiatric pedagogy and classification, including Wilhelm Mayer-Gross and Erwin Stengel: the latter would have a pivotal role at the World Health Organisation after the war. For more

Outline of the Study

The history of the Table of the Forms presented in this volume is divided into three main parts. The first section is an assessment of the conditions that allowed the Table of the Forms to come into being in 1845 and led to the concepts developed by Pinel becoming the standard used in medical statistics—these are charted in Chapter 2 and Chapter 3 respectively. The second section provides critical assessments of the first two debates on standardisation of diagnostic terms in asylum admissions procedures and statistics. The first set of debates that led up to the 1882 Revision is assessed in Chapter 4, and the debates between 1902 and 1906 that culminated in the 1907 Revision are outlined in Chapter 5. Chapter 6 acts as a bridge between the second and the third section, and is devoted to understanding the application of the Table of the Forms in asylum medical statistics on psychological diagnosis presented in reports of the Lunacy Commission and the Board of Control. The third section is an exploration of the ways that these debates shaped classification and mental health statistics during the first half of the twentieth century, with Chapter 7 covering the deliberations that led to the 1934 Revision to the Table of the Forms, and Chapter 8 exploring the changes to the collection of mental health statistics at the outset of the NHS that led to the replacement of the Table of the Forms with the *ICD* in 1948.

Chapter 2 outlines how the diagnostic concepts that populated the first Table of the Forms issued by the Lunacy Commission in 1845 came into being. The first iteration of the document bore the mark of the French school of medical psychology that had developed in the wake of Philippe Pinel's (1745–1826) work on psychological diagnosis published at the start of the nineteenth century. The story of how Pinel developed his categories and how they came to become commonplace within medical discourse sets the scene for the arguments over classification that are explored throughout this volume. Pinel's work initially faced a hostile reaction from British medical circles, with reviewers considering his nosography Cartesian and unbecoming of medicine. By drawing on the nosologies of William Cullen and Alexander Crichton,

on the impact of German émigrés on British psychiatry during the interwar period, see Rhodri Hayward, 'Germany and the Making of 'English' Psychiatry: The Maudsley Hospital 1908–1939' in *International Relations in Psychiatry: Britain, Germany and the United States to World War II*, edited by Volker Roelcke, Paul J. Weindling and Louise Westwood, University of Rochester Press, 2013, pp. 67–90.

the chapter traces the transnational exchanges on classification that helped to define psychological diagnosis during the early decades of the nineteenth century. Despite the initial British reception to Pinel's work being largely unfavourable, Pinel's ideas became popular and were recommended for use in psychological diagnosis in the first report of the Lunacy Commission published in 1845.

Chapter 3 outlines how the work of James Cowles Prichard (1786–1848) determined the popularity of ideas emerging from France. Prichard was a crucial figure in the establishment of Pinel's concepts as the standard that were used in asylum medical statistics throughout the rest of the nineteenth century, mainly due to his involvement in the early years of the Lunacy Commission. In addition, the simplicity and practicality of Pinel's ideas appealed to British alienists, whose lack of a specialist training and poor working conditions meant that ease of use and application was demanded from a standard set of diagnostic terms. Yet, despite these qualities, the hopes for a scientific classification grew as mental science matured into a medical specialism. Calls emerged from medical societies like the MPA for a classification that would allow diagnosis to be based upon mechanical, somatic and causal explanation for mental disorders. The third chapter ends by focusing on one classification that would arise to be a contender to the symptomology promoted by the Lunacy Commission; that of David Skae, whose work sought to explain the different forms of insanity through bodily processes and conditions, and sparked interest in how the causes of insanity could be incorporated into a standard Table of the Forms for use in asylum medical statistics.

The debates outlined in Chapter 4 chart the first clashes over classification that commenced in 1864 and were resolved in 1882. They are characterised by a clash between the symptom-based descriptions of mental disorder that had become dominant with the transmission of French approaches to classification, and a physicalist view that is most clearly seen through the work of Skae. He and his classification would become the figureheads for a movement that was determined to re-establish the Table of the Forms on the foundations of physical aetiology. This chapter looks at disagreements between those who wanted Skae's work to become the new standard, and those who were not convinced by the scientific credentials of Skae's work. Those against Skae's classification of aetiology acknowledged the shortfalls of the Table of the Forms introduced by the Lunacy Commission, but valued its clinical effectiveness and efficiency. As the century wore on, and the breakthroughs hoped for in anatomy and the physical causes of insanity did not materialise, these arguments over the classification to use in medical statistics intensified as they came to be viewed as the new hope for yielding insights into the nature of insanity.

Chapter 5 examines changes to the Table during a set of revisions that took place between 1902 and 1906 that led to the publication of the 1907 Revision to the Table of the Forms. What started out as an exercise to revise the concepts used in statistical tables led to discussions taking place about what the classification of the forms of insanity of the MPA should look like. This was in the hope of improving medical data and using more 'modern' concepts to understand the kinds of insanity that were being admitted to asylums. What began as an exercise in improving data would lead to a series of crucial questions being posed about the role of a psychiatric classification, including what function it should serve, and what it should look like.

Chapter 6 looks at the practical application of the Table of the Forms in asylums statistics between 1845 until the commencement of the next set of revisions in 1929. The chapter presents a detailed picture of the development of statistics on psychological diagnosis published in reports of the Commissioners in Lunacy. These developments are linked to the discussions included in the fourth and fifth chapters, with the introduction in 1867 of national statistics on psychological diagnosis to make sense of admissions. The development of statistics on diagnosis fits into a broader picture of the development of medical statistics in public reports and saw a gradual development until the first decade of the twentieth century. The reports of the Lunacy Commission between 1900 and 1913 see greater space devoted to national figures on psychological diagnosis, with lengthy passages of analysis and attempts to visualise the data in the final set of reports published by the Lunacy Commission. The handing over of powers to the Board of Control in 1913 leads to an abrupt end to the development of asylum statistics—this chapter attempts to make sense of this development and explain it through the impact of the Great War on asylums, and changes surrounding statistical theory that occurred around the turn of the century. The studies conducted by the leading proponents of mathematical statistics based in the Galton Laboratory of National Statistics in UCL used as a grounding assumption the notion that insanity did not need to be broken down into different forms within statistical enquiry. Drawing on the work of Karl Pearson and David

Heron, I outline in this chapter how attitudes towards insanity demonstrated by these studies had an influence upon ending the development of asylum medical statistics on psychological diagnosis during the era of the Board of Control, which ran from 1914 until the beginning of the Second World War.

Chapter 7 explores developments during the first decades of the twentieth century that would shape the last set of revisions to the Table of the Forms. These commenced in 1929 and ended with the publication of the 1934 Revision. The chapter argues that the revisions were a response to broader changes surrounding psychiatric treatment since the end of the First World War. It charts developments during the interwar period to critically assess these revisions and how they influenced the interwar revisions to the Table of the Forms. It will focus its analysis on a set of forms that were added to the Table, including neurosis, schizophrenic psychosis, psychopathic constitution and emotional and affective psychoses. The chapter finishes by discussing the hostile reception that these changes received from prominent members of a divided British psychiatric community, as expressed in textbooks and pages of medical journals of the time. The conversion of many asylums to military hospitals during the First World War caused major disruptions to the asylum system, and during the 1920s mental health classification and statistics were side-lined to some extent because of more pressing matters: these included the recovery from the disruptions of the war, and drawing up responses to the 1919 War Office Report on Shellshock, the findings of which had implications for clinical treatment. Changes to asylum administration were included in the recommendations of The Report of the Royal Commission on Mental Disorder, which was published in 1926, some of which were implemented into the 1930 Mental Treatment Act. Asylum superintendents feared the changes introduced through the act would curtail the powers of asylum superintendents, making them subordinate and answerable to local health authorities. As pressures began to be alleviated towards the end of the 1920s, focus turned again to the Table of the Forms, and a committee was appointed in 1928 to make new revisions to the document. Unfortunately, the records for this period are less complete than the ones for the first two sets of debates and this is somewhat significant in itself: committees during earlier sets of revisions had presented their work to members of the Association in annual general meetings, with detailed minutes of the proceedings being captured and published in the Association's publication, the *Journal of Mental Science*.

In contrast, deliberations were not conducted in the kind of open public forums of general meetings for the last set of revisions to the Table of the Forms, perhaps for fear of igniting the sort of debate that had waged over, cumulatively speaking, at least three decades of deliberations up until that point. It concludes by showing how the work of the revisions committee was not well-received, with their version of the Table being met with heavy criticism from both modernisers like David Henderson, as well as those steeped in the asylum tradition.

This account of the decline of the Table of the Forms ends by charting how it gradually faded into obscurity as war approached. It would be formally replaced during the restructuring of the health services that occurred immediately after the Second World War, primarily because of the work of the eugenicist and psychologist Carlos Patton Blacker, and Galton Laboratory geneticist Lionel Penrose. The final chapter of this book argues that the end of the Table of the Forms was due to psychiatry moving closer to general medicine on conceptual and institutional levels, and the war functioned as a catalyst for radical shifts that enabled psychiatry to become a part of general medicine. It focuses on the revisions to admissions procedures that were designed for the National Health Service, and their impact upon the collection of data on psychological diagnosis. The prominent eugenicist Carlos Patton Blacker and the statistician Lionel Penrose were in charge of a project to reform the admissions system which would improve the collection of mental health statistics. The diagnostic system they decided to use was the *International Classification of Diseases* (ICD). Ultimately, this spelled the end of the troubled history of the Table of the Forms that was drafted by the MPA, and would usher in a new, global era of mental health classification.

CHAPTER 2

Cross-Channel Exchanges and the Beginnings of the Forms of Insanity

In the first Report of the Commissioners of Lunacy for England and Wales in 1845, a set of terms of psychological diagnosis were recommended for use in asylum statistics, which would be modified in 1882 and replaced entirely only in 1907. These were based on those initially offered by the French physician Philippe Pinel: dementia, idiocy, melancholia and mania. These forms of insanity became the core pillars of Victorian diagnosis partly because of the report's recommendations that these be used to record the diagnosis of a patient admitted to an asylum in statistical paperwork. The conciseness of Pinel's classification, or nosography as he termed it, meant it continued to be used well into the late nineteenth century, with some of the terms even remaining in use during the first half of the twentieth century. Pinel's sub-class of mania without delusions, for example, known as moral insanity in the Anglophone world, had become central to discussions surrounding the dividing line between insanity and criminal responsibility from the mid-nineteenth century onwards. Pinel's method of formulating diagnostic concepts through the description of observable behavioural symptoms and changes in emotion—a symptomology—became the norm during the age of the asylum. The terms enjoyed longevity because Pinel had limited his work on diagnosis to describing observable symptoms, and had not offered a theory of causation that could be disproven through developments in medical science.

K. M. Jones, *Psychological Classification and Diagnosis in Asylum Statistics, 1800–1948*, Mental Health in Historical Perspective,
https://doi.org/10.1007/978-3-031-46154-5_2

Despite the categories introduced by Pinel being used in asylum medical statistics for much of the nineteenth century, the lack of a theory of physical causation to his classification became a recurrent criticism of diagnostic concepts based on symptomology. Symptomology alone, without a theory of physical causation, came to be viewed as an inappropriate basis for medical diagnosis as the nineteenth century rolled on. Their widespread usage as the common currency of Victorian diagnosis due to the role they played in medical statistics did not detract criticism, and many considered Pinelean terms of psychological diagnosis tired and old by the final quarter of the nineteenth century. As medical psychology developed into a mature discipline during the 1870s and 1880s, criticisms of symptomology intensified.

Some of the first British reviews of Pinel's nosography articulated criticisms of symptomology, with it receiving a hostile reception in the United Kingdom from the very beginning. A scathing review of the English translation of Pinel's textbook appeared in the *Edinburgh Review* in 1803 and dismissed any possible contribution it could make to medicine.[1] Its writer, the English physician Henry Reeve (1780–1814), deemed Pinel's work to be self-satisfied and intellectually bankrupt plagiarism, which had failed to offer any novel insight into madness or its causes:

> ...to medical readers in this country, many of our author's remarks will appear neither new nor profound, and to no-one will his work appear complete. It is a general view of madness, under all its deplorable forms, not a minute and philosophical investigation of any particular species. It may be considered as a sketch of what has already been done [...]; though [Pinel] seems frequently to wonder, with a smile of self-approbation, at what he thinks [of] his own discoveries.[2]

According to Reeve, Pinel's dilettantism was apparent in the Frenchman's tendency to drop names from the cannon of Western philosophy for little apparent reason. The reviewer went as far as to doubt whether Pinel had really understood the work he cited by the likes of John Locke and Étienne Bonnot de Condillac, and accused the Frenchman of plagiarising the British nosologists William Cullen and Alexander Crichton. He thought these characteristics were signs of deeper problems with Pinel's

[1] Henry Reeve, 'Philippe Pinel's 'Traité Medico-Philosophique sur l'Aliénation Mentale ou la Manie"' in *The Edinburgh Review*, vol. 2, April–July 1803, pp. 160–172.

[2] Ibid., p. 161.

method, which had sacrificed detail for generality.[3] This approach had corrupted the entire nosography for Reeve, with superficial and vague descriptions of the forms of insanity that were not distinct, but rather 'only varieties of the same affection'.[4] Reeve held that the symptoms the Frenchman had employed to distinguish between the different forms of insanity were often encountered in the same patient and therefore the nosographie offered by Pinel served no useful purpose:

> At different times [the patient] passes through all the gradations, from furious phrensy [sic] to complete fatuity. The four species [of insanity], as [...] defined by our author, [are] so very general, that it would include a great part of the authors quoted in our *Review*; every transitory excels of passion, and every eccentricity or peculiarity of conduct in society.[5]

The vagueness of Pinel's diagnostic concepts meant that any and all could feasibly be diagnosed with any of the forms of insanity he described. Reeve considered them unbecoming of a medicine that dealt in material facts and not the kind of shadowy Cartesian metaphysics that Pinel was pushing. As he went on to attack Pinel for having 'little sagacity and precision', he described in dramatic terms how the distinctions the Frenchman drew between the forms of insanity were unfounded and 'absurd'.[6] Opining Pinel's vagueness, Reeve thought 'the only valid distinctions which can be made, appears to be between melancholia, mania, and idiotism' and that two of Pinel's disorders, *manie sans délire* and dementia, were useless, and should be removed from any classification of insanity.[7]

What motivated Reeve's vitriol is difficult to say for certain. As we will see, some of the problems can be put down to the quality of the translation of Pinel's work: at the time of writing this historical study, there still remains no accurate English translation of *Traité médico-philosophique sur l'aliénation mentale; ou la manie*.[8] Pinel's symptomology and omission of bodily causes for the insanities he described also clashed with the sensationalist editorial tone of the *Edinburgh Review*, under the stewardship

[3] Ibid.

[4] Ibid.

[5] Ibid., pp. 168–169.

[6] Ibid.

[7] Ibid., p. 169.

[8] Dora Weiner, 'Betrayal! The 1806 Translation of Pinel's *Traité medico-philosophique sur l'Aliénation mentale, ou la manie*' in *Generus*, vol. 57, 2000, pp. 42–50 (p. 45).

of Francis Jeffrey, who favoured practical common sense over anything that as much as resembled speculative philosophy.[9] Reeve's background can provide further clues for the hostility, since he was an alumnus of the University of Edinburgh's prestigious medical school, an emerging centre for a brand of philosophical materialism that rejected metaphysics. Furthermore, Pinel's simple division of insanity into a handful of forms looked crude and simplistic in comparison to the lengthy itineraries of the kinds of insanity provided by William Cullen (1710–1790), who had done much to shape views on what constituted the most appropriate ways to classify disease. Cullen's materialist nosology had provided a theory of aetiology for mental disorders that was rooted in the nervous power of the body. In contrast, Pinel's reluctance to provide a definitive account of the physical causes of mental disorder was interpreted as mystical and Cartesian to a dogged materialist like Reeve. Indeed, Reeve interpreted Pinel's ambivalence as a rejection of physicalism, centring on Pinel's view that insanity was not always caused by brain lesions. For Reeve, these theoretical misjudgements made Pinel's work ill-suited to practical medicine.

Reeve's criticisms are echoed in later discussions presented in this volume and point towards persistent divisions over clinical concepts of psychological diagnosis. To better understand the link to later discussions on the terms of diagnosis used in asylum statistics, this chapter will explore how the circulation and communication of knowledge between France and England helped to formulate the psychological diagnostic concepts that became the centre of debate later in the century.[10] In doing so, this chapter will set the scene for the discussions over psychological diagnosis and asylum statistics explored throughout this volume. Reeve's remarks on vagueness and imprecision will be echoed throughout the debates covered by this study, as concepts of psychological diagnosis that did not present a physical aetiology were criticised on similar grounds.

Indeed, this shortfall of Pinel's work had been the inspiration for a materialist and physicalist alternative developed by David Skae during the 1850s and which had emerged from the medical materialism of the Edinburgh Medical School.

[9] John A. Taylor, 'The "Popular" Criticism of the *Edinburgh Review*' in *Journal of Popular Culture*, vol. 9, no. 3, 1975, pp. 672–682.

[10] James A. Secord, 'Knowledge in Transit' in *Isis*, vol. 95, no. 4, 2004, pp. 654–672.

This chapter outlines how Pinel's work became popular in the United Kingdom despite its initial critical reception. It argues that it was through the textbooks of James Cowles Prichard that French ideas became palatable and led to their popularity in the United Kingdom. Prichard had adapted the ideas on diagnosis that had emerged from French alienism and adapted them to a British sensibility that valued observation and concision, especially appealing to doctors posted in the Georgian madhouse.[11] Despite facing accusations that his divisions of the insanities were also Cartesian and not grounded in physiology, Pinel's classification held some appeal to British alienists because they were concise and relatively easy to learn during a period when specialised training for asylum medical practice was lacking.[12] Prichard came to be a channel of communication of French ideas on diagnosis because he had a first-hand acquaintance with French medical psychology, albeit long after Pinel had ended his professional life. His works function as the most faithful rendition of the ideas coming from France, and he used his position as Lunacy Commissioner to promote the forms of insanity Pinel had developed. Prichard's role in the early years of the Lunacy Commission would be one of the reasons why Pinel's forms of insanity were recommended for use in asylum statistics in the first Report of the Commissioners in Lunacy of 1845. It was this development which overwhelmingly contributed to them becoming the first set of standard terms of psychological diagnosis in asylum medical statistics published by the Lunacy Commission.

Neurosis, Derangement and Species of Insanity: Crichton, Cullen and Arnold

Philippe Pinel's background combined the man of letters and the clinician. This blend was vital in shaping both his medical writings on general nosology and his work on the classification of mental disorder. He was prevented from practising in Paris due to his training in Toulouse, which was deemed unfit for the elite medical schools in the capital. Pinel's reliance on income from translations and reviews led him to becoming acquainted with medical literature from the United Kingdom, rendering into French medical textbooks by William Cullen

[11] Pinel also adopted terminology that was already familiar to English physicians familiar with Cullen and Crichton's work, as we will see during the course of this chapter.

[12] Polina Merkulova, Pedagogy and the Building of British Psychiatry at the Age of Asylum, 1792–1914, PhD thesis, University of Leeds, 2021.

and Alexander Crichton (1763–1856).[13] Before the French revolution, Pinel had considered emigrating to North America for the sake of his career, such was its stagnation, but by the 1790s he had been appointed chief physician of the Bicêtre hospital in Paris and later the prestigious Salpêtrière. He drew upon experience of these and the private sanatorium he had worked in prior to these appointments when articulating the forms of insanity included in *Traité médico-philosophique sur l'aliénation mentale; ou la manie*.[14] Before publishing his work on madness, Pinel had published an encyclopaedia of medical nosology, or nosography as he termed it, and a 'Memoire on Madness' that called for careful observation and interviewing of patients before arriving at a diagnosis.[15] In line with the empirical character of his works on general medical nosology, Pinel classified mental disorders on the basis of the symptoms that presented themselves to the physician, and conceived mental alienation as having four main forms or appearances: *la simple melancholie* (melancholia), *la manie* (mania), *la demence* (dementia) and *l'idiotisme* (idiotism). These four disorders comprised a spectrum of acuteness or severity of mental disorder: melancholia was *délire partiel* (partial insanity), manias were *délire généralisé* (general insanity), dementia was *affaiblissement intellectuel généralisé* (generalised intellectual weakening) and idiotism was rendered as *abolition totale des fonctions de l'entendement* (total obliteration of the functions of the understanding).

Due to this background as a translator and reviewer, Pinel could read English, and in the *Traité* he responded to the works of British physicians who had previously made attempts to classify mental disorder.[16] These included Thomas Sydenham (1624–1689), Cullen, Crichton, and

[13] Dora Weiner, 'Mind and Body in the Clinic: Philippe Pinel, Alexander Crichton, Dominique Esquirol, and the Birth of Psychiatry' in *The Languages of Psyche: Mind and Body in Enlightenment Thought*, edited by G.S. Rousseau, UC Berkley Press, 1990, pp. 331–403 (p. 334).

[14] Henceforth referred to as 'Pinel's *Traité*' when referring to the French, and 'Pinel's *Treatise*' when referring to the English.

[15] Pinel's choice of the word nosography instead of the nosology is an interesting question and invites speculation on the intentions behind its use. *Nosologie* was in use in French as the time, and Francois Boissier de Sauvages used the term in the title to his *Nosologia methodical* of 1772: Lester S. King, 'Boisser de Sauvages and 18th Century Nosology' in *Bulletin of the History of Medicine*, vol. 40, no. 1, January 1966, pp. 43–51.

[16] Dora Weiner, 'Mind and Body in the Clinic: Philippe Pinel, Alexander Crichton, Dominique Esquirol, and the Birth of Psychiatry' in *The Languages of Psyche: Mind

Thomas Arnold (1742–1816). Pinel had translated work by Cullen into French, as well as a set of papers from the *Philosophical Transactions of the Royal Society*.[17] Cullen's 1769 *Synopsis Nosologie Methodicae* was an important influence on Pinel, apparent from the way the French physician, like Cullen, classified illnesses on the basis of symptoms. Many of the details included in Cullen's nosology were based on his twenty-five-years' experience working in teaching hospitals in Glasgow and Edinburgh.[18] Cullen was amongst the first of the medical classifiers to place nervous disorders into a category of their own, by conceptualising them as forms of neurosis (*versanie*) which Cullen thought were generated when an imbalance occurred in the brain's 'nervous power'.[19] Imbalances in nervous power were the starting point for disorders of the nervous system, and this theory of causation was used to separate different kinds of mental disorders. Imbalances could be caused by lesion on organs, or fevers due to diseases that were contracted from the miasmas, or foul and unhealthy smells. Cullen used the notion of imbalances in nervous power to explain a great number of pathologies, with the specific nature of the illness depending on which part of the nervous system was affected. Cullen believed the nervous system played a central role in the generation of the *versaniae*: in fact, two-thirds of his lectures on general pathology were devoted to the nervous system. Cullen included twenty-nine disorders in this category, which he grouped into four orders in the 'Neurosis' section of his general nosology.

As we can see in Table 2.1, within the class of the neuroses, Cullen created a specific sub-class to differentiate mental disorders, or the *versaniae*, from other kinds of nervous disorders. Cullen understood mental disorders to be problems with the mind that were not accompanied by

and Body in Enlightenment Thought, edited by G.S. Rosseau, UC Berkley Press, 1990, pp. 331–403 (p. 334).

[17] Aubrey Lewis, 'British Psychiatry in the First Half of the Nineteenth Century: Philippe Pinel and the English' in *Proceedings of the Royal Society of Medicine*, vol. 48, February 1955, pp. 581–586 (p. 582).

[18] Christopher Lawrence emphasises Cullen's desire to contribute to the development of medical teaching in *Medicine as Culture: Edinburgh and the Scottish Enlightenment*, PhD Thesis, University of London, London, 1984.

[19] F. Clifford Rose, 'William Cullen' in *History of British Neurology*, Imperial College Press, 2011, pp. 67–68.

any type of fever or delirium.[20] His theory of causation was influenced by the Scottish physician Robert Whytt's (1714–1766) notion of sentient and sympathetic nervous power, which animated and co-ordinated the body, transmitting sensation from the organs of the body to the brain.[21] Cullen drew upon Whytt's theory of the functioning of the nerves to group the disorders within his classification, yet when it came to differentiating the different forms of *versanie*, Cullen used the observation of symptoms in patients.

Cullen's student Thomas Arnold published *Observations on the Nature, Kinds, Causes, and Prevention of Insanity, Lunacy, or Madness* in 1782. Arnold's work differed from Cullen's in one important respect: he did not provide a theory of the causes of the mental disorders, but rather stressed that his work attempted to efficiently and practically classify madness based simply upon the observation of clinical symptoms.[22] Table 2.2 shows how Arnold divided insanity into two classes.

Arnold's notion of *ideal insanity* described conditions which affected the thought processes of the patient and interfered with their ability to reason. He divided the second class of *notional insanities* according to specific psychological states, such as excessive *vanity* or *impulsiveness*. Notional insanities were distinct from ideal insanities because they affected the person's emotions, and consequently, their capacity to act morally. Arnold's division of insanity according to the faculty of the mind afflicted by disturbed thought processes was perhaps due to his education in Edinburgh and the popularity of faculty psychology in the Scottish capital. The application of faculty psychology to the classification of mental disorders foreshadowed a similar strategy that was adopted by Pinel nearly twenty years later: to use a limited set of diagnostic concepts for practicality's sake, which had helped Arnold's classification gain some degree of popularity amongst doctors working in British asylums.[23]

[20] German Berrios, *The History of Mental Symptoms: Descriptive Psychopathology Since the Nineteenth Century*, Cambridge University Press, 1996 (p. 174).

[21] Julius Rocca, 'William Cullen and Robert Whytt on the Nervous System' in *Brain, Mind and Medicine: Neuroscience in the 18th Century*, edited by Harry Whitaker, C.U.M. Smith, and Stanley Finger, Springer, 2007, pp. 85–98.

[22] Peter K. Carpenter, 'Thomas Arnold: A Provincial Psychiatrist in Georgian Britain' in *Medical History*, vol. 33, 1989, pp. 199–216.

[23] Peter K. Carpenter, 'Thomas Arnold: A Provincial Psychiatrist in Georgian Britain' in *Medical History*, no. 33, 1989, pp. 199–216.

Table 2.1 William Cullen's nosology of neurosis (nervous diseases)[24]

Order I	
Comata	Sophrose Diseases
Apoplexia	Apoplexy
Paralysis	Palsy
Order II	
Adynamie	Defect of Vital Power
Syncope	Fainting
Dyspepsia	Indigestion
Hypocondriasis	Low Spirits
Chlorosis	Green Sickness
Order III	
Tetanus	Universal Cramp, or lockjaw
Convulsio	Convulsion
Chorea	St Vitus's Disease
Raphania	Spasms of the Joint
Epilepsia	Epilepsy
Palpitatio	Palpitation of the Heart
Asthma	Asthma
Dysponea	Difficult Breathing
Pertussis	Hooping Cough
Pyrosis	Water Brash
Colica	Colick
Cholera	Vomiting and Purging
Diarrhoea	Purging
Diabetes	Excessive, discharge of urine
Hysteria	Hysterics
Hydrophobia	Canine Madness
Order IV	
Versaniae	Mental Diseases
Amentia	Idiotism
Melancholia	Melancholy
Mania	Madness
Oneirodynia	Night Mare

[24] William Cullen, *Synopsis Nosologiae Methodicae*, translated by William Jackson, W. Jackson, 1827, pp. 11–12.

Table 2.2 Thomas Arnold, 'A Table of Species of Insanity'[25]

A Table of the Species of Insanity	
One Genus – Insanity.	
Two Divisions, – Ideal–*and*–Notional Insanity.	
I. Ideal Insanity.	1. Phrenitic Insanity.
	2. Incoherent.
	3. Maniacal.
	4. Sensitive.
II. Notional Insanity	5. Delusive.
	6. Fanciful.
	7. Whimsical.
	8. Impulsive.
	9. Scheming.
	10. Vain, or Self-important.
	11. Hypochondriacal.
	12. Pathetic.
	13. Appetitive.

[25] Thomas Arnold, *Observations on the Nature, Kinds, Causes, and Prevention of Insanity, Lunacy, or Madness*, G. Ireland, 1782 (p. 124).

Medicine saw much development during the late eighteenth century, and this made Arnold's work look dated by the dawn of the new century, less than twenty years after its initial publication. Arnold's *Observations* drew criticism from those who published their own textbooks on mental disease. Most prominent of these was the English physician Alexander Crichton, who in the preface to his 1797 *Inquiry into the Nature and Origin of Mental Derangement* attacked Arnold's approach to dividing insanity according to the contents or characteristic features of psychological states.[26] Crichton thought that Arnold's strategy had led to conceptual confusions, singling out the principle of differentiating disorder on the basis of characteristics such as *scheming*, *vanity* or *whimsy*. Crichton thought this would, if taken to its extreme, create an endless list of forms of insanity that would be too complicated for practical use. Crichton instead thought that classification should be based on the somatic symptoms that were presented in each patient, including

[26] Alexander Crichton, *An inquiry into the nature and origin of mental derangement: comprehending a concise system of the physiology and pathology of the human mind and a history of the passions and their effects*, Cadell Jr. & Davies, 1798, p. 5.

tics, states of catatonia and excitement. He focused his attention on thought processes, and abstract concepts of emotion. As Dora Weiner notes, these features of Crichton's work had left an impression on Pinel, with numerous citations of his work in the Frenchman's *Traité*.[27] In particular, Crichton's vitalism and animism, influences acquired during his time training in Leiden, Paris, Vienna and Berlin, had left an impression on Pinel.[28] Louis Charland claims that whilst Crichton's ideas had been an influence, Pinel had taken Crichton ideas on the relationship between emotion and social issues in a different and more abstract direction fitting of the scientific materialism of the post-revolutionary French Republic.[29] Whatever may be the case, Pinel's work had been informed by ideas over classification and diagnosis emerging from the United Kingdom, with Edinburgh being a particular source of inspiration.

Traité médico-philosophique sur l'aliénation mentale: Translating Pinel's Forms of Mental Alienation

Pinel's *Traité médico-philosophique sur l'aliénation mentale* was first published in 1800, with a second edition appearing in 1808.[30] It was a part of a wider project to develop his *Nosographie Philosophique*, that itself was published in multiple editions between 1798 and 1818. As mentioned, the *Traité* was translated into English only once during the nineteenth century.[31] Its publication is widely considered to mark the beginning of the modern classification of the mental disorders, with Mason and Hsin claiming that it was the first self-conscious attempt to break from the botanical model of disease classification that had informed

[27] Dora B. Weiner, *Comprendre et soigner: Philippe Pinel (1745–1826): La médecine de l'esprit. Penser la Médecine*, Paris: Fayard, 1999.

[28] German Berrios, '"Mind in General" by Sir Alexander Crichton' in *History of Psychiatry*, vol. 17, no. 4, pp. 469–486.

[29] Loius Charland, 'Alexander Crichton on the Psychopathology of the Passions' in *History of Psychiatry*, vol. 19, no. 3, pp. 275–296.

[30] D. Mason and H. Hsin, ''A More Perfect Arrangement of Plants': The Botanical Model in Psychiatric Nosology, 1676 to the Present Day' in *History of Psychiatry*, vol. 29, no. 2, 2018, pp. 131–146.

[31] Dora Weiner, 'Betrayal! The 1806 Translation of Pinel's *Traité´ medico- philosophique sur l'Aliénation mentale, ou la manie*' in *Generus*, vol. 57, 2000, pp. 42–50.

the medical classifications of Sydenham, Carl Linnaeus (1707–1778), François Boissier de Sauvages (1706–1767) and Cullen. He utilised concepts from Cullen's classification of the versanies but replaced the Latin-derived term amentia with the French *la demence*.[32] Although the symptoms that Pinel described and associated with dementia very closely resembled Cullen's description of amentia, it is unclear why he chose dementia for his nosology. Berrios argues that it was because the term *la demence* had a long tradition in the French language, whereas the term amentia was typically used in English clinical literature: he cites as an example William Battie's (1703–1776) employment of amentia in his 1758 *Treatise on Madness*.[33] The use of *la demence* by Pinel helped to make it a standard term in French, with dementia coming to be the standard within English language medical literature as seen in James Cowles Prichard's (1786–1848) *Treatise on Insanity* published in 1835.[34] As a result, Pinel's term *dementia* gradually came to be used instead of *amentia*, although there are notable exceptions to this trend. Thomas Laycock (1812–1876) and David Skae (1814–1873), both of whose work would prove to be influential in Britain in the second half of the nineteenth century, employed *amentia* in versions of their classifications published from the 1850s onwards, partly to differentiate their work from Pinelean symptomology.

Pinel employed the term *melancholie*, yet the symptoms he referred to were different to Cullen's. Pinel had made melancholie a broader category, and had used a larger collection of symptoms than Cullen had to describe it.[35] For Pinel, melancholia was not limited to 'sadness' or forms of depression, but included a number of other behaviours including delusions and obsessive behaviours.[36] Pinel included emotional disorders, like

[32] Philippe Pinel, *Traité médico-philosophique sur l'aliénation mentale*, Chez J. Ant. Brosson, 1800, p. 130.

[33] German Berrios, 'Dementia During the Seventeenth and Eighteenth Century' in *Psychological Medicine*, vol. 7, no. 4, 1987, pp. 829–837 (p. 834).

[34] Hannah Franziska Augstein, 'JC Prichard's Concept of Moral Insanity—A Medical Theory of the Corruption of Human Nature' in *Medical History*, vol. 40, 1996, pp. 311–343 (p. 314).

[35] German Berrios, 'Mood Disorders: Clinical Section' in *A History of Clinical Psychiatry: The Origin and History of Psychiatric Disorders*, edited by German Berrios and Roy Porter, London, 1995, pp. 384–408. (p. 389).

[36] Ibid., p. 384.

the feeling of sadness and despair that Cullen understood it to be, but he also included certain manias and delusions, as well as chronic psychotic states.[37] It would not be until the work of Jean-Étienne Dominique Esquirol (1772–1840), whose work is discussed in more detail later in this chapter, that melancholia as a form of depression of the emotions would begin to be separated from disorders that affected the intellectual capacities, and he achieved this by developing the concepts *lypemania* and *monomania*.

Pinel intended some overlap in the categories of his nosography, with the concepts not being mutually exclusive. A patient could be diagnosed with both mania and melancholia since Pinel thought that it was possible to exhibit symptoms of both at different times: this could be a day, a week or several months apart. Pinel was not attempting to classify natural kinds with his *nosographie* and he therefore did not provide a theory of the physical causes of insanity, such as the sympathetic nervous power developed by Whytt and Cullen. He was not attempting to describe different kinds of insanity, or anything like Arnold's 'species' of insanity. Instead, his nosography sought to develop a descriptive account of the manifestations of insanity through behavioural symptoms that he had observed during his practice. The concepts of diagnosis he developed clustered sets of behavioural symptoms and linked them to diagnostic labels.[38] Pinel intended them to be useful guides in medical practice, and not as descriptions or representations of natural diseases.[39] Pinel's famous conviction on the social causes of insanity, or the mental alienations, proved decisive in making his nosography diverge from Cullen and Crichton's: for instance, he had divided Cullen's amentia into dementia and idiotism to differentiate between gradual forms of degenerative mental alienation, and hereditary or congenital diseases. He had cordoned off the mental alienations of *melancholia*, *dementia*, the *manias* and *idiotism* from other

[37] Judith Misbach and Henderikus J. Stam, 'Medicalizing Melancholia: Exploring Profiles of Psychiatric Professionalization' in *Journal of the History of the Human Sciences*, vol. 42, no. 1, 1996, pp. 41–59 (p. 45).

[38] K.S. Kendler, 'Philippe Pinel and the Foundations of Modern Psychiatric Nosology' in *Psychological Medicine*, vol. 50, no. 16, 2020, pp. 2667–2672.

[39] Woods and Carlson claim that Pinel's work had marked a division in the study of cognitive and mental disorders due to neurosis not being recognised by Pinel as a form of mental alienation: Evelyn A. Woods and Eric T. Carlson, 'The Psychiatry of Philippe Pinel' in *Bulletin of the History of Medicine*, vol. 35, no. 14, 1961, pp. 14–25.

Table 2.3 Pinel's forms of insanity[40]

La simple mélancolie (délire partiel)
La manie (délire généralisé)
La demence (affaiblissement intellectual généralisé)
L'iditotisme (abolition totale des fonctions de l'entendement)

[40] Philippe Pinel, *Traité médico-philosophique sur l'aliénation mentale*, 2nd edition, Chez J. Ant. Brosson, 1809.

nervous diseases, which were included in the same category in Cullen's nosology (Table 2.3).

Although he did not subscribe to the causal theory of nervous power presented by Cullen, Pinel had sought to develop the Scottish physician's classification of the *neuroses*, albeit parsed by Pinel as mental alienations.[41] Like Cullen, Pinel based his division of the insanities on observable symptoms including behaviours, tics and convulsions, providing detailed behavioural trends associated with each disorder. He did not however attempt to explain physical causes, and had devoted space in the *Traité* to criticise positions that strongly linked brain lesions to mental alienation.[42] He had also entertained the possibility that certain forms of mania could exist without a brain lesion. In rejecting Cullen's theory of nervous power and not providing an alternative theory of physical causation, Pinel restricted his work to being a symptomology. Crichton's faculty psychology had also left its mark on the nosography, and provided the basis of Pinel's *manie sans délire*, a disorder which he thought affected the emotional, but not the intellectual, faculties of the mind. The preface to the *Traité* praises elements of Crichton's classification, concurring with the criticisms of Arnold's use of psychological content, such as nightmares and reverie, to differentiate forms of insanity from one another.[43]

[41] Ibid.

[42] Ibid., p. 156.

[43] Dora Weiner, 'The Madman in the Light of Reason. Enlightenment Psychiatry: Part II. Alienists, Treatises, and the Psychologic Approach in the Era of Pinel' in *History of*

For the purposes of this chapter, then, it is possible to make conclusions at this point. Firstly, the concepts in the *Traité*, although modified, were informed by Cullen's classification of the neuroses, but differed in that Pinel did not provide a theory of causation. Returning to Reeve's review, we can see now that his representation of Pinel's attitudes on the relationship between afflictions of the body and the mind was somewhat unreasonable, although not completely unjustified. The Frenchman's speculation that some forms of insanity may have no physical basis in the form of a brain lesion and instead may find their root in the mental faculties particularly angered Reeve. He accuses Pinel of Cartesianism, but whilst there is a rather a modest call for nosologists to refrain from offering speculative theories of causation, there is little evidence that substance dualism informed the Frenchman's work. Pinel acknowledged that physical causes for mental disorders may exist, but until they could be proven, a worthwhile division of the insanities should be restricted to observable physical symptoms. In other words, Pinel thought it wise to make looser connections between bodily and behavioural symptoms, at least until the links were better understood. Pinel even speculated that certain forms of insanity could be caused by the mental faculties alone, with thoughts and emotions being a causing agent that ought to be taken into consideration in diagnosis. As Huneman notes, the influence of vitalist medicine played a role in shaping Pinel's view of the emotions being a disturbance of the soul by the body as a result of an 'animal economy' that was comprised of both the physical and the moral capacities.[44] A reticence to draw strong connections between the conditions of the mind and body was interpreted by Reeve as a sign of a dangerous kind of dualist metaphysics, but Pinel was in fact a committed materialist in many ways and thought it possible to explain the conditions of the mind through the afflictions of the body. However, he did not view the thought processes affected by the passions as distinct from the body, and as such, any theory of causation must consider the role of psychological processes in the development of the mental alienations. Reeve's suspicions motivated his harsh judgement of Pinel's division of the insanities, describing them as imprecise and unwieldy, and devoid of any possible value, for

Psychiatry and Medical Psychology: With an Epilogue on Psychiatry and the Mind–Body Relation, edited by Edwin R. Wallace and John Gach, pp. 281–304 (p. 294).

[44] Philippe Huneman, 'Montpellier Vitalism and the Emergence of Alienism in France (1750–1800): The Case of the Passions', *Science in Context*, vol. 21, 2008, pp. 615–647.

natural medicine.[45] Reeve rounded off his scathing piece by warning his readers that the *Traité* and the forms it presented had no place in the practice of medicine in the British Isles.[46]

Reeve's criticisms of Pinel's dualism were also driven by a natural philosophy that demanded natural histories of natural kinds, as he wrote that the 'want of an accurate history of the several kinds of insanity, has often been felt and acknowledged'.[47] The intensity of his criticisms are partly borne from the unfair demands he placed on Pinel's nosographie to provide an account of the natural kinds of insanity from a work that sought to present the *forms* of insanity, or a symptomology. Pinel's nosography did not aim to provide an authoritative and natural representation of the divisions of insanity, but was designed as a tool for clinical use. The clearest evidence for this is in Pinel's own descriptions, which describe trends and tendencies, and are in no way deterministic. Furthermore, his simple division of insanity into six disorders shows his desire to keep the list simple and the labels loose. It is the minimal quality of Pinel's division of insanity that also contributed to its lasting appeal.[48]

Reeve missed this point in his demand from Pinel that the behaviours he associated with different forms of insanity be tied to brain lesions. Reeve demanded from Pinel something that the French physician had not aimed to provide: a description of the natural kinds of insanity that would be drawn along the lines of pathology, prognosis and causation. Pinel

[45] Ibid.

[46] Philippe Pinel, 'Traité Medico-Philosophique sur l'Aliénation Mentale ou la Manie' in *The Edinburgh Review*, vol. 2, April–July 1803, pp. 160–172 (p. 164).

[47] Ibid., p. 160.

[48] See in particular the following remarks included in a letter to the Congrés des Medicins Alientistes et Neurologistes de France et des Pays de Langue Francaise drafted by Reginald Worth marking the centenary of Pinel's death: 'The Members of the Royal Medico-Psychological Association [RMPA], in acknowledging their indebtedness to Pinel, feel that they have faithfully carried on the great tradition that he created. They also feel that they are associated with him in no ordinary way. It was Pinel who translated into French the medical works of Prof. Cullen of Edinburgh—himself a great psychiatrist. Our academic courses of lectures on psychiatry were directly inspired by Esquirol—first the pupil and then the friend of Pinel [...] On this memorable occasion, which recalls the glorious and epoch-making work of a great French alienist, the RMPA sends its congratulations to those now assembled, whose brilliant achievements have advanced psychiatry to the high position it now occupies among the medical sciences'. Reginald Worth and Donald Ross, 'Centenary of the Death of Philippe Pinel' in *JMS*, vol. 72, no. 299, October 1926, p. 718.

grouped together symptoms commonly associated with one another to formulate the concepts of mania, melancholia, idiotism and dementia, but did not attempt to explain them through natural or mechanical processes; he provided accounts in the *Traité* which spoke of the damage to the *mental faculties*, the different parts of the mind, and not the attrition to the organic matter of the brain.

The initial reception of Pinel's *Traité* amongst British physicians was, as Reeve's review indicates, less than enthusiastic, and there is little to suggest Pinel's work on the mental alienations caught on amongst British physicians upon their initial publication at the beginning of the nineteenth century.[49] In addition to a poor translation, it is possible the prohibition of printed material entering the United Kingdom from France as a result of the Napoleonic Wars may have also played a role in obstructing the transmission of French clinical ideas.[50] Pinel's lack of adherence to a strictly causal and physical explanation of insanity would, as we will see especially in the next three chapters, continue to reverberate throughout Victorian psychiatry and the age of the asylum. Another critical review of Pinel's division of insanity, published in 1803 in *the Monthly Review*, also called into question the practical use of the nosography:

> With regard to the practical utility of his division, (which, it is to be remarked, by no means entirely belongs to the present author) it may be doubted to what extent it may reach. The distinctions are far from being constant, even in the same individual; nor are the means of cure always dependent on the particular place which may be allotted in nosology to the combination of existing symptoms.[51]

[49] Aside from the lack of reviews lauding Pinel's work, a remark made by Victorian social campaigner Ellice Hopkins wrote in *Fraser's Magazine* also suggests that Pinel's influence in the United Kingdom was slow to take hold: 'Not only was the spread of Pinel's principles extremely slow, so that as late as 1836, when, as we shall afterwards see, Charlesworth and Hill, in England, were abolishing the last vestige of mechanical treatment...' Hopkins, 'The Moral Treatment of Insanity' in *Fraser's Magazine*, vol. 15, no. 88, 1877, pp. 444–459 (p. 449).

[50] Jonathan Topham, 'Science, Print, and Crossing Borders: Importing French Science Books into Britain, 1789–1815' in *Geographies of Nineteenth-Century Science*, edited by D.N. Livingstone and C.W.J. Withers, University of Chicago Press, 2011, pp. 311–344.

[51] It is important to note that whilst this review did not value Pinel's nosography, it did hold in esteem Pinel's moral treatment and the observations from his case notes. 'Book review' in *Monthly Review, Or, Literary Journal*, vol. 42, 1803, pp. 526–532 (p. 530).

Once again, the vagueness and broadness of Pinel's work did not rest easy, although the impression this reviewer had that the forms of mental diseases were not constant, or particularly steadfast, may not have been helped with the French 'la demence', Pinel's technical term for dementia, being translated as simply 'madness' in this review and in the only translation available of the textbook.[52]

The unenthusiastic reception to Pinel's nosography can be partly explained through the imprecision of the first English translation of the work, carried out in 1806 by the Sheffield-based physiologist David Daniel Davis (1777–1841).[53] The title given to the translation itself demonstrated a major divergence from Pinel's original, with Davis opting for *A Treatise on Insanity in Which are Contained the Principles of a New and More Practical Nosology of Manical Disorder*—a more faithful translation would be *A Medical Philosophical Treatise on the Mental Alienations, or the Manias*. The differences in the titles is no small point, because it reflected Davis's tendency to translate the French 'manie' as 'insanity' throughout the 1806 translation, which introduced a number of key ambiguities, such as 'Manie intermittente' (intermittent mania) being translated as 'periodical insanity', 'le traitement de la Mànie' (the treatment of mania) being rendered by Davis as 'treatment of insanity' and 'Les accès de Manie' (outbursts of mania) being rendered in the translation as 'paroxysms of insanity'.[54] Most serious of all these liberties was Davis's rendering of 'manie sans délires' as 'mania without delirium': with the original French 'délires' being a clinical term that described delusions, hallucinations, false beliefs and distortions in chains of reasoning. Davis's 'mania without delirium' was inaccurate, with the English *delirium* suggesting the kind of transitory hallucinations and delusion seen in fevers and intoxication. Further inconsistencies included Thomas Arnold being lauded in the translation, despite Pinel having

[52] Ibid.

[53] In addition, a second expanded edition published by Pinel in 1809 was not translated until 2018, leaving a rather shoddy and inaccurate translation of the earlier edition of his work as the only one available to English readers. Dora Weiner suggests that this has had a profound impact upon the understanding of Pinel amongst Anglophone scholars; Dora Weiner, 'Betrayal! The 1806 Translation of Pinel's *Traité' medico- philosophique sur l'Aliénation mentale, ou la manie*' in *Generus*, vol. 57, 2000, pp. 42–50.

[54] Philippe Pinel, *A Treatise on Insanity, in Which Are Contained the Principles of a New and More Practical Nosology of Maniacal Disorders*, translated by D.D. Davis, W. Todd, 1806, p. 43 and p. 25.

criticised him in the original French textbook.[55] The style of writing employed by Davis was florid and complicated, a stark contrast to Pinel's clinical and austere French.[56] It is difficult to say for certain what may have led to these inconsistencies, but the quality of the translation could perhaps be explained by Davis's lack of experience working in an asylum, and therefore the intricacies of alienism, or wider political differences between England and France at the time.[57]

The basic forms of insanity presented in Pinel's original *Traité* were preserved to some degree in the translation, albeit with different guises. The quality of Pinel's prose in Davis's translation of the foundational principles informing the work had suffered, and created ambiguities which may also account for the harsh reviews it received. Davis's translation was far away from the more precise clinical style that characterised Pinel's own writing.[58] For instance, 'les diverses lesions des facultes intellectuelles ou affectives' [the various lesions of the intellectual and emotional faculties] was rendered by Davis as the 'the various lesions of the intellectual and active faculties'.[59] It is unclear why Davis opted for 'active' instead of 'affective' or 'emotional', either of which would have been a more accurate translation. It may have been that Davis construed intellectual faculties as being a passive feature of the mind, and emotional faculties as being active, but whatever may have been the case, a fundamental distinction of Pinel's nosography was obscured by this mistranslation. Davis's translation went on to infer this distinction when he wrote that 'the powers of perception and imagination are frequently disturbed without any excitement of the passions' and that 'the functions of the understanding are [...] often perfectly sound, while the man is driven by his passions to acts of turbulence and outrage'.[60] However, the use of passions lacked the abstraction and neutrality that emotions offered; from

55 Ibid.

56 Ibid.

57 Ibid.

58 Dora Weiner, 'Betrayal! The 1806 Translation of Pinel's *Traité´ medico- philosophique sur l'Aliénation mentale, ou la manie*' in *Generus*, vol. 57, 2000, pp. 42–50 (p. 45).

59 Philippe Pinel, *A Treatise on Insanity, in Which Are Contained the Principles of a New and More Practical Nosology of Maniacal Disorders*, translated by D.D. Davis, W. Todd, 1806, p. 135, and Philippe Pinel, *Traité médico-philosophique sur l'aliénation mentale*, 2nd edition, Chez J. Ant. Brosson, 1809 (p. 136).

60 Davis, p. 135.

Davis's translation it appeared that Pinel was narrowing this to furious passions, with the distinction between affective faculties and intellectual faculties again becoming obscured.

A further peculiar move taken by Davis was in the section of the work that discussed the terminology Pinel had decided to use to describe each of the forms of the mental alienations. Pinel wrote that the Ancient Greeks had only offered terms for acute forms of delirium that were seen in severe illnesses, but lacked a language which described the human understanding.[61] Pinel then stated:

> Il fallut donc revenir sur mes pas, et faire entrer dans l'ordre de mes études les écrits de nos Psycologistes modernes, Locke, Harris, Condillac, Smith, Stewart, etc., pour saisir et tracer toutes les variétés comprises dans la dénomination générique d'aliénation de l'esprit.[62]

Pinel here was saying that it was necessary to retrace steps in his studies and return to reassess the work of modern psychologists to find, apprehend, collect and trace all the varieties of alienation of the mind that they had described. Pinel's aim for research was more vaguely put by Davis in his translation:

> But the history of insanity, being inseparable from that of the human understanding, is necessarily found in a very imperfect state in the writings of the ancients. I have, therefore, felt the necessity of commencing my studies with examining the numerous and important facts which have been discovered and detailed by modern pneumatologists.[63]

Aside from not including the names of the thinkers that Pinel invoked, adding to the sense of vagueness that was criticised by Reeve in the English translation, Davis's substitution of psychology for pneumatology placed the work firmly in the previous century and amplified any Cartesian undertones: although pneumatology was used to describe the functioning of the human mind and was a precursor to *psychology*, it still held mystical and supernatural connotations. Pinel's footnotes to this section

[61] Philippe Pinel, *Traité médico-philosophique sur l'aliénation mentale*, 2nd edition, Chez J. Ant. Brosson, 1809, p. 136.

[62] Ibid.

[63] Davis, p. 135.

are completely omitted from the English version, yet in the French they provided lengthy and illustrative elaborations in the form of nuanced descriptions of the details of each of the alienations, often invoking specific cases for further elaboration.[64]

Despite the imprecision of Davis's translation, and the omission of a great deal of material from the original text, the main forms of the mental alienations were preserved. Melancholia's different forms are given in the translation: Melancholia with delirium was split into the two forms that Pinel gave it, with those that are characterised by symptoms of despair and other forms which are accompanied by exalted delusions of grandeur.[65] Intellectual forms of melancholia Pinel had described as patients building obsessions but without any accompanying delusions, which he considered to be a form of *versanie*, or neurosis. In addition, Davis described forms of melancholia that were connected to suicide, but again in less precise terms. 'Mania without delirium' and 'with delirium' were included in Davis's translation, in addition to 'periodical mania', and 'dementia, the abolition of the thinking faculty', and 'dementia, marked by ideas unconnected amongst themselves, and without relation to external objects'.[66] The forms of mental alienation that Pinel presented in the first edition of his *Traité* were preserved in the English translation, but Davis lost much of the nuance, and the quality of his translation contributed to his ideas receiving an unenthusiastic initial reception in the United Kingdom.

Prichard's Textbooks and the Introduction of the Pinelean System to the British Isles

In lieu of an authentic translation of Pinel's work, the ideas of French psychiatry had a somewhat limited influence in the British Isles during the first decades of the nineteenth century.[67] It was not until the work of

[64] Philippe Huneman, 'Écrire le cas–Pinel aliéniste', *Philosophie*, vol. 120, no. 1, 2014, pp. 67–94.

[65] Philippe Pinel, *Traité médico-philosophique sur l'aliénation mentale*, 2nd edition, Chez J. Ant. Brosson, 1809, p. 142.

[66] Ibid., pp. 140–165.

[67] Pinel was regarded in high esteem in British medical journals such as the Lancet during the 1920s as result of his contributions to general medicine and his asylum management: there is little evidence to suggest his nosographie receives much attention until at least the late 1820s.

Prichard that they began to exert some influence. Prichard served a pivotal role in bringing French ideas on insanity to the British Isles during the 1830s. As we have seen, the ideas in Pinel's *Traité* failed to gain traction upon their initial publication partly because of a poor translation, but also because of hostility towards Pinel's views on the relationships between body and mind. Prichard took advantage of the improved relations between Britain and France after the end of the Napoleonic Wars to spend time in Paris and come into first-hand contact with the French School of medical psychology. Because of his time spent in Paris and his ability to read the original French manuscripts of both Pinel and Esquirol, Prichard's textbooks would capture an authenticity not seen in previous translations. They would serve as the main conduit for ideas on medical psychology developed in France, bringing the spirit of French psychological classification and diagnosis to English language readers. Furthermore, Prichard's influence as a medical authority on the Lunacy Commission helped to make these concepts a common currency in the United Kingdom, with the Commission recommending the concepts developed by Pinel for use in statistical returns that recorded the forms of insanity of admissions. This development would prove a decisive factor in making Pinel's categories the standard language used in asylum diagnosis and medical statistics from 1845 onwards. The use of these diagnostic terms in Victorian medicine is often taken for granted, but as this study shows, a contingent set of clinical, legal and administrative developments made melancholia, dementia, idiocy, moral insanity and mania the standard categories of psychological diagnosis employed in Victorian asylum medical statistics.

Along with an interest in anthropology and geology, Prichard was to become a prominent figure in British medicine and lunacy administration, as well as an influential legal theorist.[68] Textbooks published under his name from the mid-1830s onwards helped to popularise diagnostic concepts that had been developed in France in the wake of Pinel. He had spent time working at Esquirol's hospital in Ivry, near Paris, gaining first-hand knowledge that allowed him to become the English

[68] H.F. Augstein, 'James Cowles Prichard's Anthropology: Remaking the Science of Man in Early Nineteenth Century Britain' in *Clio Medica*, vol. 52, 2016.

language interpreter of French ways of classification.[69] The context in which Prichard published his textbooks, the 1830s and 1840s, was one that saw a wane in interest in phrenology, opening the door for a classification such as that of Pinel which did not rely on a theory of physical causation. It also placated any possible ill-feeling from the clergy, who viewed the notion of thought as an organ of the brain as challenging the notion of an immaterial soul.[70] Prichard's amiability and Quaker background made him an appealing choice for public office, and he served as the mental health specialist for the Lunacy Commission, the body that emerged from the Metropolitan Commissioners in Lunacy and which was formally established in 1845 to regulate and monitor asylums across England and Wales. The appointment provided him with a great deal of influence in a period that was pivotal in the formulation of the rules and regulations that would govern asylum psychiatry during the Victorian period. These rules and regulations shaped the bureaucracy and administration of asylums, determining the paperwork used to record admissions, discharges and transfers, as well as the procedures used to collect statistical information from institutions. Prichard's work with the Lunacy Commission, albeit cut short by his death in 1848, would have wide implications for the history of diagnostic categories used in medical statistics, as it were the diagnostic terms developed in France after Pinel that were recommended as the standard to be used in asylum statistics in the first report of the Commissioners in Lunacy, issued in 1845. As a result, they would become foundational to debates over the Table of the Forms during the latter half of the nineteenth century.

A brief look at Prichard's own intellectual development points towards broader trends in the development of ideas surrounding psychological diagnosis during the first half of the nineteenth century. His first textbook on mental disorder, *A Treatise on Diseases of the Nervous System*, was published in 1822 and bore the mark of Cullen's aetiology and Arnold's descriptions of psychological symptoms. His later textbook, *A Treatise on*

[69] H.F. Augstein, 'J C Prichard's Concept of Moral Insanity—A Medical Theory of the Corruption of Human Nature' in *Medical History*, vol. 40, no. 3, 1996, pp. 311–343; and J.C. Prichard, 'Temperament' in *The Cyclopaedia of Practical Medicine vol. 4*, edited by John Forbes, Alexander Tweedie and John Connolly, with revisions by Robley Dunglison, Lea and Blanchard, 1845, pp. 349–363 (p. 362).

[70] Elfed Huw Price, 'Do Brains Think? Comparative Anatomy and the End of the Great Chain of Being in 19th-Century Britain' in *History of the Human Sciences*, vol. 25, no. 3, 2012, pp. 32–50.

Insanity, was published in 1835 and had been informed by the work of French medical psychology, and postulated that there were distinct forms of mental disorder that had different behavioural manifestations.[71] This is quite different to his earlier work, with his 1822 textbook holding that insanity was one disease which had different manifestations depending on a person's constitution and at what point they were in the course of the disease.[72] Prichard held in his earlier textbook that the essence of insanity was the mind's inability to distinguish reality from illusion, with the two becoming confused due to damage to the faculties of memory and imagination.[73] When writing about the confusion between recollection and fantasy, Prichard employed Arnold's notion of *reverie* to describe how a patient 'mist[ook] the [intellectual] ideas of *reverie* for the impressions of memory and reflection'.[74] Insanity's essence in memory and self-reflection was the metaphysical foundation for Prichard's theory of the causes of madness:

> To sum up this account in a few words, the character of madness seems to consist in the circumstance that the impressions of reverie are so modified by the disease as to be no longer distinguishable from those of attentive and active reflection.[75]

Prichard held in his earlier work that all forms of insanity had this same essence. His division of mania also bore the influence of Arnold, distinguishing between forms where patients experience symptoms of daemonomania, or when patients talk to imaginary or fantastical beings, and those who have maniacal hallucinations. Prichard's early ideas on madness not only pay tribute to the work of both Cullen and Arnold, but also criticise work on classification emerging from France: *A Treatise*

[71] James Cowles Prichard, *A Treatise on Diseases of the Nervous System*, Thomas and George Underwood, 1822.

[72] Denis Leigh, 'James Cowles Prichard' in *Proceedings of the Royal Society of Medicine: Section of Psychiatry with Section of the History of Medicine*, 1955, pp. 586–590; James Cowles Prichard, 'Chapter IV: A General Description of Madness' in *A Treatise on Diseases of the Nervous System*, Thomas and George Underwood, 1822, pp. 113–116 (p. 113).

[73] James Cowles Prichard, *A Treatise on Diseases of the Nervous System*, Thomas and George Underwood, 1822.

[74] Ibid., p. 122.

[75] Ibid., p. 126.

on the Nervous System rejected Pinel's notion of *manie sans délire*, and provided an alternative explanation for manic symptoms in patients who seemed to be in full possession of their intellectual faculties:

> ...such a phenomena [sic] as that of a man rushing with eagerness to commit the most atrocious of murders, under the influence of ungovernable fury, without any impression on his mind that is calculated to excite anger, even without any fancied ground of offence against his unfortunate victim, cannot be imagined to result from the operation of *any natural causes*. Such a maniac must be literally possessed by a daemon: his action is not *that of a human being*, however insane. Yet M. Pinel describes this as the proceeding of a man who, in the common sense of words, must be called *sane*, as being in full possession of his intellectual faculties.[76]

In identifying sanity with rational capabilities, Prichard ignores Pinel's distinction between emotional and intellectual forms of mental alienation.[77] Instead, his own explanation for behaviours Pinel associated with *manie sans délire* was rooted in his theory of the essence of insanity, and that manic states were periods of temporary confusion between reality and illusion. For Prichard, this was a more plausible explanation for a rational being committing atrocious acts, as the individual could appear to be in full possession of their intellectual faculties 'free from any maniacal illusion, and are hence supposed to have an undisturbed possession of their intellectual faculties', yet they could 'fall at certain periods under the influence of some sudden hallucination, which excites their rage to a vehement degree'.[78] Those suffering from *manie sans délire* were therefore not suffering an emotional disturbance that was distinct from their rational capacities, as Pinel would have it, but instead suffering from intermittent delusions that led them to commit violent or indecent acts.[79]

Pinel's work on classification set the standard for French medical psychology during the first half of the nineteenth century. He was a towering figure during this period, creating division and debate, with

[76] Ibid., p. 136 [Italics added for emphasis].

[77] Prichard's uncharitable reading of Pinel could be due to his reliance on Davis's translation: the sole footnote citing Pinel in Prichard's *A Treatise on Nervous Diseases* was made to the English translation, and not the original French which Prichard would cite in his later works on insanity; ibid., p. 132.

[78] Ibid., p. 137.

[79] Ibid., p. 140.

much critical discourse centring around the validity of his concept of *manie sans délire*. Some, like François-Emmanuel Fodéré (1764–1835) and Étienne-Jean Georget (1795–1828) welcomed the notion, but there were others including Jean-Pierre Falret and Jean-Etienne-Dominique Esquirol who cast a more sceptical eye.[80] After writing a medical thesis that offered an explanation for *manie sans délire* that resembled Prichard's early position, Esquirol came to accept Pinel's distinction between the emotional and intellectual faculties and devoted much of his writing to developing Pinel's nosography. His 1810 textbook *De la monomanie* stands as one of the most striking examples, in which he distinguished between two forms of melancholia: monomania and lypemania.[81] The devotion to further clarification of one concept is a neat example of Esquirol's approach, since he was not a system builder like Cullen, Arnold or Crichton, and unlike Pinel, his oeuvre does not contain a magnum opus containing his ideas on psychiatric classification. Instead, his piece-meal approach to refining existing categories was reflected within shorter monographs that had a narrower scope of enquiry, as well as entries in medical dictionaries, often in those that he himself had edited.[82] He served as an editor of the *Dictionnaire des Sciences Médicales*, a prestigious work in medical classification, and had written the entry on monomania for the 1819 edition.[83] One of Esquirol's aim in developing lypemania and monomania was to demarcate between emotional disorders and intellectual disorders: lypemania was an emotional form of melancholia that was characterised by sadness, melancholy and sorrowful feelings, whereas *monomania* was an intellectual disorder associated with an obsession over one idea, thought, memory or action. For Esquirol,

[80] Y. Trichet and A. Lacroix, 'Esquirol's Change of View Towards Pinel's mania Without Delusion' in *History of Psychiatry*, vol. 27, no. 4, 2016, pp. 443–457.

[81] Roy Porter, 'Psychiatry' in *The Greatest Benefit to Mankind: A Medical History of Humanity from Antiquity to the Present*, Harper Collins, 1997, pp. 493–524 (p. 502).

[82] R. Huertas, 'Between Doctrine and Clinical Practice: Nosography and Semiology in the Work of Jean-Etienne-Dominique Esquirol (1772–1840)' in *History of Psychiatry*, vol. 19, no. 2, 2008, pp. 123–140. https://doi.org/10.1177/0957154X07080659.

[83] Rafeal Huertas, 'Esquirol: Between Doctrine and Clinical Practice' in *History of Psychiatry*, vol. 19, no. 2, 2008, pp. 123–140.

the division between the two was presented in Pinel's work on melancholia but had not been clearly articulated.[84] Researchers associated with the large Parisian hospitals followed in Esquirol's wake in attempting to divide monomania and lypemania into further sub-types on the basis of the symptoms presented, making further distinctions between emotional and intellectual disorders.[85]

By the time it came to writing his later textbook, *A Treatise on Insanity*, published in 1835, a shift had occurred in Prichard's attitudes towards French psychology, with a more favourable attitude to Pinel's ideas characterising the work. This is partly due to the time he had spent in Paris gaining first-hand acquaintance of practices of diagnosis within large state asylums. During his time there, he had met Esquirol, and was now able to read to French, giving him access to untranslated works of French medical psychology. These included the second edition of Pinel's *Traité* that had not been translated into English, and articles by Esquirol.[86] This allowed Prichard to understand and capture the spirit of Pinel's work for an English readership, and how it had been developed in subsequent decades. Prichard incorporated the ideas of Esquirol into his nosography of insanity with his addition of *monomania*, as we can see from the four main categories of Prichard's nosology shown in Table 2.4.

Prichard's nosography did not signal an uncritical acceptance of the ideas of French psychology. Idiocy, for instance, was not included because Prichard believed it was unnecessary as a separate disease category to dementia and including it would make the classification overly complicated for practice within English asylums. Despite the influences from France, Prichard still held on to the notion of unitary insanity:

> ...the practical advantages of a definition [of insanity] can, in this instance, only be attained by stating what are in reality those disturbances which the

[84] D.B. Weiner, 'Betrayal! The 1806 Translation of Pinel's *Traité' medico- philosophique sur l'Aliénation mentale, ou la manie*' in *Generus*, 2000, vol. 57, pp. 42–50 (p. 45).

[85] German Berrios, 'Mood Disorders: Clinical Section' in *A History of Clinical Psychiatry: The Origin and History of Psychiatric Disorders*, edited by Berrios and Porter, Athlone, 1995, pp. 384–408 (p. 389).

[86] James Cowles Prichard, *A Treatise on Insanity and Other Disorders Affecting the Mind*, Sherwood, Gilbert, and Piper, 1835, p. 14.

Table 2.4 Prichard's nosography as included in his *Treatise*[87]

1. moral insanity;
2. monomania or 'partial derangement of the understanding';
3. *mania*, or raving insanity
4. *dementia*, or incoherence.

[87] James Cowles Prichard, 'Nosography of the Four Forms of Insanity' in *A Treatise on Insanity and Other Disorders Affecting the Mind*, Sherwood, Gilbert, and Piper: London, 1835, pp. 6–7.

> mental operations sustain in cases of insanity, [but] these disturbances [...] present very different phenomena in different forms of the disease.[88]

Prichard wrote that moral insanity was the least acute form of insanity because it was a disorder of the 'feelings' and not the intellect, whereas monomania was a partial form of intellectual derangement that only affected the understanding when the mind was engaged in harmful thought patterns. Mania was a 'general', or complete intellectual derangement that affected the rational capacities of the sufferer, with dementia being the most severe form of insanity because rational associations between ideas were completely broken down, leading to a complete obliteration of a patients' intellectual capacities.[89] It was within his concise nosography of mental illnesses that Prichard believed 'all varieties of madness may find their place'.[90]

Prichard's *Treatise* introduced the term moral insanity to the Anglophone world and had been modelled on Pinel's mania without delusions, with Prichard defining it as a 'perversion of moral disposition'.[91] By the time it came to writing the textbook, he had gained an understanding of

[88] Ibid.

[89] Ibid.

[90] Ibid., p. 7.

[91] Ibid., and German Berrios, 'Introduction to J.C. Prichard and the Concept of 'Moral Insanity'' in *History of Psychiatry*, no. 10, 1999, pp. 111–126 (p. 111).

'délire' that was closer to Pinel's original French and not simply as 'delirium' as it had been translated by Davis. 'Delire' referred to a degradation of the powers of reasoning and the cognitive faculties. Prichard wrote of moral insanity:

> ...[it is] madness consisting in a morbid perversion of the natural feelings, affections, inclinations, temper, habits, moral dispositions, and natural impulses, without any remarkable disorder or defect of the intellect or knowing and reasoning faculties, and particularly without any insane illusion or hallucination.

Prichard wrote that moral insanity was accompanied by symptoms which demonstrated a distortion of the emotions, whilst intellectual faculties remained intact. This form of madness was distinctly important for him because the other forms of insanity in his nosography all involved a degree of damage to the intellectual capacities of the mind.[92]

One notable absence from Prichard's classification was melancholia, which had been replaced with Esquirol's monomania. Prichard did not use lypemania that Esquirol employed to describe a form of melancholia characterised by depressive states. Instead, he incorporated lypemania into monomania, which functioned in his nosography to refer to all partial insanities and replaced the term melancholia. This is because Prichard believed that the obsessive thought processes of monomania gave rise to the symptoms that had been associated with melancholia in Cullen and Pinel's work, as he described:

> Monomania, or partial insanity, in which the understanding is partially disordered or under the influence of some particular illusion, referring to one subject, and involving one train of ideas, while the intellectual powers appear, when exercised on other subjects, to be in a great measure unimpaired.[93]

[92] It is also important to note here that Prichard followed Pinel in employing the term 'nosography' instead of 'nosology': this demonstrates that he intended his diagnostic criteria to be an empirical representation of the behavioural symptoms of mental disorders, and not to be a theory-based nosology. See James Cowles Prichard, *A Treatise on Insanity and Other Disorders Affecting the Mind*, Sherwood, Gilbert, and Piper, 1835, p. 131.

[93] Ibid.

Prichard had thus eventually come to employ the descriptions of disorders from Pinel and Esquirol but took a departure from their work by continuing his earlier emphasis on the links between perception, memory and madness in his description of monomania. The thought processes that Esquirol associated with monomania then, for Prichard, also explained lypemania and melancholia, thereby eliminating the need for a separate disease category.

Prichard's description of mania or 'raving madness' drew further upon the work of Pinel when he wrote in the *Treatise* that it constituted:

> ...the understanding [being] generally deranged; the reasoning faculty, if not lost, is confused and disturbed in its exercise; the mind is in a state of morbid excitement, and the individual talks absurdly on every subject to which his thoughts are momentarily directed.[94]

Accepting Pinel's thesis that the intellectual and reasoning faculties of the mind are damaged in cases of mania signalled a further departure from Prichard's earlier rejection of the distinction. Mania was thought of as a general state of insanity that should be understood in contrast to monomania, which Pinel and Prichard both considered a partial insanity because the patient would only experience spells that would accompany certain 'thought patterns'.[95]

The severest form of insanity then was dementia, although Prichard frequently used the term incoherent insanity which had also been used by Arnold. Although preferring this term to Pinel, Prichard still relied on the Frenchman's work to formulate his description of dementia:

> Rapid succession or uninterrupted alternation of insulated ideas and evanescent and unconnected emotions; continually repeated acts of extravagance; complete forgetfulness of every previous state; diminished sensibility to external impressions; abolition of the faculty of judgement; perpetual activity.[96]

[94] Ibid., p. 6.

[95] Ibid., p. 6.

[96] Pinel quoted and translated by Prichard in ibid., p. 6.

Prichard placed great emphasis on the need for a classification system to be concise for it to be of practical use. However, there was no compromise to pragmatics or concision at the expense of scientific value for Prichard: in borrowing Pinel's 'nosography' as the term for his classification, Prichard assumed a realist and empirical position on the way his classification represented mental disorders. In his own words, Prichard attempted to provide:

> an accurate and tolerably complete description of the phenomena of insanity [...and] in this description, while I avail myself of the aid afforded by the best practical writers of different countries, it will be my aim to avoid the admission of any circumstance or feature of disease which I have not in more or fewer instances actually observed.[97]

In addition to its practical utility, Prichard justified the forms presented in his nosography with empirical evidence in the form of clinical observations and detailed notes on example cases.

Prichard sold the practicality of his nosography by contrasting it to the classification developed by Johann Christian Heinroth.[98] Heinroth had divided the drives of the human into basic ones of the body, and higher ones of the ego. Disorders in the latter were caused by behaviours that are considered by many religions to be sins. The mind communicated with the body through the soul, and so the sins of the mind could lead to illnesses in the body.[99] This indicated to Heinroth humanity's *telos* or purpose, albeit one which was based upon a form of Christian morality. Like Prichard, Heinroth's attitudes towards mental health were informed by his research in anthropology, and by his vision of the development of human civilisation. Despite apparent affinities between the two, Prichard dismissed Heinroth's classification as 'singular and absurd in some of its fundamental principles', and criticised it for being too complex for use in practice.[100] He distinguished it from his own work as

[97] Ibid.

[98] Ibid., p. 18.

[99] Holger Steinberg, 'The Sin in the Aetiological Concept of Johann Christian Heinroth' in *History of Psychiatry*, vol. 5, no. 4, December 2004, pp. 299–344.

[100] James Cowles Prichard, *A Treatise on Insanity and Other Disorders Affecting the Mind*, Sherwood, Gilbert, and Piper: London, 1835, p. 18.

being 'theoretical and speculative [rather] than the result of actual observation and experience'.[101] Although the theory that Heinroth used to deduce the existence of the disorders in his classification system resembled a form of faculty psychology, Prichard thought that the disorders of the classification were over-determined by his teleological theory. Although Prichard found some worth in the theoretical component of Heinroth's work, Prichard ultimately considered it empirically flawed, with the lack of evidence in the form of case notes and observations being the clearest sign of this shortcoming.[102] Prichard concluded that Heinroth had provided 'the most elaborate and comprehensive' of the classifications of mental disorders that had so far been published, but whether it was useful for clinical practice is a different story.[103]

Prichard's nosography saw immediate popularity, with the concepts quickly becoming used by asylum medical superintendents for the purposes of classification. In 1839, only four years after the publication of the first edition of the *Treatise on Insanity*, the most popular diagnosis for patients at Ticehurst House was moral insanity, and by the 1860s it became a common diagnosis in asylums across the British Isles.[104] The adoption of Prichard's classification indicates that alienists valued a nosology that was of simple and practical use, over and above the scientific value of the concepts that were presented. Instead of a complex classification such as that of Heinroth's that sought to make subtle distinctions between the forms of insanity, the classification offered by Prichard included broad groups which could be easily learnt and quickly used in practice.[105] Practical considerations were especially important to those working in asylums in the 1830s, who at this point were without professional representation in the form of an official body that

[101] Ibid.

[102] Ibid.

[103] Ibid.

[104] Charlotte Mackenzie, *A Family Asylum: A History of the Private Madhouse at Ticehurst in Sussex, 1792–1917*, PhD thesis, UCL, 1986, p. 139. For wider considerations on moral insanity, see David W. Jones, 'Moral Insanity and Psychological Disorder: The Hybrid Roots of Psychiatry' in *History of Psychiatry*, vol. 28, no. 3, pp. 263–279.

[105] John Walton, 'The Treatment of Pauper Lunatics in Victorian England: The Case of Lancaster Asylum, 1816–1870' in *Madhouses, Mad-doctors and Madmen*, edited by Andrew Scull, Athlone, 1981, pp. 166–200.

would represent their interests. They were often overworked and practising their profession in poor conditions. The 1840s was a crucial decade in the development of asylum psychiatry, with the rules and regulations that would define practice for a great proportion of the era of the asylum being enshrined in the Lunacy Act and the Country Asylums Act, both passed in 1845. The concepts that were used in the diagnosis of those admitted to asylums would be caught up in this context of reform, and Prichard's classification of the forms of insanity would be, from 1845, established as the recommended standard terms of psychological diagnosis used in asylum medical statistics for the next half of the nineteenth century.

Despite an initial negative reception, the concepts developed by Pinel and Esquirol, and channelled through the work of Prichard were recommended for use by the Lunacy Commission for the purposes of diagnosis upon its establishment through the Lunacy Act and the County Asylums Act in 1845.[106] Prichard's work would help to establish the Table of the Forms of Insanity in the United Kingdom until the end of the nineteenth century. Prichard was central to the operations of the first Lunacy Commission due to his role as one of the medical experts appointed to the regulatory body, and the only one who had written a textbook on psychological diagnosis. He promoted the classification that he had developed in response to Pinel and Esquirol's work.[107] This was not an easy task for there was much disagreement on the concepts that should be used in diagnosis. For example, the renowned John Charles Bucknill wrote that he frequently disagreed with the diagnoses given by Poor Law medical officers.[108]

Conclusion

It is commonly assumed that melancholia, mania and dementia, the most common of the Victorian diagnostic categories, were preserved from antiquity. Although the Victorians were preoccupied with the history of

[106] Earl of Shaftesbury et al., 'Forms of Disease, Medical Treatment, Diet, and Classification' in *The Report of the Metropolitan Commissioners of Lunacy*, Bradbury and Evans Printers, 1844, pp. 102–128.

[107] D.J. Mellett, 'Bureaucracy and Mental Illness: The Commissioners in Lunacy 1845–1890' in *Medical History*, vol. 21, 1981, pp. 221–250 (p. 228).

[108] Bill Forsythe and Joseph Melling, *The Politics of Madness*, Routledge, 2006, p. 51.

medicine since ancient Greece, the concepts employed in medical statistics were very much a modern construct, and the result of channels of circulation between France and the British Isles. The concepts introduced by Pinel would eventually become popular in the United Kingdom, but a poor translation and initial hostility including accusations of Cartesianism stymied the initial influence of Pinel's work in the British Isles. This was until Prichard captured the spirit of French medical psychology in his textbooks, and Pinelean diagnosis gained quick popularity because Prichard conveyed the empirical and practical dimensions of Pinel's work. These were especially important for British asylum medical superintendents during the early years of alienism. Furthermore, their popularity was partly because Pinel's nosography did not offer a theory on the pathology or aetiology of insanity, and therefore remained adaptable to empirical findings. Pinelean diagnosis appealed to the intuition of many because it described symptoms that most asylum superintendents had encountered in some form, and did not rely upon a complicated aetiological theory. Prichard's adaptation of Pinel's work became widely used before the advent of psychiatry as an established discipline with training facilities, and during a period of rapid expansion of the asylum system. As we will see in subsequent chapters, Pinel's classification played a vital role in the communication of clinical knowledge from the 1840s onwards within asylum statistical reports, medical textbooks and pedagogical practices. The concision of Prichard's nosography and its intuitive appeal was partly behind its widespread use. Pinel's work on diagnosis, channelled through Prichard's later textbook on insanity, was a step in establishing medical psychology as a discipline distinct from other branches of medicine; previously, concepts of mental disorder had been included in general nosologies of medicine, such as those of Cullen. In addition, Pinel established the notion of moral, or emotional, insanity, an application of faculty psychology to the clinic. Like the nosography, this would become very influential throughout the nineteenth century, causing controversy as it came to be viewed as medicalising immorality.

In exploring how Prichard captured the spirit of the ideas of French medical psychology, this chapter has attempted to chart the exchanges between France and Britain, and the wider implications they have for the history of psychological diagnosis. After Prichard had published his *Treatise on Insanity*, the concepts of Pinel, with the addition of

Esquirol's monomania, began to be employed by the Lunacy Commission, who recommended that the symptom-based classifications formulated by Prichard be used to record the form of mental disorder that every person admitted to an asylum suffered. Legal developments imposed the requirement to arrive at a diagnosis at the point of entry to the asylum as well as accurate record-keeping practices. The concepts that Pinel developed established the diagnostic concepts that Victorian alienists would use for psychological diagnosis, and as we will see in subsequent chapters, became the standard used in asylum medical statistics. Because of their use in asylum statistical returns, French nosography was tantamount to being the standard used for diagnosis within the Victorian asylum.

CHAPTER 3

The Bureaucratic Origins of the Table of the Forms of Insanity

National asylum statistics were a result of wider reforms made to lunacy administration during the mid-nineteenth century. The 1845 Lunacy Act set up the board of Commissioners in Lunacy, a body comprised of physicians, barristers and non-professionals that were responsible for overseeing asylums. This included county, borough and private asylums, privately run and licensed madhouses, public lunatic hospitals and retreats established by charitable and religious organisations. The linked 1845 County and Asylums Act made it a requirement for counties in England to establish a lunatic asylum to reduce reliance upon private asylums and madhouses: these had attracted a reputation for low standards fuelled by administrators more concerned with financial gain than the care of patients.[1] Although there had been a steady increase in the number of county asylums since the turn of the century, they rapidly expanded in number after the passing of the 1845 lunacy laws, which would also establish the frameworks and legal mechanisms that regulated asylum care during the second half of the nineteenth century. Legislation passed since the beginning of the century had brought legal requirements to keep basic records on admission, discharges and deaths, but calls were made during

[1] William Parry-Jones, *The Trade in Lunacy: A Study of Private Madhouses in England in the Eighteenth and Nineteenth Centuries*, Routledge, 1973.

K. M. Jones, *Psychological Classification and Diagnosis in Asylum Statistics, 1800–1948*, Mental Health in Historical Perspective,
https://doi.org/10.1007/978-3-031-46154-5_3

the 1830s to increase the level of oversight by expanding the data on patients collected from asylums. In his report on the mortality of lunatics in 1836, William Farr (1807–1883) called for changes to be made:

> I would therefore suggest that by some modification of the present system of inspection, the circumstances of every lunatic confined should be investigated personally by a crown officer, and recorded previous to committal, at the expiration of every quarter of a year after admission, and at the time of dismissal. The sex, and age, the stage, form and complications of insanity should be registered, on entering and leaving the several institutions, by impartial officers. This would be a protection to lunatics, and to the public; the deaths and recoveries would be registered on a uniform plan, and an invaluable statistical check on the results of treatment would be obtained.

Moreover, Farr envisaged that this would not just be a bureaucratic exercise that would impose regulation upon asylums, since the information collected could prove to be of scientific value:

> We may then discover the causes of insanity, the laws which regulate its course, the circumstances by which it is influenced, and either avert its visitations, or mitigate their severity; perhaps, in a later age, save mankind from its inflictions, or, if this cannot be, at any rate ensure the sufferers merciful treatment.[2]

Farr's remarks link asylum reform to medical science through the use of mechanisms of oversight and data collection to provide insights into insanity and its different forms.

Statistics gathered from asylum paperwork recording diagnoses were inextricably linked to the formation of concepts of psychopathology.[3] Medical certificates and admissions books formulated the basis of asylum medical statistics, which constituted the main source of data for Victorian statistical research into insanity. Medical statistics were a growing concern for health administration from the 1830s onwards as the public health

[2] William Farr, 'Report Upon the Mortality of Lunatics' in *Journal of the Statistical Society of London*, vol. 4, no. 1, April 1941, pp. 17–33.

[3] Åsa Jansson, 'From Statistics to Diagnostics: Medical Certificates, Melancholia, and 'Suicidal Propensities' in Victorian Psychiatry' in *Journal of Social History*, vol. 46, no. 3, Spring 2013, pp. 716–731.

and sanitary movements came into being partly in response to the expansion of towns and cities during the first phases of the industrial revolution. The General Record Office (GRO) was established in 1837, and its work for a great period was characterised by the involvement of Farr, who acted as Superintendent of Statistics from 1842 until 1879. The GRO played an important role in the establishment of demographics, and the development of epidemiology. Along with the founding of the Statistical Society of London in 1834, there was a growing political will to develop statistical understandings of public health issues. Farr in particular had been involved in the accumulation of statistics relating to insanity before the establishment of the Lunacy Commission, making it a concern of the GRO during his stewardship.[4] Responsibility for collecting statistics on insanity would fall under the jurisdiction of the Lunacy Commission upon its establishment in 1845. Aside from centring medical statistics on insanity around the asylum, this move would mark a separation between the collection of statistics relating to lunacy and general medical statistics that would last nearly a century, as mental health statistics would come to be placed back in the hands of the GRO in 1948 with reforms to medical statistics developed during the planning phases of the National Health Service.[5]

The 1845 Lunacy Act required detailed information on patients to be logged and submitted annually to the Commissioners in Lunacy. Numbers based upon information collected during asylum admissions procedures were submitted by asylum medical superintendents to the Lunacy Commission in annual statistical reports. The recording of a psychological diagnosis in asylum records became a legal requirement under the terms of the act, and provided the basis for medical statistics on diagnosis. This development did not lead to fully developed asylum medical statistics on psychological diagnosis overnight; as Elaine Murphy notes, the Lunacy Commission did not completely fulfil its aims of bureaucratic centralisation during its early years, although its annual reports had been influential at least inasmuch as they 'set the moral tone

[4] William Farr, 'Report upon the Mortality of Lunatics' in *Journal of the Statistical Society of London*, vol. 4, no. 1 April 1841, pp. 17–33.

[5] For a detailed exploration of the development of asylums statistics on diagnosis, please see Chapter 6.

and care standards for a generation of asylums'.[6] The sixth chapter of this volume shows how despite developments associated with the 1845 acts, national statistics on psychological diagnosis would not become the norm until the 1870s. Problems with standardisation and crude computational methods adopted by the Lunacy Commission had hindered progress after the passing of the act.[7] Despite the slow movement in publishing data on diagnosis, the passing of the 1845 Lunacy Act had established the mechanisms and structures for the collection and collation of data on diagnosis from asylums across England and Wales by a centralised medical bureaucracy.

The statistical returns opened up the possibility for medical data to be collected, and as large amounts of data came to be returned from asylums, new questions arose. One that captured attention both from those within health circles as well as the wider public was whether insanity was on the increase, and if so, where was this was occurring and what was the cause. Much was written warning of the increase in insanity, with much speculation on the causing factors taking place. Some thought the pressures of modern life caused by industrialisation was responsible, with others pointing to anxieties over financial instability and some believing new technologies were responsible for increasing numbers of asylum admittances. Asylum medical statistics, including those on psychological diagnosis, could help to answer these questions.

This chapter will further develop one of the central arguments of the study: that the bureaucratic frameworks that enabled asylum statistics on psychological diagnosis to be collected and published motivated debates over psychiatric classification and the standardisation of terms of psychological diagnosis. The assembly of a bureaucracy that collected patient data was a pivotal factor in the formalisation of psychological diagnosis.[8] This chapter will commence by outlining the introduction of legislation that placed legal obligations to collect medical data within records and

[6] Elaine Murphy, 'The Administration of Insanity in England 1800 to 1870' in *The Confinement of the Insane: International Perspectives, 1800–1965*, edited by Roy Porter and David Wright, Cambridge University Press, 2003, pp. 334–349 (p. 341).

[7] Simon A. Hill and Richard Laugharne, 'Mania Dementia and Melancholia in the 1870s: Admissions to a Cornwall asylum' in *Journal of the Royal Society of Medicine*, vol. 96, no. 7, 2003.

[8] Charles Rosenberg, 'The Tyranny of Diagnosis: Specific Entities and Individual Experience' in *the Milbank Quarterly*, vol. 80, no. 2, June 2002, pp. 237–260.

submit yearly asylum statistical returns of patient data. It will then discuss the ways medical organisations responded to these legal requirements with early attempts to standardise the concepts of psychological diagnosis during the early years of the Medico-Psychological Association (MPA). Finally, the chapter will outline how the classification of David Skae would arise as a serious contender to replace the common currency of Victorian psychological diagnosis that had been shaped by Pinelean symptomology.

The Beginnings of the Statistical Tables 1840–1868

Lunacy reform was part of the wider context of the expansion of the bureaucratic state in Victorian Britain, with the aim being to document and understand the public health crisis that had emerged in many British towns and cities.[9] As Dorothy Porter notes, the expansion of public health in the British Isles can be interpreted as displaying tensions between liberal, laissez-faire politics that favoured a minimal state, Malthusian-style population control, and an emerging utilitarian view of health policy to potentially increase quality of life and a general happiness of the social body.[10] Upon the passing of the Lunacy Act in 1845, a national Lunacy Commission was established which would function as a regulatory body, appointing commissioners who would carry out visits to oversee conditions in asylums throughout the British Isles. Some historians argue that legal justification for a person's admission to an institution has been one of the principal functions for the development of psychological classification and diagnoses. Jan Goldstein, for instance, claims that the act of classification was carried out by alienists in order to justify their activity as medical men, whereas in reality, their 'treatment' was no more advanced than the consolation provided by religious orders before the French Revolution.[11] Georges Canguilhem claimed that the boundary between what is deemed normal and what is considered pathological in biology and medicine is historically contingent, with it arising during the early nineteenth century not only due to scientific discoveries but also thanks to a complex set

[9] Dorothy Porter, 'Public Health and Centralisation: The Victorian British State' in *Health, Civilisation and the State: A History of Public Health from Ancient to Modern Times*, Routledge, 1998, pp. 117–127.

[10] Ibid.

[11] Jan Goldstein, *Console and Classify: The French Psychiatric Profession in the Nineteenth Century*, Cambridge University Press, 1988.

of technological, political and social changes that include the expansion of the bureaucratic state and the emergence of paper technologies such as the statistical returns issues by the Lunacy Commission to collect and collate information.[12] Following in a similar vein, Foucault offered the view that psychiatry was a concealed and sophisticated form of social control, and that the moral treatment that emerged from the Quaker Retreat in York replaced the physical chains that had hitherto confined the insane.[13] Foucault's work, hugely significant in stimulating scholarly interest in the history of psychiatry over the last fifty years, has influenced many later writers, including Andrew Scull and Nikolas Rose, who both place clinical knowledge within its wider social context, attempting to understand how the dominance of the medical model of mental disorder has shaped society and psychological subjects.[14]

Internment in an asylum was a sensitive issue, with concerns about wrongful confinement, standards of care and low discharge rates being motivating factors behind the establishment of the powerful nationwide Lunacy Commission.[15] Failure to record and submit information through statistical returns could lead to fines being imposed on the asylum by the commission and its chief medical officer being held personally accountable.[16] Records would then be reviewed by members of the Lunacy Commission upon their inspection of the institution. The legal requirement that the diagnosis of a patient be recorded on admission shows how the law surrounding mental health did not merely constrain and regulate clinical practice, but in fact had a role in formulating clinical knowledge.[17]

[12] George Canguilhem, *The Normal and the Pathological*, translated by Carolyn R. Fawcett, MIT Press, 1991.

[13] Michel Foucault, *Madness and Civilisation: A History of Insanity in the Age of Reason*, translated by Richard Howard, Routledge, 1989.

[14] Nikolas Rose, *Governing the Soul: Shaping of the Private Self*, Free Association Books, 1999; Andrew Scull, 'The Social History of Psychiatry in the Victorian Era' in *Mad Houses, Mad Doctors and Madmen: The Social History of Psychiatry in the Victorian Era*, edited by Andrew Scull, Athlone, 1981.

[15] Kathleen Jones, 'Law and Mental Health: Sticks or Carrots' in *150 Years of British Psychiatry*, edited by Berrios and Freeman, Gaskell, 1991, pp. 89–102.

[16] Ibid., p. 93.

[17] Roger Smith, 'Legal Frameworks for Psychiatry' in *150 Years of British Psychiatry*, edited by Berrios and Freeman, Gaskell, 1991, pp. 137–151.

Like Farr, many viewed admissions data as holding potential for the development of mental science.[18] Mental health statistics were a growing concern, and from the 1850s until the end of the century, the pages of the *Journal of Mental Science*, the publication of the Association of Asylum Medical Officers (AAMO) and later the Medico-Psychological Association (MPA), became increasingly populated with studies that aimed to draw correlations between social background and the prevalence of insanity. Data from admissions could help to answer questions that were attracting interest from the medical profession, public health bodies and the wider public. These included concerns over rates of insanity, whether rapid urbanisation and industrialisation were responsible for any increase, and if the conditions in larger cities were somehow to blame. Alarmist views appealed to statistics to make claims that rises in the rates of madness were early signs of a forthcoming degeneration of human civilisation.[19] More sober commentators were interested in knowing whether certain forms of insanity were linked to material conditions in the workplace and the family, whether there were different rates amongst men and women, or if there were any significant differences in trends in the rate of psychological diagnosis between urban and rural asylums. Asylum medical statistics were frequently used in attempts to settle these debates. For example, the chairman of the Metropolitan Lunacy Commission, the progenitor of the Lunacy Commission, remarked in 1840 that:

> the most ample means exist in the records of the commission for determining the age and previous occupations of the lunatics, with a view of ascertaining whether any particular time of life, or any one occupation more than another, be characterised by mental affections; but I have been utterly debarred from embarking in such a minute and laborious enquiry

[18] The end to the pursuit of these statistics is a matter of considerable debate. Theodor Porter claims that since the establishment of the association, alienists had been interested in asylum statistics primarily to understand the heredity of mental disorder since the establishment of the MPA. Whilst there certainly was a strong current of interest in heredity within the British context, this claim requires important caveats. Information was routinely collected on the family background of a patient admitted to an asylum, and whether there had been bouts of insanity within the immediate family. At the same time, much information on the social background of a patient was also collected, such as their religion, occupation and their level of literacy. Alienists were interested in social and environmental factors that gave rise to insanity at least as much as heredity.

[19] Daniel Pick, *Faces of Degeneration: A European Disorder c.1848–c.1918*, Cambridge University Press, 1993.

> by the want of leisure; but the day may come when a paper on the statistics of the [Metropolitan] Lunacy Commission, more worthy than the present, may be presented to the notice of the Society.[20]

The exchange of statistical information was also a priority for the MPA from its very beginnings in 1841. A preliminary meeting to: establish the association made it a founding principle that to:

> ensure a correct comparison of results of treatment in each [asylum] it is strongly recommended that uniform registers be kept, and that tabular statements upon a uniform plan be circulated with the Annual Report of each hospital, or when this be not practicable that it be otherwise transmitted to the Association.[21]

When charting the history of the association, T. Outterson Wood remarked in 1896 that the pledge to bring about the standardisation of medical data was one of the organisation's fundamental purposes.[22] Prominent Lunacy Commission members were in attendance at these formative meetings, including James Cowles Prichard and his successor as Lunacy Commissioner, Samuel Gaskell.[23]

Despite these lofty aims at standardisation, asylum medical statistics remained somewhat rudimentary immediately after the passing of the 1845 Acts. In lieu of standardised statistics on diagnosis from a number of institutions, medical superintendents used data on diagnosis from large individual asylums. For example, John Webster's paper on the statistics of insanity at Bethlem provided a breakdown of admissions according to gender, and compared the number of 'cured' to 'deaths'.[24] Reports from asylums varied in the level of detail, with the admissions statistics of the Lancaster County Asylum for 1841 being broken down according to

[20] Lieut.-Col. Sykes, 'Statistics of the Metropolitan Commission in Lunacy' in *Journal of the Statistical Society of London*, vol. 3, no. 2, July 1840, pp. 143–160.

[21] T. Outterson Wood, 'The Early History of the Medico-Psychological Association' in *JMS*, vol. 42, no. 177, 1896. pp. 241–260.

[22] Ibid., p. 245.

[23] Ibid.

[24] John Webster, 'Statistics of Bethlem Hospital with Remarks on Insanity' in *Medico-Chirurgical Transactions*, vol. 26, 1843, p. 374–416.

occupation, level of literacy, religion and the suspected cause of insanity.[25] The Dorset County Lunatic Asylum provided details on the form of insanity diagnosed amongst its 108 admissions for the year 1840, and these were also broken down according to gender (see Table 3.1).[26] In contrast, the Murray Royal Asylum in Dundee for that same year provided scant information in its annual report of its inmates.[27]

In the 1844 Report of the Metropolitan Lunacy Commission, statistics were published which classified admissions as private or pauper patients, and as epileptics, idiots, homicidal patients and suicidal patients.[28]

As discussed in the last chapter, the classification recommended by the Lunacy Commission for the purposes of diagnosis adopted the terminology devised by French medical psychology. It followed Pinel's method of clustering behavioural symptoms associated with cases admitted to an asylum, and drawing them under disease concepts.

The concepts recommended by the Lunacy Commission played a role in establishing the forms of insanity outlined in Table 3.2 as the nearest to a standard set of psychological diagnostic categories the United Kingdom would have during the second half of the nineteenth century. As well as these recommended set of diagnostic categories, the report also included a detailed description of each disorder, which happened to closely resemble the descriptions in Prichard's textbook; it differentiated between acute forms of mania and melancholia, and the partial insanities, which included less severe forms of melancholia, monomania and moral insanity. The legal requirement to provide a diagnosis was described in the 1845 Lunacy Act:

> every Physician, Surgeon, or Apothecary signing such Certificate shall specify therein any Fact or Facts (whether arising from his own Observation or from the Information of any other Person) upon which he has

[25] Edward De Vitre and Samuel Gaskell, Report of the Medical Officers of the Lunatic Asylum for the County of Lancaster, C. Barwick, 1841.

[26] James A. Templar, Report of the Visiting Justices of the County Lunatic Asylum Forston, 1841, Dorset, T. Patch, 1841.

[27] David Dron, Fourteenth Annual Report of the Directors and Physician of James Murray's Royal Asylum for Lunatics. 1841.

[28] John Thurnam, Essays on the Statistics of Insanity: including an inquiry into the Causes influencing the Results of Treatment in Establishments for the Insane. To which are added, the Statistics of the Retreat, near York. London: Simpkin and Co., 1845.

Table 3.1 Dorset County Lunatic Asylum, psychological diagnosis in admissions[29]

Table 1: Forms of Disease in the Cases of the 108 Patients at Present in the Asylum.			
	Males	Females	Total
Mania	10	17	
With Epilepsy	4	2	
With Paralysis	2	0	
	16	19	35
Melancholia	5	6	
With Epilepsy	0	1	
With Paralysis	0	1	
With Occasional Violence	0	6	
Suicidal	1	2	
	6	16	22
Hypochondriasis	0	1	
	0	1	1
Incoherence	5	14	
With Epilepsy	0	1	
With Paralysis	1	0	
With Occasional Violence	5	4	
Suicidal	0	1	
	11	20	31
Imbecility	3	0	
Congenital	0	1	
	3	1	4
Dementia	10	2	
With Epilepsy	1	0	
With Paralysis	1	0	
	12	2	14
Idiotcy [*sic*]	2	0	
	2	0	2

formed his Opinion that the Person to whom such Certificate relates is a Lunatic or Insane Person, or an Idiot, or a Person of Unsound Mind.[30]

[29] James A. Templar, Report of the Visiting Justices of the County Lunatic Asylum Forston, 1841, Dorset, T. Patch, 1841, p. 7.

[30] Section 46, Lunacy Act, 1845.

Table 3.2 Forms of disease, medical treatment, diet and classification recommended by the Metropolitan Commissioners in Lunacy[31]

I.	Mania
	1. Acute Mania, or Raving Madness
	2. Ordinary Mania, or Chronic Madness of a less acute form
	3. Periodical, or Remittent Mania, with comparatively lucid intervals
II.	Dementia, or decay and obliteration of the intellectual faculties
III.	Melancholia
IV.	Monomania
V.	Moral Insanity

Form II, IV and V sometimes being comprehended under the term Partial Insanity.

VI.	Congenital Idiocy
VII.	Congenital Imbecility
VIII.	General Paralysis of the Insane
IX.	Epilepsy

To these heads may perhaps be added 'Delirium Tremens' since it is mentioned, as a form of Insanity, in the Reports of some Lunatic Asylums.'

Asylum registers from the period immediately after the passing of the Act show that medical superintendents often followed the recommendations of the Lunacy Commission. From 1845 to 1880, the Devon County Asylum also diagnosed the vast majority of patients entering the asylum according to the classification concepts of mania, dementia, melancholia and idiotism.[32] During the 1870s, the Cornwall County Asylum diagnosed the vast majority of patients with mania (38%), dementia (35%) or melancholia (26%).[33] The Buckinghamshire Asylum also employed elements of Prichard's classification for admissions, with all but a very few patients passing through its doors being classified as suffering from

[31] 'Forms of Disease, Medical Treatment, Diet, and Classification' in *The Report of the Metropolitan Commissioners of Lunacy*, Bradbury and Evans Printers, 1844, pp. 102–128.

[32] Bill Forsythe and Joseph Melling, *The Politics of Madness*, Routledge, London, 2006, p. 62.

[33] Simon A Hill, and Richard Laugharne 'Mania Dementia and Melancholia in the 1870: Admissions to a Cornwall Asylum' in *Journal of the Royal Society of Medicine*, vol. 96, no. 7, 2003.

mania, dementia, idiocy or melancholia.[34] Although many asylums used the basic concepts of the classification proposed by the Lunacy Commission that had been drafted by Prichard, there were divergences, with some choosing to use their own terms of psychological diagnosis in admissions records. Needless to say, this hampered and delayed efforts to publish national statistics on psychological diagnosis.

Standardisation was driven by aims to develop bureaucratic procedures that would facilitate lunacy administration and oversight. Although oversight was the main motivating factor behind the introduction of the bureaucratic processes and statistical returns that collected asylum medical data, the MPA, like Farr, wanted to develop these procedures to allow them to be utilised by scientific research. As Farr articulated during the early phases of public health administration, it was frequently the case that bureaucratic frameworks were developed so that they would eventually furnish researchers with statistical data. In the case of psychological diagnosis, public health officials and medical psychologists hoped that data recorded by the statistical tables, including the Table of the Forms of Insanity and the Table of the Causes of Insanity would yield statistically significant correlations that may point towards the causing factors of different manifestations of madness.

In John Charles Bucknill and Daniel Hack Tuke's *A Manual of Psychological Medicine*, the authoritative textbook for the English-speaking world since its publication in 1858, terminology used by Pinel and Esquirol was employed in its chapter on diagnosis:

> Idiocy, Cretinism and Imbecility
> Dementia
> Melancholia
> Emotional Insanity (Moral, Homicidal, Suicidal, Kleptomania, Erotomania, Pyromania, Dipsomania)
> Mania.[35]

[34] David Wright, 'Delusions of Gender?: Lay Identifications and Clinical Diagnosis of Insanity in Victorian England' in *Sex and Seclusion, Class and Custody*, Clio Medica, 2003, pp. 149–176 (p. 161).

[35] John Charles Bucknill and Daniel H. Tuke, *A Manual of Psychological Medicine*, Blanchard and Lea, 1858.

In the preface the authors stated their intention to provide 'a systematic treatise on insanity' which would serve as a definitive guide to the diagnosis and treatment of mental health disorders.[36] They acknowledged the influence of Pinel, noting that at the time of their writing his nosographie was out of print, and that Prichard's work served as the main conduit for the ideas of French medical psychology.

Bucknill's chapter on diagnosis was also published in the *Journal of Mental Science*, so would have certainly been circulated to all members of the MPA; in it he wrote that the purpose of diagnosis was to distinguish a state of mental pathology from a state of healthiness, and to distinguish one form of mental disease from another.[37] A clear set of concepts which distinguished diseases from one another was therefore deemed vital for the correct diagnosis of a mental disorder, with the concepts employed once again resembling those of Prichard, Pinel and Esquirol. Bucknill cautioned that complications could arise with the misidentification of certain disorders for one another during admissions procedures, with acute melancholia and acute mania being the most commonly confused because:

> Between acute mania and acute melancholia, no distinct line of demarcation can be drawn. The domains of the two diseases overlap so much, that in practice, cases not unfrequently present themselves, which may with equal propriety be referred to the one or to the other; cases which we may call acute mania with melancholic depression, or acute mania with maniacal excitement. The typical forms of the two diseases are however sufficiently distinct.[38]

Diagnosis might become confused in extreme cases because, Bucknill claimed, of the overlap in symptoms in acute cases. In typical cases of both *melancholia* and *mania*, the forms of the diseases were distinct from one another. Bucknill thought that both *mania* and *melancholia* were distinct diseases, but there existed symptoms that were common to both forms of the disease, at least in acute cases.

[36] Ibid.

[37] Ibid.

[38] John Charles Bucknill, 'The Diagnosis of Insanity' in *The Asylum Journal of Mental Science*, vol. 3, no. 20, May 1957, pp. 141–185.

Prichard's role on the Lunacy Commission in drafting the forms of insanity recommended in their first report contributed to the concepts of French medical psychology becoming embedded as the standard used in asylum admissions procedures. The diagnostic concepts employed by Pinel and Esquirol thus came to be central to the practice of psychiatry in the British Isles during the age of the asylum, with the system they developed being valued by alienists and medical psychologists principally for its efficiency, ease of use and practical utility.

Forms of insanity were included in statistical tables that were introduced at the very establishment of the MPA in 1841. During its second meeting in 1842, a classification of the forms of insanity was approved for the purposes of statistics, and due to this preceding the establishment of the Association's journal, the *Journal of Mental Science*, it saw itself published in the form of John Thurnam's 1845 textbook, *Observations and Essays in the Statistics of Insanity*.[39] The forms of insanity presented in this work did not diverge much from the forms of insanity which had been recommended by the Lunacy Commission as described in the last chapter, but Thurnam included a number of sub-classes (Table 3.3).

Thurnam followed the plans of the earlier Metropolitan Lunacy Commission by including sub-divisions of the forms of mania but made the perhaps over-optimistic statement that the Table of the Forms presented to the AAMO in 1842 was 'perhaps as complete and as scientifically accurate as any which is ever likely to be adopted in classifying the cases of mental disorder admitted into asylums'.[40]

The Lunacy Commission did not use the same table to the line and letter that was adopted by the AAMO, and which was published in Thurnam's textbook, but there were similarities: both the Lunacy Commission and the AAMO used the same main classes of *dementia*, *mania*, *melancholia*, *moral insanity* and *idiocy*, for instance. However, there were important divergences, with the Table devised by Thurnam including both *dementia* and *amentia*, a distinction which served to differentiate between degenerative disorders that were considered to only exist in

[39] John Thurnam, *Observations and Essays in the Statistics of Insanity: Including an Inquiry into the Causes Influencing the Results of Treatment in Establishments for the Insane; To Which Are Added the Statistics of the Retreat, Near York*, London: Simpkin Marshall, 1845, pp. 39–40.

[40] Ibid., p. 39.

Table 3.3 Forms of mental disorder presented in John Thurnam's *Observations and Essays in the Statistics of Insanity*[41]

Partial Insanity

i. Moral Insanity

ii. Monomania

iii. Melancholia

General Insanity

I. Mania

1. Acute Mania (raving madness)

2. Ordinary Mania (chronic madness of a less acute form)

3. Periodical or Remittent Mania (with comprehensively lucid intervals)

II. Dementia (decay and obliteration of the intellectual faculties)

1. Imbecility (acquired)

2. Fatuity (confirmed dementia)

III. Amentia

1. Idiocy (congenital)

2. Imbecility (congenital)

IV. Delirium Tremens (when, as in the United States, this is regarded as a form of insanity, and is treated in hospitals for the insane)

old age and congenital disorders, respectively.[42] It also did not include *General Paralysis of the Insane* (GPI).[43] The association did not have a journal until 1853, when the *Asylum Medical Journal* was established,

[41] John Thurnam, *Observations and Essays in the Statistics of Insanity: Including an Inquiry into the Causes Influencing the Results of Treatment in Establishments for the Insane; To Which Are Added the Statistics of the Retreat, Near York*, London: Simpkin Marshall, 1845, pp. 39–40.

[42] Ibid.

[43] C. Lockhart Robertson, superintendent of the Sussex asylum and secretary of the by now renamed AAMO to the Medico-Psychological Association, in an 1860 report concepts that were recommended for use by the Lunacy Commission replacing by the ones proposed by Thurnam and adopted as the classification of the MPA; C. Lockhart

and thus Thurnam's medical textbook would have been the only means via which the nosology was circulated. This had a smaller circulation than the reports of the Lunacy Commission, which may explain why the concepts approved by the Commission were more widely used and came to be adopted as the standard set.[44] Since the Commission led the way during the 1850s on the collection of statistics, very little occurred in the development of asylum statistics within the MPA until Lockhart Robertson published an 1860 report that recommended the following concepts be used for the diagnosis of asylum admissions, with the aim of strengthening the consistency of data by establishing a standard set of diagnostic concepts (Table 3.4).

Lockhart Robertson proposed a simpler classification of the forms of insanity than that presented in Thurnam's textbook, which was at that

Table 3.4 Forms of mental disorder presented in Lockhart Robertson's 'Suggestions Towards an Uniform System of Asylum Statistics [...]'[45]

1. Mania
2. Melancholia
3. Monomania
4. Moral Insanity
5. Dementia – Under the two heads of imbecility and fatuity
6. Congenital Idiocy

Criminal Lunatics should be further distinguished as such.

Robertson, 'Suggestions Towards an Uniform System of Asylum Statistics (with Tabular Forms)' in *JMS*, vol. 7, no. 36, January 1861, pp. 195–211 (p. 195).

[44] It is worth reminding ourselves here that whilst the Lunacy Commission recommended that concepts of the forms of insanity were employed to be used in asylum admissions, they did not force them to be so used. It seems for the most part that superintendents complied with their recommendations.

[45] C. Lockhart Robertson, 'Suggestions Towards an Uniform System of Asylum Statistics (with Tabular Forms)' in *JMS*, vol. 7, no. 36, January 1861, pp. 195–211 (p. 199).

point the classification that had been adopted as the standard by the MPA. His goal was to bring about greater uniformity, and one of the strategies he adopted was to make the classification simpler by following the Table of the Forms drafted by Prichard during his time on the Lunacy Commission. In addition, Thurnam's sub-class of amentia was merged into dementia in Lockhart Robinson's proposed draft. Unlike Thurnam, Lockhart Robertson's concern was to standardise data as opposed to presenting an exhaustive classification of the forms of insanity. In so doing, he wanted to create a concise set of diagnostic concepts that were easier to standardise and would help to improve the integrity of the statistical data that was collected by the MPA and the Lunacy Commission. Lockhart Robinson did not provide much explanation to accompany the choice of diagnostic concepts, and this was because the report that he drew up was not restricted to the forms of insanity, with it proposing wholescale revisions to improve the efficiency of most of the tables in the statistical returns issued by the association. These included information relating to asylum personnel, finances, dietary information, recovery rates, discharge data and the duration of the disorder prior to a person's admittance to an asylum.[46] The sheer number of changes proposed meant that the Table of the Forms of Insanity became lost in the details, not gathering so much attention from members of the MPA. For instance, during the 1860 annual meeting, members of the Association appeared to be more concerned with discussing Lockhart Robertson's recommendations to standardise the financial data than discussing the proposed changes to the Table of the Forms of Insanity.[47]

At the 1864 AGM, the MPA appointed a Committee on Asylum Statistics to further consider how the association could bring about uniformity in the recording of asylum data.[48] At this stage, the MPA relied on the Lunacy Commission for patient and asylum management data. Amongst the membership of the MPA, there was a growing desire for detailed information to be collected on pathology and mortality, and how to effectively link these numbers to data on psychological diagnosis. One member, Dr

[46] Ibid.

[47] 'Association of Medical Officers for the Asylums and Hospitals for the Insane: Official Report of Proceedings at the Annual Meeting held at the Freemasons' Tavern, Thursday, July 5th, 1860' in *JMS*, Vo. 7, no. 35, pp. 23–49.

[48] 'Annual Meeting of the Association of Medical Officers of Asylum and Hospitals for the Insane' in *JMS* vol. 10, no. 51, October 1864, pp. 448–469 (p. 468).

Wood, complained that the 'statistics present[ly] rendered were of very little value' and Thurnam himself expressed concern about the paucity of data collected about admissions, stating 'that the [data] returned in some of the tables were so incomplete that even the distinction of sex was not marked'.[49] Lockhart Robertson, following up on Thurnam's earlier call for uniformity, introduced a bill which called for another committee to be appointed that would consider ways to analyse the data returned from asylums to identify trends and inefficiencies that could provide clues on how to improve asylum management. Lockhart Robinson himself cites a discovery that he had made towards this end, albeit after a great deal of work:

> In one case he had discovered that a great element of economy was the marvellously small cost of the beer consumed, so that instead of spending £1000 a year, as asylums of similar size did, on beer, the establishment in question expended only £400, making a difference of fourpence on the rate.[50]

This was no small saving considering the stretched resources of large county asylums. Despite Lockhart Robinson's discovery, Wood voiced concerns that some medical superintendents may be unwilling to adopt any plan to increase uniformity; a concern born out of a fear of an increased workload and suspicion of possible interference from the Lunacy Commission in daily management of the institution.[51] Regardless of these concerns, Wood acknowledged the value of statistical uniformity, and the discussion at the 1864 annual meeting finished with the appointment of a committee who were placed in charge of drawing up a set of uniform statistical tables.[52]

It took the committee one year to return their report, and they recommended that the collection of financial data relating to the day-to-day running of the asylum be left as it was, and that if any adjustments be made, they should be carried out by the Lunacy Commission, ideally

[49] Ibid.

[50] Ibid.

[51] Ibid.

[52] Ibid.

through a change in legislation.[53] Putting these concerns to rest, the committee paid attention to the ways medical information was collected, and recommended that a new set of tables be introduced which would provide additional data on admissions, re-admissions, discharges and deaths. At this point, it did not recommend that information on the forms of insanity suffered by patients admitted to asylums be implemented into these statistical tables, although they recommended that 'maniacal and melancholic exhaustion or decay' and 'general paresis' were included as causes of death.[54] It also concurred with the judgement of the Royal College of Physicians when it came to the forms of insanity, writing that 'the concepts may be subject to revision in light of the publication of the Report of the College of Physicians on "Medical Nomenclature"'.[55]

In 1866 and only one year later, a motion was proposed by Lockhart Robertson to act on a recommendation made in the *1865 Annual Report of the Lunacy Commission* to reappoint the Committee on Asylum Statistics so that the statistical tables could be revised to allow more data on admissions to be gathered and returned. This included information on the form of insanity suffered by a patient and the diagnosis they had received upon admission to the institution.[56] In the Lunacy Commission's report of that year that was cited by Lockhart Robertson, a call was made for '[u]niformity in recording the ages of patients on admission, the duration of the existing attack, and the form of mental disorder under which they labour', and he reported that the Commission 'hoped that the medical officers of asylums may see great importance of coming to some agreement on these points'.[57]

[53] 'The Medico-Psychological Association Proceedings at the Annual Meeting of the Association, held at the Royal College of Physicians, on Thursday, July 13th, 1865' in *JMS*, vol. 11, no. 55, October 1865, pp. 383–427 (p. 403).

[54] Ibid., p. 410.

[55] Ibid.

[56] 'The Medico-Psychological Association: Proceedings at the Annual Meeting of the Association, held at the Rooms of the Royal Society, Edinburgh, on Tuesday, July 31st, 1866' in *JMS*, vol. 12, no. 59, October 1866, (p. 425).

[57] Ibid.

Aspirations to a Scientific Classification: The Aetiological Classification of David Skae

The potential for agreement had been thrown into doubt in 1863 when the Scottish physician David Skae delivered an address as president of the association that consisted of a sustained attack on Prichard's standard terms of diagnosis. His speech marked the beginning of a set of debates over classification that would span nearly two decades, ending in 1881. Skae argued that the classification of aetiology he had developed when teaching medical students in Edinburgh asylums was superior to the Table of the Forms imposed on alienists by the Lunacy Commission. He contrasted his own diagnostic terms with those in use, focusing in particular on the notions of mania and of melancholia. He thought that the lack of a physiological basis to both undermined their usefulness in clinical practice, making them vague and unbecoming for medical science. He argued that a precise and reliable classification system ought to be based upon an aetiology rooted in bodily conditions, along with what he described as the natural history of an illness. He considered the forms then in use to not be fit for purpose, and argued that the widespread practice of basing diagnosis solely on symptoms had led to confusion. Monomania, dementia and other forms of mania were easily confused with one another, according to Skae, with patients also being frequently misdiagnosed with moral insanity.[58] When describing his experience training medical students in the methods of psychological diagnosis, he noted:

> it has always struck me, that the moment [that these students] came into contact with the insane, all their preconceived notions of Insanity [that were] derived from our systematic works were found to be vague, misty, and purely conventional descriptions of what they actually saw.[59]

Training students with categories based upon symptomology alone had led, in Skae's view, to students emerging from medical school ill-equipped to make a precise diagnosis. The problem had become endemic to medical

[58] David Skae, Of the classification of the various forms of insanity on a rational and practical basis: being an address delivered at the Royal College of Physicians, London, at the annual meeting of the Association of Medical Officers of Asylums on 9th July 1863, Royal College of Physicians, 1863.

[59] Ibid., p. 6.

practice, leading to a wholesale corruption of psychological classification that had seeped into alienism's very foundations. The problem was particularly apparent in the diagnosis of mania, which was frequently confused with other forms. He described acute mania as a 'transient and babbling excitement of a harmless and frightened, but dirty, nudifying, and destructive patient'.[60] Mania was very hard to differentiate from other forms of insanity, since attacks were intermittent and the diagnosis a patient received depending on the symptoms apparent at the time of an inspection.[61] This was a problem for Skae; he thought symptoms fluctuated during the course of an illness, with the diagnosis received largely depending upon a patient's condition at the time of inspection. He used the examples of melancholia and mania to highlight his point: during a period of stupor, a patient could be diagnosed with melancholia, yet if they were examined and admitted during a period of particular agitation, then they could just as easily be diagnosed with mania. Skae deemed forms of insanity like acute mania to be based upon a limited set of clinical observations, which were inadequate because 'the form of Insanity [*sic*] varies within very short periods of time [...] [and] [w]hat was a few days ago a case of *mania*, is now one of monomania or dementia, in any of their forms or degrees'.[62] Continuity or blur between the handful of forms offered by Prichard's Table confounded matters, leading Skae to the conclusion that the judgement and habits of any inspecting officer were unacceptably influential in determining the diagnosis granted to a patient. Skae thought that this was not helped by concepts like idiocy and dementia being so broad that they ended up becoming meaningless, claiming that every degree of mental impairment could be found amongst these classes of patients, 'from simple loss of memory and slight childishness, to total fatuity, and obliteration of all the mental faculties'.[63] Similarly with monomania, with Skae questioning the main criterion for the category, namely a patient being obsessed with one thing, but otherwise having a sane mind:

60 Ibid.

61 Ibid., p. 8.

62 Ibid.

63 Ibid., p. 7.

> Among the so-called Monomaniacs, they found very few who were Monomaniacs at all: most of them were insane on several subjects, although presenting some more salient feature, such as the fear of poison, hanging, or eternal damnation, or the belief of exalted rank or enormous wealth or power.[64]

Skae's views echo the many critics of the symptom-based concepts developed by French medical psychology, which prompted numerous efforts across Europe to develop a means of dividing and classifying mental disorder that aspired to scientific rigour. The work carried out in the emerging research clinics of the German-speaking lands in the middle decades of the century had inspired British alienists in this endeavour. In particular, Skae and Thomas Laycock, his colleague at the University of Edinburgh's medical school, would publish work that paid testament to Wilhelm Griesinger, who had also attempted to connect psychological forms to physical aetiology and somatic pathology.[65] Griesinger presented a detailed nosology of mental diseases he hoped would improve the accuracy of psychological diagnosis by moving away from an over-reliance on symptoms when differentiating diseases from one another.[66] The nosology was split into three parts: the first were states of depression, which included forms of melancholia including those associated with stupor, self-harm and hypochondria.[67] The second class described states of 'exaltation' that included mania and monomania, with the third class being forms of 'mental weakness' including dementia and idiocy. Despite not breaking entirely from the symptom-based terms like those employed by Pinel and followers, Griesinger, like Skae, rejected the notion of moral insanity, claiming that it lacked real evidence, and even went as far as to say that Pinel's establishment of the term had had a lasting detrimental impact on the mental sciences.[68] Griesinger's harsh judgement was based on his dismissal of the fundamental distinction between the moral and intellectual faculties that had informed moral insanity; he thought it impossible

[64] Ibid., p. 6.

[65] Roy Porter, 'Psychiatry' in *The Greatest Benefit to Mankind*, Harper Collins, 1997, p. 507.

[66] Wilhelm Griesinger, *Mental Pathology and Therapeutics*, translated by C. Lockhart Robinson and James Rutherford, The New Sydenham Society, 1867.

[67] Ibid., p. 301.

[68] Ibid., pp. 301–302.

for the intellectual faculties to remain intact in an acute disorder, and that corruption of the emotional faculties would inevitably be linked to damage in the intellectual faculties. He considered Pinel's *manie sans délire* to be a non-existent category of mental disorder that confused two different 'morbid mental states':

> on the one hand actual periodic attacks of fury with very little delirium, and on the other hand and principally, to those moderate states of mental exaltation [...] in which the patient performs foolish actions and shows perversity of demeanour, but [is] also in a position to justify and explain their conduct [with] coherent reasoning which lies within the bounds of possibility.[69]

He went on to attack 'disciples of Pinel' in France, who, like Prichard, had mistakenly categorised many other conditions, such as the 'moderate degree[s] of melancholia with violence' seen in moral insanity.[70] Griesinger's rejection of moral insanity led him to develop a number of new categories which had hitherto been conceptualised as forms of moral insanity.[71] Griesinger, then, thought that the intellectual faculties could not remain unaffected and 'perfectly free from any disorder' and that 'in *all* attacks of fury, clear, calm, healthy thought is quite impossible'.[72] Karl Kahlbaum (1828–1899) and Ewald Hecker (1843–1909) would develop Griesinger's criticisms, claiming that such terms described temporary and transient conditions as opposed to referring to natural kinds, or diseases.[73]

French psychiatrists also developed ways to augment symptom-based classification. Jules Baillarger's 1853 'Essay on a Classification of Different Genera of Insanity' called for greater accuracy in diagnosis through links to physical symptoms.[74] Baillarger was a defender of phrenology, and argued that the division between Pinel's partial and general insanities

69 Ibid.

70 Ibid.

71 Ibid.

72 Ibid.

73 Ewald Hecker, cited in Kenneth Kendler and Eric Engstrom, 'Kahlbaum, Hecker, and Kraepelin and the Transition from Psychiatry Symptom Complexes to Empirical Disease Forms' in *American Journal of Psychiatry*, vol. 174, no. 2, February 2017, pp. 102–109.

74 German Berrios and Jules Baillarger, 'Classic Text no. 75: Essay on a Classification of Different Genera of Insanity' in *History of Psychiatry*, vol. 9, no. 3, pp. 358–373.

corresponded to 'partial and general lesions' of the parts of the brain responsible for the intellectual, moral and emotional faculties.[75] These lesions resulted in delusions, hallucinations, unusual impulses, excitation of the intellect and depression of the moral and intellectual faculties.[76] Baillarger differed somewhat from Griesinger because he still agreed with Pinel's fundamental idea of partial insanity, and that emotional disorders could exist without affecting the intellectual capacities. He argued for a stronger connection between physical lesions and different forms of insanity, and that a classification of mental disorder should be structured according to which faculty of the mind was affected by a lesion. Melancholia, for instance, was understood by Baillarger as a 'paralysis of the moral and intellectual faculties that abolishes strength and will' caused by a lesion.[77] Correct identification of the physical source of the mental disorder would prevent confusion and misdiagnosis with disorders that had similar behavioural symptoms, including monomania and certain forms of mania.

Further criticisms of symptomology ensued. Jean Pierre Falret published an essay only a year later that sought to argue against the existence of monomania.[78] Falret, who did not subscribe to faculty psychology, had argued against the existence of Pinel's *manie sans délire* since writing his medical thesis, and his 1854 essay also argued against the idea that the mind was divided into discrete faculties.[79] As a result, at least according Falet, any diagnostic concept which presumed the empty abstractions of intellect and emotion was not of clinical use. Although Falret's target was monomania in this instance, he was concerned with the theoretical basis of the prevalent symptom-based classification system because he did not think that this provided a scientific basis to the formulation of disease concepts. Falret's criticisms of monomania spelled the beginning of its end as a disease category. To add to these critical voices, when the French psychiatrist Bénédict Augustin Morel published his 1860 *Treatise on Mental Diseases*, he did not consider melancholia and mania as

[75] Ibid.

[76] Ibid.

[77] Ibid.

[78] '"De la non-existence de la monomania" by Jean-Pierre Falret', translated by Thomas Lepoutre and Tom Denning, in *History of Psychiatry*, vol. 23, no. 3, 2012, pp. 356–370.

[79] Ibid.

'essential forms' since 'depression and excitation are but symptoms which can be found in any form of madness'.[80] Like Falret, Morel rejected the formulation of mental disease concepts solely on the basis of observed symptoms, and instead sought to establish his own classification on the foundations of pathology.[81] In 1861, the *Edinburgh Medical Journal* reported that Morel's classification was a contender for the German Society of Psychiatrie and Juridical Psychology's competition on 'What is the Classification of Mental Disturbances which is likely to prove the Most Serviceable in Regard to Practical Medicine?'[82] Summarising the contenders for the one hundred thaler prize, the review focuses on how Bénédict Augustin Morel's system was split into four categories based not on symptomology but on aetiology: heredity, toxins, other nervous disorders, and 'morbid conditions of some other part of the body than the brain'.[83] Although praising the classification system offered by Morel, the review criticised his approach for being overly reliant on biological aetiology in the form of heredity, and for not taking into account the moral and psychological aspects of mental illness, such as anger, grief, shame, love or jealousy.

At the same time, some still held that a nosology based on symptomology held a great deal of practical value, despite any scientific shortcomings. Henry Monroe, writing in the *Asylum Journal of Mental Science* in 1856, thought that the symptom-based classification provided a useful description of behaviours associated with insanity, without being overly theoretical, therefore being of use to non-specialists as well as asylum medical superintendents.[84] Yet for Monroe, these strengths also led to its weaknesses, in that the terms employed by the nosology were inaccurate and superficial, often leading to misdiagnosis. Monomania was doubted by Monroe on the grounds that the symptoms were inaccurate, and indeed he claimed that instead of being fixated on one notion

[80] John C. O'Neal, 'Understanding and Interpreting Confusion: Philippe Pinel and the Invention of Psychiatry' in *Lumen*, no. 26, 2007, pp. 243–258.

[81] Pierre Pichot, 'Nosological Models in Psychiatry', in *British Journal of Psychiatry*, vol. 164, no. 2, February 1994, pp. 232–240.

[82] 'Reports of Societies: Royal Medical and Chirurgical Society, Tuesday, May 14, 1861', in *Medical Times & Gazette*, May 25th, 1861, pp. 562–565 (p. 565).

[83] Ibid.

[84] Henry Monroe, 'One the Nomenclature of the Various Forms of Insanity' in *The Asylum Journal of Mental Science*, vol. 2, no. 17, April 1856, pp. 286–305.

or idea, the monomaniac's 'characteristic is rather an invincible and generally melancholic persistence in the erroneous notions'.[85] As such, Monroe thought that the term, 'monomelancholia', would be a more suitable description of the condition. Monroe offered some suggestions to improve the accuracy of the terminology in any symptom-based classification but he thought that even if these adjustments were made, the classification of Pinel and Esquirol could not continue to be used because it relied upon the groundless claim that there were distinct intellectual and emotional faculties of the mind. Monroe, like his French counterpart Falret, considered these to be redundant metaphysical categories that ought to be abandoned. Instead, diagnosis needed to be based upon harder empirical evidence in the form of physiological aetiology. The popularity of Skae's classification was partly down to it harmonising with criticisms like those made by Monroe, who thought Prichard's Table of the Forms had preserved the Cartesian metaphysics originally introduced by Pinel. In opposition to Pinel's ghostly metaphysical entities, Skae considered his classification to be a natural and materialist one: he introduced his classification in the 1863 presidential address of the association with the announcement that '[f]or the facility of reference, I sum up the various natural orders I have thus sketched out in the following tabular form' (Table 3.5).

Skae was motivated partly in response to phrenology, and although a vociferous critic of Johann Spurzheim, the movement had inspired him to develop a materialist division of insanity that was rooted in bodily conditions.[86] To avoid confusing one disease with another, Skae thought that 'the Natural History of the disease' should be traced, and this could be found by observing the progression of mental and physical symptoms during the course of an illness. The term 'natural history' echoes Alexander Crichton, who in his 1797 *Inquiry into the Nature and Origin of Mental Derangement* employed the terms 'natural history of the mind' and 'morbid history of the mind' to describe the progression of mental

[85] Ibid.

[86] Michael Anthony Finn. The West Riding Lunatic Asylum and the Making of the Modern Brain Sciences in the Nineteenth Century, PhD Thesis, University of Leeds, 2012, p. 98.

Table 3.5 Skae's classification included in his lecture on the classification of the various forms of insanity[87]

<table>
<tr><td>Idiocy</td><td rowspan="2">Moral and Intellectual</td><td colspan="2" rowspan="2">Senile Mania</td></tr>
<tr><td>Imbecility</td></tr>
<tr><td colspan="2">Insanity with Epilepsy</td><td colspan="2">Phthistical Mania</td></tr>
<tr><td colspan="2">Insanity of Masturbation</td><td colspan="2">Metastatic Mania</td></tr>
<tr><td colspan="2">Insanity of Pubescence</td><td colspan="2">Traumatic Mania</td></tr>
<tr><td colspan="2">Satyriasis</td><td colspan="2">Syphilitic Mania</td></tr>
<tr><td colspan="2">Nymphomania</td><td colspan="2">Delirium Tremens</td></tr>
<tr><td colspan="2">Hysterical Mania</td><td colspan="2">Dipsomania</td></tr>
<tr><td colspan="2">Amenorrhoeal Mania</td><td colspan="2">Mania of Alcoholism</td></tr>
<tr><td colspan="2">Post-connubial Mania</td><td colspan="2">Post-Febrile Mania</td></tr>
<tr><td colspan="2">Puerperal Mania</td><td colspan="2">Mania of Oxaluria and Phosphaluria</td></tr>
<tr><td colspan="2">Mania of Pregnancy</td><td colspan="2">General Paralysis with Insanity</td></tr>
<tr><td colspan="2">Mania of Lactation</td><td colspan="2">Epidemic Mania</td></tr>
<tr><td colspan="2" rowspan="2">Climacteric Mania</td><td rowspan="2">Idiopathic Mania</td><td>Sthenic</td></tr>
<tr><td>Asthenic</td></tr>
<tr><td colspan="2">Ovario-Mania (Utero-Mania)</td><td colspan="2"></td></tr>
</table>

diseases.[88] The notion of a disease having a natural history provided the foundation for Skae's classification, and through questioning the patient, their family and their friends, its pre-history, so to speak, could be discovered. Skae proposed that information on the background of the patient be used to draw up the categories that would populate any worthwhile clinical classification of mental disorders because it would provide some indication of the future course of the disease. In making his argument for the importance of understanding the natural history of a mental disorder,

[87] David Skae, Of the classification of the various forms of insanity on a rational and practical basis: being an address delivered at the Royal College of Physicians, London, at the annual meeting of the Association of Medical Officers of Asylums on 9th July 1863, Royal College of Physicians, 1863, p. 15.

[88] Alexander Crichton, *An Inquiry into the Nature and Origin of Mental Derangement: Comprehending a Concise System of the Physiology and Pathology of the Human Mind and a History of the Passions and Their Effects*, Cadell Jr. & Davies, 1798.

he drew a comparison between typhus and typhoid fevers, asking the question:

> Why should we attempt to group and classify the varieties of Insanity by the mental symptoms, and not, as we do in other diseases, by the bodily disease, of which those mental perversions are but the signs?[89]

Michael Barfoot puts Skae's adoption of the term 'natural history' down to an attempt to use language that would strike a chord with fellow medical physicians.[90] Charlotte Mackenzie on the other hand claims that Skae's concern with the link between certain forms of insanity and the 'life-cycle' suggests his alignment to the degenerationist ideas of Morel.[91] There is little evidence however to suggest Skae used the term natural history to gain an audience or took Morel seriously enough to base his classification on degenerationist principles. Rather, natural history had its origin in the *naturphilosophie* of German romantic philosophy, an attempt to dispel the dualism inherent in post-Cartesian thought. The ailments of the human mind could be explained through natural laws, and any medical psychology that wanted to be a science had to cast off any remainder of a corrosive dualism.

Likewise, fellow Edinburgh physician Thomas Laycock attempted to provide an aetiological classification of mental disorders in his *Principles and Methods of Medical Observation and Research*.[92] Like Skae, he thought that an aetiological classification of mental disorder would help to improve accuracy in diagnosis and be more becoming of a clinical science. Laycock attempted to provide an exhaustive nosology of medical disorders of the body and mind, and included a section on mental diseases, although he considered them to have the same kind of causation as other nervous and bodily diseases. Laycock's system of classification was lengthy

[89] David Skae, Of the classification of the various forms of insanity on a rational and practical basis: being an address delivered at the Royal College of Physicians, London, at the annual meeting of the Association of Medical Officers of Asylums on 9th July, 1863, Royal College of Physicians, 1863.

[90] Michael Barfoot, 'David Skae: Resident Asylum Physician; Scientific General Practitioner of Insanity' in *Medical History*, 2009, no. 53, pp. 469–488 (p. 482).

[91] Charlotte Mackenzie, *Psychiatry for the Rich: A History of Ticehurst Private Asylum*, Routledge, 1992, p. 177.

[92] Thomas Laycock, *The Principles and Methods of Medical Observation and Research*, MacLachlan & Stewart, Edinburgh, 1863.

and elaborate, but its central concern was quite simple, and followed Skae in attempting to find ways of differentiating between the forms of insanity by focusing on physical causes. In the section of his textbook devoted to 'The Naming and Classifications of Diseases', Laycock wrote that 'the development of any department of science may be measured by the copiousness and precision of its terminology'.[93] Like Skae, he held that understanding the physical causes of the different forms of insanity could go some way to enabling this precision.[94] Laycock also posed the philosophical question of what constituted a disease, with his answer being that diseases caused irregularity in behaviour and hindrance of function. To classify these irregularities, Laycock argued that a classification of the insanities should be based on observations that linked the breakdown of 'tissues' and breakdowns of psychological function. This led him to conclude that it was ultimately useless to classify diseases by psychological symptoms alone. Laycock's classification was an attempt to return to the spirit of Cullen's work; like his Edinburgh predecessor, he employed the Latin *versaniae* to describe mental disorders and thought that they were caused almost exclusively by problems in the nervous system. This principle of aetiology should form the basis for a nosology not only of insanity, but all diseases. By appealing to the concepts of Cullen, both Laycock and Skae both sought to overturn the dominance of the symptom-based classification system established by Pinel which had become the standard used in psychological discourse and statistics by the second half of the nineteenth century.

Conclusion

Pinel cast a shadow over psychological classification and diagnosis throughout Europe for at least the entirety of the nineteenth century. The eventual adoption of his concepts of the mental alienations as the

[93] Ibid., p. 219.

[94] Laycock also thought the problem of classification had a linguistic dimension. He criticised the English language as having 'so degenerated in its inflexions as to become unpliable' for the purposes of scientific classification. He thought instead the German language ought to be adopted when attempting to classify the objects of scientific study, especially when developing science like medical psychology. This was because according to Laycock, the fixed structure of the English language meant that the references of terms would be too wide, and the terms could not be modified to adjust for slight differences in the manifestation of diseases.

standard in the United Kingdom by the middle of the century was not a certainty but was the result of a contingent set of factors linked to the development of lunacy administration during the early years of the AAMO. The appeal of Pinel's symptom-based classification lay in it not being encumbered by a metaphysics of causation, limiting itself to describing symptoms of asylum inmates without an elaborate theory of aetiology. The longevity that the nosography enjoyed was down to the absence of a theory of physical causes that could be disproven, with its simple structure holding appeal to those immersed in asylum practice sixty years after its initial publication. Pinel's forms traced recurring patterns of behaviour in patients, providing some indication of the prospects of patients and commonly associated psychological symptoms. In opposition stood figures like Skae who wanted a scientific classification of the insanities that would be linked to physical causes, representing natural divisions that would help to determine the prognosis of a patient. Symptomology functioned well-enough in practice but did not quench the Victorian thirst for evidence and scientific rigour. A classification based upon the disorders of the body came to be seen as the next step in the development of the mental sciences because it would represent mental disorders and psychological symptoms as being determined by laws of nature. The challenge to lay the path for this step forward in clinical knowledge was taken up by many, but as we will see in the next chapter, it would be Skae's that became the serious contender for use in asylum medical statistics.

In charting the divisions that occurred in approaches to dividing insanity, this chapter has attempted to tell a broader story of the tension between those satisfied with symptomology, and those who wanted to further the mental sciences by developing diagnostic categories that were natural, subject to physical laws and rooted in bodily causes. Both the project of symptomology and natural history were stages in the development of the *medical gaze*, with the classification of the insanities, inspired by the botanical sciences, being initially restricted to categorising collections of behavioural symptoms.[95] When the gaze went beyond the surface, and into the patient's body, alienists sought to find the concealed,

[95] In *Birth of the Clinic*, Michel Foucault discusses the reorganisation of discourse that framed the medical patient, and which led to a change in how the patient was conceptualised, a development that was fundamental to clinical knowledge: *The Birth of the Clinic: An Archaeology of Medical Perception*, translated by A.M. Sheridan, Routledge, 1989.

internal and mechanical bodily processes linked to insanity. The link was generally understood as being a causal one as this adhered to the increasingly dominant scientific worldview that had permeated Victorian culture. Representations of psychological disorders within classifications that aimed to be works of natural science placed the mind within a determinist worldview under the banner of eradicating artificial Cartesian divisions between spiritual and material substance. Symptomatology was an empirical exercise, but it remained at the surface level, and did not cohere to the metaphysics of natural philosophy that sought to explain all physical phenomena through causation. Although appearing to conform to a scientific ideal by explaining the mental through the physical, materialists like Skae were themselves putting forward a metaphysical view of causation, often in the same breath they accused Pinel's symptomology of containing unacceptable Cartesian metaphysics. The causal links offered by figures like Skae were speculative and conformed to a doctrinaire metaphysics of natural cause. In contrast, despite accusations of being tainted by Cartesian metaphysics, symptomology was in fact a purer empirical exercise since figures like Pinel and Prichard had limited themselves to describing the observable through detailed descriptions of behavioural symptoms. The logic of arch-materialists risked being self-consuming, and as in the example of Skae's aetiology, the grounding assumption that bodily conditions caused distinct forms of mental disorder committed him to the odd conclusion that each physical state gives rise to a particular kind of insanity. In other words, whereas Pinelean concepts could easily diagnose two people in different bodily states and with different genders with melancholia, Skae's attempt to fuse psychological diagnosis with aetiology meant that the melancholia suffered by a pregnant woman and a male labourer would be essentially different. This was no small point, with the infinite regress of dividing insanity according to physical states and the potential absurdity that could follow being picked up by critics of Skae when his classification became a candidate for use as the standard in asylum medical statistics. As we will see in the next chapter, some thought that far from giving medical knowledge a firm foundation, Skae's classification of aetiology would be entirely contingent on empirical findings that themselves could be revised upon further investigation.

Differing approaches to classification signalled the beginning of the divergence of clinical views. On the one hand, there was an approach that prioritised the pragmatic value of divisions for the purposes of diagnosis that ordered forms of insanity according to observations of symptoms, and on the other were aspirations for a scientific classification of the *kinds* of insanity, ordered according to categories of aetiology and the natural history of a disease. As we have seen, those who took up the challenge were motivated not only by the glory of making this step forward in scientific progress, but by concerns over imprecision and misdiagnosis that could have an impact on the treatment of a patient and the quality of medical statistics. For some, reliable diagnoses would only be made once madness was classified according to its aetiology, yet the limitations of psychiatric knowledge in its then current state meant that the aspiration for this sort of classification would never be fully realised, at least in the period covered by this study. By the second half of the nineteenth century, many began to view the dominance of the classification offered by Pinel as an obstruction to the ideal of a natural, scientific classification. The fact that only one could be chosen for use in asylum medical statistics meant that aetiology was put against symptomology as the ideal means of dividing insanity, and this issue acted as the catalyst for discussions on classification amongst the thought collective (*denkollektiv*) of British psychiatrists.[96] As we will see in the next chapter, the toing and froing between symptomology and aetiology would do much to define the debates that surrounded psychiatric classification, and in lieu of the knowledge that would allow a scientific classification, a Pinelean symptom-based classification of the forms would remain as the standard used for asylum medical statistics.

[96] A thought collective (*Denkkollektiv*) is a term that according to Ludwik Fleck describes the ways in which scientific communities come together to produce knowledge based upon a shared set of values and customs. As will become apparent during the pages of this volume, British psychiatrists shared fundamental assumptions on mental disorder—primarily that it was an illness that could be understood and treated medically—and fundamental assumptions like these provided structure to the debates. Although assumptions like this served to draw lines around the debates, divergence existed within these boundaries, which come alive when reading the minutes of the MPA that capture the debates surrounding the revisions. See: Ludwik Fleck, *Genesis and Development of a Scientific Fact*, translated by Fred Bradley, Robert K. Merton, and Thaddeaus J. Trenn, University of Chicago Press, 2008.

CHAPTER 4

Uniformity in Asylum Statistics: The 1882 Revisions to the Table of the Forms of Insanity

In October 1875, James Crichton-Browne (1840–1938), then the asylum medical superintendent of the West Riding Lunatic Asylum, made a spirited defence of the standard classification introduced by the Lunacy Commission and adopted by the Medico-Psychological Association (MPA) in the pages of the Journal of Mental Science (JMS).[1] This was in the face of the classification of aetiology developed by David Skae (1814–1873) having become a candidate to replace the Table of the Forms of Insanity. Skae's classification had attempted to provide psychological diagnosis with a foundation in conditions of the body by combining psychological and physical symptoms, with the implication being that specific physical states gave rise to particular forms of insanity. Many found Skae's work appealing because it held the promise of providing clearer distinctions between the insanities by differentiating illnesses according to causes, and the natural history of a disorder. With its foundation being in physical states and natural processes, the classification promised a more objective common ground than the symptomology that had provided the foundation for the Table of the Forms drafted by James Cowles Prichard. By attempting to link states of the body to

[1] James Crichton-Browne, 'Skae's Classification of Mental Diseases: A Critique' in *JMS*, vol. 21, no. 95, October 1875, pp. 339–365.

K. M. Jones, *Psychological Classification and Diagnosis in Asylum Statistics, 1800–1948*, Mental Health in Historical Perspective,
https://doi.org/10.1007/978-3-031-46154-5_4

states of the mind, Skae satisfied a widely held demand amongst alienists for a mechanistic and physiological classification that resembled other branches of medicine. Indeed, a great number of Skae's former Edinburgh medical school students had thrown their weight behind the cause to make his classification the standard used in asylum diagnosis and statistics. For its supporters, Skae's system realised aspirations for a scientific classification of the insanities that would lend legitimacy to psychological diagnosis, with many hoping that it could improve the reliability of diagnosis amongst admissions, and the quality of medical data being returned from asylums through yearly statistical returns.

Crichton-Browne did not think Skae's classification lived up to its scientific aspirations. He considered the classification of aetiology to be lacking, with the links drawn by Skae between psychological conditions and bodily states being dubious at best. He thought the idea that there were specific kinds of insanity linked to physical conditions such as pregnancy and paralysis ridiculous, and the concepts introduced by Skae risked causing more confusion than remedy. He thought Skae's classification was overly complicated, with questionable categories such as insanity of lactation and paralytic insanity. Clarity was not helped by it being a multi-axial system of sorts, that noted the main diagnosis, whether it was a case of mania or melancholia, and what prominent symptoms were presented, for example, hallucinations, stupor or chorea. The introduction of this experimental and potentially confusing system, which for Crichton-Browne was based on unfounded speculation about the causes of insanity, risked rendering useless the data on diagnosis collected by asylum statistical returns. His fears were far from unfounded, since only two years previously, John Archibald Campbell, a former student of Clouston, had recommended Skae's aetiological classification be used as the standard in the MPA's statistical tables.[2] Crichton-Browne was not a committed supporter of Prichard's Table of the Forms of Insanity which like Skae he also considered vague and unscientific. At the same time, he thought that the forms were the best available as the standard for asylum statistics and served some limited purposes until the mental sciences reached a greater level of maturity and sophistication. Crichton-Browne's attitudes are partly explained by, in the words of Janet Oppenheim, the 'uneasy

[2] J.A. Campbell and J. Todd, 'Uniformity in Public Asylum Reports' in *JMS*, vol. 19, no. 85, April 1873, pp. 67–78 (p. 69).

co-existence of physiological and psychological interpretations' of psychological disorders that are emblematic of broader tensions in Victorian psychiatry.[3] Although a committed subscriber to physical explanations of mental disorder in theory, in practice he contested the introduction of Skae's classification of physical causation, writing that adopting it as the standard used in statistical tables could hinder the development of mental health statistics and could hinder progress in the mental sciences. For him, the forms in use at least had the benefit of being familiar, with their meaning being defined largely by convention and usage. They were also concise, as opposed to Skae's system, which appeared convoluted and unnecessarily complicated. Since major breakthroughs enabling a scientific understanding of the causes of insanity were yet to materialise, Crichton-Browne thought those recommended for use in asylum statistics were the best available. The over-reductive nature of Skae's classification irked Crichton-Browne as he viewed the classification of Skae as being emblematic of the somatic dogma that had gripped medical psychology during the second half of the nineteenth century. Furthermore, the work required to introduce Skae's system into statistical returns offered little pay-off or prospects of improving the state of asylum medical statistics.

On a more profound level than administrative complexities, Crichton-Browne thought the existing Table of the Forms captured the flux of insanity, and that imposing causal connections between its forms, especially unproven ones, would not capture its amorphous character.[4] As discussed in the last chapter, one of the motivations for Skae was that he found continuity and overlap between disease concepts unacceptable, primarily because he feared it would open the door to subjective judgements and the possibility of misdiagnosis. Skae thought that confusion over diagnosis was widespread and had seeped into the foundations of medical science, bringing with it grave implications for the quality of asylum medical statistics on psychological diagnosis. Skae believed it to be the duty of medical science to incorporate physical states into psychological diagnostic categories, seeking to describe natural entities with his classification of aetiology. In contrast, Crichton-Browne thought that

[3] Janet Oppenheim, 'Sir James Crichton-Browne' in *"Shattered Nerves": Doctors, Patients, and Depression in Victorian England*, OUP, 1991.

[4] James Crichton-Browne, 'Skae's Classification of Mental Diseases: A Critique' in *JMS*, vol. 21, no. 95, October 1875, pp. 339–365.

some degree of overlap between diagnostic concepts was an unavoidable part of practice, especially in medical psychology, and this needed to be accepted for what it was instead of imposing artificial boundaries between disorders. He thought that until indubitable evidence was found to prove links between psychological and physical conditions, classifiers of insanity should limit themselves to describing appearances of visible symptoms, flawed as an approach to classification based on symptomology may be. His fear was that the state of the art did not allow Skae's causal connections to be established with certainty, and that asylum statistics could be corrupted by metaphysical speculation. The fundamental choice that framed the debates outlined in this chapter was essentially whether the *forms* of insanity recommended by the Lunacy Commission should be retained for the purposes of medical statistics, or if the ***natural kinds*** described by Skae should be introduced to replace them.

The exchanges were not just conducted on the philosophical level, with divisions drawn along professional interests and practicalities, both administrative and clinical. The stakes were high as the scientific potentials of asylum medical statistics were recognised by many of those engaged in these discussions. At times they descended into ill-feeling and open conflict between MPA factions. Crichton-Browne for instance described Skae's supporters as 'disciples' whose judgement had been blinded by devotion to their master. He thought their 'bungling' and 'divergent opinions' proved a threat to the quality of asylum statistics then being collected from across the country.[5] The most outspoken of Skae's followers was his former student Thomas Clouston (1840–1915). The Edinburgh physician had led a push for the classification of aetiology to be used as the standard in asylum medical statistics. Crichton-Browne's attack on Skae's followers came towards the end of a set of debates over classification that engulfed the MPA throughout the 1870s, which constitute the focus of this chapter. They were resolved in 1881 with a classification that attempted to combine the existing Table of the Forms with Skae's work. The discussions presented in this chapter show how administrative matters and statistics from admissions procedures triggered debates over clinical classification, and how record-keeping played an important role in the development of psychological diagnostic categories used in mental health statistics. In analysing the debates and reactions

[5] Ibid., p. 350.

to the work of revisions committees, this chapter will demonstrate how the categories 'into which people could conveniently fall in order to be counted' were developed in relation to bureaucratic procedures and record-keeping practices that led to efforts to standardise diagnosis for national medical statistics.[6]

Revisions to the Statistical Tables: 1869–1880

Up until the 1860s, the terms of diagnosis used in asylum medical statistics were principally based on symptomology, or the observations of patient behaviours, with some predictions on outlook. David Wright notes in his analysis of admissions to the Buckinghamshire County Asylum that concepts of psychopathology based on symptomology were the 'standard classifications in the mid-Victorian period', as does Michael J. Clarke in his assessment of intellectual cultures informing Victorian psychiatry.[7] Efforts to standardise diagnosis and asylum medical statistics were part of a wider context in public health administration to bring about consistency in relief and welfare.[8] Classifications of symptomology used in administration came into conflict with an increasing desire to have terms of psychological diagnosis that were linked in some way to the organic roots of insanity. Revising diagnosis in this direction came to be viewed as the ideal by the end of the 1860s, principally because perfecting asylum statistics in psychological diagnosis in accordance with the cutting edge of the mental sciences was viewed as one of the ways to progress knowledge. Prior to the first set of revisions to the Table that are outlined in this chapter, information on the physical causes of insanity was kept distinct from psychological diagnosis and was collected from asylums in a

[6] Ian Hacking, *The Taming of Chance*, Palgrave, 1990, p. 15.

[7] David Wright, 'Delusions of Gender?: Lay Identifications and Clinical Diagnosis of Insanity in Victorian England' in *Sex and Seclusion, Class and Custody: Perspectives on Class and Gender in the History of British and Irish Psychiatry*, edited by Jonathan Andrews and Anne Digby, Rodopoi, 2004, pp. 149–171; and Michael J. Clarke, 'The Rejection of Psychological Approaches to Mental Disorder in Late Nineteenth Century British Psychiatry' in *Mad Houses, Mad Doctors and Madmen: The Social History of Psychiatry in the Victorian Era*, edited by Andrew Scull, Athlone, 1981.

[8] Elaine Murphy, 'The Administration of Insanity in England 1800 to 1870' in *The Confinement of the Insane: International Perspectives, 1800–1965*, edited by Roy Porter and David Wright, Cambridge University Press, 2003, pp. 334–349.

separate statistical table. Those in favour of introducing Skae's classification to the statistical tables thought the time had come to combine the two and thereby provide firm physical foundations to psychological diagnosis. Although the aspiration to base psychological diagnosis on physical causes had been in existence since at least the late eighteenth century in William Cullen's writings on nervous disorders, it gained traction during the second half of the nineteenth century as psychiatry developed into a medical specialism. As the techniques and equipment used to understand the body of the insane patient became increasingly sophisticated many hoped that firmer foundations for diagnosis through a classification of aetiology would help to develop the field of medical psychology and asylum statistics.[9]

Asylum medical statistics were increasingly becoming seen as a problem that needed to be fixed, and due to the plethora of different terms used by doctors and the confusion surrounding their application, data on psychological diagnosis was seen as a particularly thorny problem. Lunacy statistics found themselves at the centre of a complex set of links between asylum administration, public health reform and mental health care. Since the introduction of the Table of the Forms in 1845, work by MPA members including David Skae and Thomas Laycock had attracted an appreciative audience. Work from continental Europe including that of Jean-Pierre Falret (1794–1870), Wilhelm Griesinger (1817–1868), Joseph Guislain (1797–1860) and Karl Ludwig Kahlbaum (1829–1899) had made the diagnostic terms then in use seem dated, and much in need of revision. Although phrenology was somewhat old hat by the turn of the 1870s, its legacy was seen in attempts to pinpoint the location of

[9] Jennifer Wallis, *Investigating the Body in the Victorian Asylum Doctors, Patients, and Practices*, Palgrave Macmillan, 2017.

lesions in the brain, and find links to psychological symptoms.[10] Degenerationist thought, inspired by Bénédict Morel and Jean-Baptiste Lamarck's ideas on heritability, also informed calls to revise the statistical tables, with prominent members of the MPA voicing strong views on the hereditary causes of insanity.[11] Although the widespread assumption held by a great deal of members was that the best psychiatric classification was the one that would carve insanity at its natural joints, debates raged over whether this would be realised through heredity, symptomology or aetiology.

In July 1869, a committee was appointed by the MPA to revise the statistical tables, with the Table of the Forms of Insanity taking centre stage. Skae and his former students Thomas Clouston and John Batty Tuke sat on the committee, with Robert Smith, James Howden and John Sibbald comprising the rest of the members. The first revisions committee unsurprisingly, given its constitution, presented a classification that bore the mark of Skae's work when it returned its report in January 1870. It proposed a classification system that combined Skae's aetiology with symptomology. The primary categories were for the most part lifted from Skae's classification, with most of them having sub-categories of mania and melancholia. Post-febrile fever was included in both the revised classification and Skae's original, as were the many forms of insanity Skae thought were caused by sexual activity and reproduction, with the inclusion of insanity of masturbation and climacteric insanity, although satyriasis and nymphomania did not make it on to the table proposed by the committee. Skae's fixation on pregnancy and insanity is apparent when we consider that four out of the fifteen main categories of his classification are linked to reproduction: insanity of childbirth, insanity of pregnancy, insanity from uterine disorder and insanity of lactation. As with satyriasis

[10] According to Cooter, physicalists like Skae were motivated to eliminate psychological considerations in reaction to the influence of phrenology. Skae had formed a career of long hostility towards phrenology, with his Royal Medical Society dissertation arguing against the existence of phrenological classification in favour of the Kantian division of the mind into faculties. He associated the symptomatic approach to the ties it had had to phrenology, which had enjoyed widespread popularity during his training: influential members of the MPA such as W.A.F. Browne (1805–1885), Crichton-Browne's father, subscribed for a time to phrenology, enthusiastically promoting the potential contributions it held towards advancing the newly established moral treatment: Roger Cooter, 'Phrenology and British Alienists c.1825–1845: Part II: Doctrine and Practice' in *Medical History*, vol. 20, no. 2, April 1976, pp. 135–151.

[11] Henry Maudsley, 'On Some of the Causes of Insanity' in *JMS*, vol. 1, no. 60, January 1867.

and nymphomania, some did not make it on to the revision committee's draft from Skae's original, including manias of oxaluria and phosphaturia: these respectively referred to insanities caused by the presence of oxalate crystals in urine, and insanities caused by abnormalities in the quantities of phosphates. The draft also showed Skae's interest in the links between intoxicating substances and insanity, with delirium tremens and insanity from alcoholism finding their way into the draft.

Bodily causes were the primary distinguishing feature between each of the main classes of insanities in the table, and as per Table 4.1, these ran along the vertical axis. Psychological symptoms included both sub-classes and a horizontal axis that allowed them to be recorded next to each of the main classes and sub-classes. This was carried out to realise Skae's goal of making clearer distinctions between the categories used in psychological diagnosis:

> In regard to classification, [the committee is] of opinion [*sic*] that the chief point to be attended to in adopting any system is to secure accuracy and definiteness of terms, so that each case may with certainty be placed in its class by different observers, and that by the same terms different observers may mean the same thing. They are of the opinion that none of the ordinary systems of classification used alone is sufficient for this purpose.[12]

Through their classification, the committee sought to bring scientific principles of reproducibility and replicability to admissions diagnosis. Skae's categories, that were defined by physical causes and their natural history, were combined with categories of symptomology. The revisions committee considered the categories from their revised statistical table to be natural kinds which would allow reliable and reproducible diagnosis to be made.[13] The hope was that the categories employed in the table would reduce the space for individual judgement, therefore making the data included in the statistical returns replicable and thereby realising the goals of greater conformity, compatibility and standardisation. With their revisions, the committee attempted to change the Table of the Forms from a table that divided insanity according to observable appearances to

[12] Ibid., p. 224.
[13] Ibid., p. 224.

Table 4.1 Classification proposed by the MPA Statistical Revisions Committee in 1870[14]

		PREDOMINANT FEATURES.									
		Acute delirium and incoherence.	Simple Excitement.	Simple Depression.	Stupor.	Hypochondria.	Strong Suicidal Impulses.	Remittency or Intermittency.	Chorea.	Hallucinations.	Enfeeblement.
CURABLE.		a	b	c	d	e	f	g	h	i	k
1. Insanity of Pregnancy*	Mania	1	1					1		1	
2. " "	Melancholia			1	1		1			1	
3. Insanity of Childbirth	Mania	1	1							1	
4. " "	Melancholia			1	1		1				
5. Insanity of Lactation	Mania	1	1							1	
6. " "	Melancholia			1	1		1			1	
7. Climacteric Insanity	Mania	1	1					1		1	
8. " "	Melancholia			1	1	1	1	1		1	
9 Insanity from Uterine Disorder	Mania	1	1					1		1	
10. " "	Melancholia			1	1	1	1	1		1	
11. Insanity from Tuberculosis	Mania	1	1							1	1
12. " "	Melancholia			1	1	1				1	1
13. Insanity from Masturbation	Mania	1	1			1				1	1
14. " "	Melancholia			1	1	1	1			1	1
15. Insanity from Alcoholism	Mania	1	1							1	
16. " "	Melancholia			1	1	1	1			1	
17. Delirium Tremens	Delirium Tremens	1			1		1			1	
18. Post Febrile Insanity	Mania	1	1					1	1	1	
19. " "	Melancholia			1	1	1	1	1	1	1	
20. Hysterical Insanity	Mania	1	1					1		1	1
INCURABLE.											
1. General Paralysis	Paralytic Insanity	1	1	1	1	1	1	1		1	1
2. Epileptic Insanity	Epileptic Insanity	1	1	1	1		1	1	1	1	1
3. Senile Insanity	Senile Dementia		1	1		1	1			1	1
4. Paralytic Insanity	Organic Dementia		1	1	1					1	1

* e g. A case could be quoted as being in class 1 (a, b, i).

[14] Skae David et al., 'Report of the Committee Appointed at a Meeting of Member of the Medico-Psychological Association, Held at the College of Physicians, Edinburgh, on 25th November, 1869, for the Purpose of Taking Certain Questions Relating to the Uniform Recording of Cases of Insanity and to Medical Treatment of Insanity into Consideration' in *JMS*, vol. 16, no. 74, July 1870, pp. 223–232.

one that used physical causes as the basis to represent natural kinds of insanity.

This vital change triggered debates surrounding the nature of insanity, as criticisms were quickly directed towards the draft classification. One of the most sustained attacks came from John Batty Tuke, the asylum superintendent of Fife & Kinross District Asylum who had trained under Skae at the Royal Edinburgh Lunatic Asylum. Despite being largely sympathetic to his former teacher's work, he had misgivings about the classification being adopted within the statistical tables. In April 1870, he published a paper which included a classification he branded as a pathological classification of mental disease.[15] Batty Tuke developed his work partly in response to Skae, but also because the Royal College of Physicians' had recently published a new nosology that included a simple and sparse classification of the insanities.[16] Batty Tuke complained that whilst the proposed nomenclature listed over 900 somatic disorders, it, like the Table of the Forms then in use, only included six forms of insanity.[17] Like Skae, Batty Tuke was no admirer of the Table of the Forms, but he argued that the committee could have found firmer ground if pathology instead of aetiology was used as the basis for his classification.[18] Batty Tuke claimed that Skae's work was confused in purpose since Skae had stated that it was a work of aetiology, but it in fact had used pathology as its foundations.[19] Echoing Crichton-Browne's criticisms, Batty Tuke claimed that Skae's classification rested on uncertain conceptual and empirical grounds, employing murky and unclear concepts that he thought confused pathology and aetiology in an attempt to make natural distinctions between different diseases. Although not included in the draft revisions, Batty Tuke used the concept of mania of oxaluria included in earlier editions of Skae's work to highlight his concern that Skae frequently confused symptoms for causes when establishing natural divisions between disorders. Mania of oxaluria was believed by Skae to be a family of insanities characterised by the existence of an excess of calcium

[15] J. Batty Tuke, 'A Pathological Classification of Mental Disease' in *JMS*, vol. 16, no. 74, July 1870, pp. 195–210.

[16] Ibid.

[17] Ibid.

[18] Ibid., p. 204.

[19] Ibid.

oxalate in a person's urine.[20] Batty Tuke thought that they 'can hardly be regarded as a natural family from the mere fact of the occurrence of the salt in certain cases, as its presence must be regarded as a consequence, not a cause, of such diseases as Climacteric or Idiopathic Insanity'.[21] For Batty Tuke, Skae had been hasty in his claim that the presence of calcium oxalate formed a natural family of insane diseases. Aside from judging Skae's work to be theoretically confused, Batty Tuke also contested his empirical findings, claiming that oxalation was 'generally found in cases where *melancholy* (not *mania*) is the leading mental symptom'.[22] The most serious of Batty Tuke's criticisms was that idiopathic insanity functioned as what scholars of science and technology studies refer to as a garbage or junk category, or to use Batty Tuke's term, a Gahenna.[23] In comparing idiopathic insanity to the biblical valley in Jerusalem where kings sacrificed their children to fire, Batty Tuke deemed patients given this diagnosis to be damned as untreatable and hopeless cases. According to Batty Tuke, this hardly allowed for the classification to be called one that divided insanity according to natural kinds, although he tried to save the face of his former teacher by making the conciliatory description of him as 'the Cullen of Psychiatric Medicine', albeit after savaging the conceptual basis of his nosology.[24]

Like Crichton-Browne, Batty Tuke thought that Skae's work was a false departure since his aetiological classification was dressing up symptom-based concepts of psychopathology in the language of natural kinds. Interestingly enough, his own pathological classification eschewed

[20] Although *Oxularia* was not explicitly reproduced in the revisions to the Table of the Forms produced by the committee, it was included under the broader category of Insanity from Uterine Disorder that was included in their report.

[21] Ibid.

[22] Ibid., p. 205.

[23] Ibid.; Skae's idiopathic insanity is what Star calls a 'garbage' category, and although her works focused on functional categories such as neurasthenia and hysteria, idiopathic insanity would seem to fulfil the model that she sets up for these categories since garbage categories function to classify cases that do not fit other categories. The success of a classification is usually judged by the number of cases that fall into the garbage category, with a larger number suggesting the classification is failing to adequately fulfil its purpose; S.L. Star, *Regions of the Mind: Brain Research and the Quest for Scientific Certainty*, Stanford University Press, 1989.

[24] Ibid., p. 205.

all categories of symptomology since he considered psychological disorders to be symptoms of, but not necessarily caused by, an underlying physical disorder. Instead of aetiology, which he thought to be an unrealistic way of formulating disease concepts due to the limited knowledge of insanity's causes and the possibility that the relationship between the body and mind was not a simple causal one, Batty Tuke called for '[p]athology [to be adopted] as the fundamental principle, without any regard to mental symptoms; that the causating [*sic*] pathological influence which induces the symptoms ought to be accepted as the ground-work of nomenclature'.[25] For Batty Tuke then, 'insanity' was not a disease in itself, but rather a symptom that pointed to an underlying physical condition. As such, insanity became a symptom 'of a disease either of the brain plasm primarily, or of a disease of the brain dependent on exoteric influences'.[26] The physicalist stance differs from that of Skae because Batty Tuke had not established linear and causal relationships between physical and psychological conditions, and instead eliminated all talk of symptomology from his classification system (Table 4.2).

Batty Tuke proposed seven main classes in his classification: *insanity from arrested development*, which incorporated acquired and congenital idiocy; *idiophrenic insanity*, caused by physical brain defects and organic problems, which included *traumatic insanity*, the traumas in these cases being impacts to the skull; *sthenic* and *asthenic* insanity, which were abundances and deficiencies in nervous energy, respectively, a term finding its origins in the work of Edinburgh physician John Brown, private tutor of Cullen;[27] *sympathetic insanity*, a vague class which included bodily processes such as *enteric* (relating to the digestive system) and emotional imbalances *post-connubial* (consummation), or *hysterical insanity*.[28] The final four main classes were: *anoemic insanity*, caused by deficiency in nutrients; *diathetic*, caused by weaknesses in physical constitution; *toxic*, caused by drugs, pollution and alcohol; and the final class, *metastatic*

[25] Ibid.

[26] Ibid., p. 206.

[27] Sean Dyde, 'Cullen, a Cautionary Tale' in *Medical History*, vol. 59, no. 2, 2015, pp. 222–240.

[28] German Berrios and J.H. Pons, 'J.H. Pons on "Sympathetic Insanity": With an Introduction by G.E. Berrios' in *History of Psychiatry*, vol. 25, no. 3, September 2014, pp. 364–376.

Table 4.2 The classification presented by John Batty Tuke in 'A Pathological Classification of Mental Diseases'[29]

	SUB-CLASSES.
Class I.—Insanity resulting from arrested or impaired development of the brain.	Idiocy, congenital and acquired.
Class II.—Idiophrenic Insanity.	Sthenic and Asthenic Idiopathic Insanity.
	Phrenitic Insanity (Inflammatory)
	General Paresis.
	Paralysis with Insanity.
	Traumatic Insanity.
	Senile Insanity
	Epileptic Insanity.
Class III.—Sympathetic Insanity.	Epileptic Insanity.
	Insanity of Masturbation.
	Insanity of Pubescence.
	Climacteric Insanity.
	Ovarian and Uterine Insanity.
	Insanity of Pregnancy.
	Puerperal Insanity.
	Post-connubial Insanity.
	Hysterical Insanity.
	Enteric Insanity.
Class IV.—Anœmic Insanity.	Limopsoitos (from starvation).
	Post-febrile Insanity.
	Insanity of Lactation.
Class V.—Diathetic Insanity.	Insanity of Tuberculosis.
	Syphilitic Insanity.
Class VI.—Toxic Insanity.	Cretinism.
	Delirium Tremens.
	Insanity of Alcoholism.
	Insanity from Opium-eating.
Class VII.—Metastatic Insanity.	Rheumatic Insanity.
	Pellagrous Insanity.
	Metastatic Insanity (from healing of long-established issues).

[29] Ibid., pp. 206–207.

insanity, referring to sets of insanity caused by a seemingly distant or unconnected condition, such as rheumatism or pellagra.

Batty Tuke's paper was read at the quarterly meeting of the association in Edinburgh, with Thomas Laycock as chairman and Skae and Clouston in attendance.[30] It gave rise to one of the longest discussions on the most appropriate means of classifying the forms of insanity yet. Laycock questioned the grounding principle of both Batty Tuke and Skae's classifications by claiming that it was not possible to come up with one singular cause or pathology for insanity. Rather, it was a composite of psychological and bodily disorders. Furthermore, Laycock criticised the basis of *insanity of alcoholism*:

> alcoholism was not a sufficiently discriminating classification. It was not a scientific term. Nobody drank alcohol, but alcohol mixed in some way – in beer for instance. [...] He was mentioning this because they were adopting the popular phraseology, when they should deal with these matters with strict attention to the facts. Of late there had been great adulteration of fermented drinks, and he thought that he had tended to insanity more than the alcohol in these liquors. Beer was a wholesome drink, let the teetotallers say what they would.[31]

Laycock claimed then that the English ordinary language term 'alcoholic' had no place in a clinical classification of insanity because it lacked the scientific precision that Batty Tuke and Skae sought. Laycock did concede that Batty Tuke's diathetic class of mental disorder had a stable pathology, remarking that even if the rest of the classification was disputable, Batty Tuke's exploratory and speculative classification could be excused if it included at least one valid category.[32]

Clouston thought that Batty Tuke's rejection of the language of symptoms was a step too far. He took issue with a fundamental feature of Batty Tuke's classification: the move to treat insanity solely as a symptom

[30] 'Report of a Meeting of Members of the Medico-Psychological Association, held at Glasgow, April 27th, 1870' in *JMS*, vol. 16, no. 74, July 1870, p. 300.

[31] Thomas Laycock, remarks in 'Report of a Meeting of Members of the Medico-Psychological Association, held at Glasgow, April 27th, 1870' in *JMS*, vol. 16, no. 74, July 1870, p. 304.

[32] Ibid.

of brain states.[33] Clouston called this a fallacy because Batty Tuke's assumption was out of sync, he thought, with the reality of being an alienist—insanity was a composite of physical states and mental states, which were both treated in asylums, not merely the underlying pathology. Clouston inferred from Batty Tuke's classification that alienists should place their emphasis on treating the body of asylum inmates and Clouston accused him of eradicating the years of accumulated knowledge of psychological forms of insanity with his classification of pathology. Clouston thought that the established forms of insanity corresponded to physical states appealing to 'certain French observers [who] had the good luck to find out that in certain cases of insanity they could lay their finger on a particular portion of the brain as the diseased part'.[34] Clouston then claimed that the forms originally described by Pinel had seen some success amongst alienists including Jean-Pierre Falret, Jean-Martin Charcot and Georges Gilles de la Tourette precisely because they had established connections between the forms of symptomology and physical states through research into anatomy. These physicians, centred around the Salpêtrière in Paris, had made discoveries since at least the 1860s that linked observable symptoms, such as facial tics and disordered speech, to disorders of the nervous system and certain areas of the brain. This tradition had been characterised by a dualism between physical and mental symptoms, but physicians sought to resolve these two different spheres with research into pathologies. Clouston argued that the successes of the French school demonstrated the need to retain symptomology, when researching the physical causes of mental disorder. He agreed with Skae that the natural history of mental diseases and aetiology needed to be implemented into diagnostic categories based on symptomology. This would help to avoid misdiagnosis and increase reliability.[35] Clouston rounded off his criticism of Batty Tuke's classification and defence of the efforts of the revisions committee by warning that a radical departure from accumulated knowledge of symptomology meant placing the future course of British psychiatric statistical research on uncertain and untested foundations. Adding his voice to Clouston's criticisms, Skae waded in

[33] Ibid., p. 305.

[34] Ibid.

[35] Thomas Clouston, *Clinical Lectures on Mental Diseases*, 3rd edition, J & A Churchill, 1892, p. 20.

and turned Batty Tuke's criticism of his system on him by claiming that he was in fact doing aetiology and not pathology, although his remarks were generally genial in their tone.[36] Skae is said to have conducted himself with the air of someone who relished disagreement and discussion on scientific physiology, even if his own work was the target of critique.[37] He adroitly observed that Batty Tuke's pathologies were, upon closer scrutiny, aetiologies since they described a single physical condition that accompanied a kind of insanity, which was tantamount to describing causal relationships.

These would come to be the last contributions Skae himself would make to the discussions on psychological diagnosis; although he would pass away less than three years later, his work would continue to exert an influence through his disciples, as Crichton-Browne called them. His last recorded remarks in these debates reveal insights into the later ideas on classification from an enigmatic yet influential figure in the history of classification:

> What [Batty Tuke] sought in his paper was to point at natural groups. They were founded on causation, but not on that alone. He described climacteric mania. He did not say that that was the cause of insanity; but that at that particular period of the life of the female, insanity occurred which ran its natural course, and they had just to look for the symptoms [psychological phenomena]. It was the same with many other causes of insanity. He could tell a case of puerperal mania the moment he saw it. He did not mean to say what caused puerperal insanity, but where it occurred there must be predisposition. He believed that predisposition existed in every case of insanity. No remarks occurred to him with regards to Dr Tuke's re-arrangement of his classification. It would require consideration but it seemed to be very good. He agreed with Dr Clouston that they could only arrange those forms of insanity he had mentioned in certain groups or natural families. He did not think that they would gain much by dividing them into seven different classes.[38]

[36] David Skae, remarks in 'Report of a Meeting of Members of the Medico-Psychological Association, held at Glasgow, April 27th, 1870' in *JMS*, vol. 16, no. 74, July 1870.

[37] 'David Skae: Obituary' in *Edinburgh Medical Journal*, vol. 18, no. 11, May 1873, pp. 1055–1056.

[38] David Skae, remarks in 'Report of a Meeting of Members of the Medico-Psychological Association, held at Glasgow, April 27th, 1870' in *JMS*, vol. 16, no. 74, July 1870.

Skae's remarks indicate that by this point he had moved away from thinking that his concepts of psychological diagnosis mapped simple causal relationships. Rather, the kinds of insanity he described were concurrent with certain physical conditions, but the causing factor may have been predisposition or hereditary constitution.

John Sibbald, by this time assistant superintendent at Morningside asylum under Skae, joined the defence of the committee's classification in the face of attacks like those of Batty Tuke.[39] He called the committee's draft 'the only one that came anything near to the truth', and that whilst even 'Dr Skae, he believed, did not consider it good himself; [...] he thought it was the most practicable classification we had yet'.[40] Clouston himself thought that it was vital to precisely differentiate forms on the firmer foundations of aetiology that Skae provided because it would allow alienists to isolate them from the 'general mass of unclassified insanity' and give a clearer understanding of the kinds of patients that were being admitted into asylums across the country.[41] However, despite these goals and the defence of the revisions that had been proposed by Clouston, Sibbald and Skae, the blows had landed and the first draft of revisions did not attract widespread support amongst members of the Association. Undeterred, Skae's disciples, led by Clouston, would continue to press for a Skae-inspired classification to replace the Table of the Forms. At the MPA's 1876 annual meeting, Clouston tabled a motion to appoint a new committee that would be responsible for the revision of the tables of statistics, which was seconded by Joseph Lalor, another Edinburgh-educated asylum superintendent. The address in which he made these calls outlined a vision to correlate the information on psychological diagnosis collected by the Table of the Forms of Insanity with data on physical inspections and autopsies to provide a rich source of research data.[42]

Crichton-Browne's attack on Skae's classification was published in the association's *Journal of Mental Science* in autumn 1875. It was a twenty-six-page hatchet job that repeated the same criticism: that upon closer

[39] 'Obituary: John Sibbald' in *JMS*, vol. 51, no. 214, July 1905, pp. 636–637.

[40] John Sibbald, remarks in 'Report of a Meeting of Members of the Medico-Psychological Association, held at Glasgow, April 27th, 1870' in *JMS*, vol. 16, no. 74, July 1870, pp. 295–306 (p. 305).

[41] Ibid.

[42] Thomas Clouston, 'Skae's Classification of Mental Disorder' in *JMS*, vol. 21, no. 96, January 1876, pp. 532–500.

scrutiny, Skae's classification was not a classification of aetiology at all, and unwittingly used the very basis of symptomology Skae criticised in the work of Pinel, Prichard and Esquirol. Crichton-Browne was motivated by concerns that Clouston's 'oecumenical council of Morningside' would achieve their aim to 'replace those classifications that have preceded it, and that are still incomparably superior to it'.[43] In his attempt to thwart their aims, he targeted the conceptual basis of Skae's classification, describing it as 'philosophically unsound, scientifically inaccurate and practically useless'.[44] During his lengthy critique of Skae's work, or at least the version included in Clouston's edited edition of Skae's Morisonian Lectures, Crichton-Browne acknowledged that Skae's task was ambitious, but judged it to be conceptually confused due to him having laid down 'no general principle to guide' an audience through his system.[45] In doing so, Skae's intial aim to develop an aetiological system had become a system based on pathology, which was speculative and unfounded. The judgement that he reached was harsh:

> [Skae's pupils] will resent the indictment of the many counts brought against it – but the sooner they realise the justice of that indictment the better will it be for British Medical Psychology. The verdict sooner or later will be that this so-called classification is no classification, for it involves no act of comparison or judgement, but trusts to hearsay testimony, and is founded on conditions numerous, venial, and inextricably entangled. Griesinger says, with true wisdom, 'Our classification [...] proceeds upon the symptomological method', and by such a method alone can any classification be effected.[46]

He went on to address the details of the concepts within Skae's system, the primary target being idiopathic insanity, a concept Crichton-Browne thought served no other purpose than being a junk category:

> there is the objection which has been before advanced by Dr Maudsley and others, that at the tail of the classification there is a miscellaneous

[43] James Crichton-Browne, 'Skae's Classification of Mental Diseases: A Critique' in *JMS*, vol. 21, no. 95, October 1875, pp. 339–365 (pp. 339–340).

[44] Ibid., p. 341.

[45] Ibid.

[46] Ibid., p. 365.

> lot – *idiopathic insanity*, a refractory ward into which are forced all the recalcitrant cases that will not submit to the discipline of classification. Into this limbo march all cases that cannot be identified as belonging to any of the other thirty-four circles of madness, and in it we may suppose there is a strange and motley mob. We are told by Dr Clouston that only one-tenth or one-twelfth of the whole number of the insane require to be placed in this group, but a medical friend of mine who tried on a small scale to apply Skae's system, and surviving the attempt, has assured me that about thirty per cent. of the asylum patients ought to be included within it.[47]

Crichton-Browne concluded that Skae's classification was logically incoherent and had failed in its attempt to provide a firmer basis for psychiatric classification. He went as far as to say that, like Batty Tuke, Skae could not decide whether to base his work on pathology or aetiology. As if this was not enough, most serious of all was his judgement that the classification of aetiology was impractical, a potentially fatal blow because of the use of the terms of diagnosis in statistical returns. Crichton-Browne was one of the most vocal opponents of the tendency of psychiatrists like Batty Tuke to reduce insanity in its various forms to being entirely a symptom of brain pathology, despite him having established a research school dedicated to investigating insanity's physical treatments and its pathological causes.[48] Crichton-Browne was also a student of Laycock, who, unlike Skae, attempted to incorporate psychological considerations as causative factors in his own classification system.[49] In contrast, the system proposed by Skae explained all mental disorders through physical causes, and in doing so relegated thought processes to being dependent on physical states.

Clouston was quick to respond to Crichton-Browne's accusations, providing a rebuke in the next issue of the Association's journal in Spring

[47] Ibid., p. 362.

[48] Michael J. Clarke, 'The Rejection of Psychological Approaches to Mental Disorder in Late Nineteenth Century British Psychiatry' in *Mad Houses, Mad Doctors and Madmen: The Social History of Psychiatry in the Victorian Era*, edited by Andrew Scull, Athlone, 1981, pp. 271–312.

[49] Joseph Melling and Bill Forsythe, *The Politics of Madness: The State, Insanity and Society in England, 1845–1914*, Routledge, 2006, p. 21.

1876.[50] He sought to address accusations of filial loyalty by stating that Skae's work was not solely supported by his former students since it had even won over those initially sceptical of his classification. In contrast to Skae's reputation for good humour at even the harshest criticisms, Clouston's response was irritable in tone. He quickly described Crichton-Browne's reasoning as that of the 'uneducated', accusing him of 'childish sophistry' that showed 'the unwisdom of its author'.[51] He considered Crichton-Browne's claim that Skae had completely rejected Pinel and Esquirol's work unwarranted, and repeated the argument he had made in response to Batty Tuke's classification of pathology that Skae's system was compatible with symptomology. At the same time, he warned that to regard the current forms of mania and melancholia as the 'true forms of mental disease was a scientific blunder', and investigations like Skae's had refined these concepts by connecting symptomology, physical causes and the natural history of a disorder.[52] Clouston's response rested on the claim that Crichton-Browne had mistaken Skae's classification to be one that classed the causes of mental disorders. The correct interpretation of it, according to Clouston, was that it should be understood as a classification that associated physical causes and psychological symptoms, with Skae using aetiology as a convenient naming practice for diagnostic concepts, and not as a means to make strong causal claims. This dubious response allowed Clouston to acknowledge the limitations of the causal connections established by Skae that were questionable in the light of empirical evidence and argue that many of Crichton-Browne's criticisms were based on the mistaken assumption that it was a classification of causes. Stating that instead the correct interpretation of Skae's system was that it rested on the foundation of the natural history of a condition, Clouston attempted to dismiss Crichton-Browne's criticisms that the causal distinctions of Skae's classification were unfounded.

Clouston continued his push to replace the existing Table of the Forms. During an address to the association's annual general meeting in July that same year he delivered the case for the classification of symptomology to be replaced by a classification of physical causes. He cited the

[50] Thomas Clouston, 'Skae's Classification of Mental Disorder' in *JMS*, vol. 21, no. 96, January 1876, pp. 532–500.

[51] Ibid., p. 534.

[52] Ibid., p. 536.

statistical work of Robert Boyd, superintendent of the Somerset asylum and another Edinburgh trained physician to support his cause. In his 1867 report, Boyd dismissed the work 'of metaphysicians of emotion' who traded in psychological categories, and instead argued for diagnostic categories that understood mental disorders as fevers induced in the stages of physical disease.[53] Boyd used this philosophy of insanity to argue for greater welfare and healthcare for the poor: if you could administer preventative medicine for bodily conditions, then asylums may cease to be clogged up with those who were in pitiful mental states that were caused by advanced physical illnesses.[54] In citing Boyd's work, Clouston appealed to committed physicalists like Batty Tuke, despite his own acknowledgement of the worth of symptomology. Statistics collated in light of these considerations would guide the future research of the MPA, and would, in Clouston's mind, be one step towards achieving the kind of aetiological classification system that his teacher Skae had sought to achieve. Clouston had his way, and he managed to get himself appointed to a committee established to revise the statistical tables in response to his motion. However, despite a great deal of preparatory work, there is no evidence to suggest the committee ever met or published any sort of report.[55] As is clear from the assessment of Lunacy Commission reports conducted in the sixth chapter of this study, the symptomatic classification of mental disorder continued to provide statistics that were used by the MPA as before.[56]

[53] Robert Boyd, *16th Annual Review of the Somerset County Pauper Lunatic Asylum, Wells, 1863.*

[54] Ibid.

[55] Ibid.

[56] D.G. Thompson, 'The Prognosis in Insanity' in *JMS*, vol. 29, no. 126, July 1883, pp. 188–205.

Revisions to the Statistical Tables: 1880–1882

Renewed calls for the improvement of the statistical tables were published in the *JMS* between 1876 and 1880.[57] In response, revisions to the tables would recommence at the beginning of the next decade with the appointment of another revisions committee. This would give rise to further debates over asylum medical statistics. The Table of the Forms increasingly became the focus of members of the MPA during the first wave of revisions of the statistical tables. In attempts to increase the quantity and quality of information gathered from asylums across the country, the forms of insanity that were employed by the Lunacy Commission were viewed as not gathering enough information on the conditions suffered by patients who were being admitted to asylums. It was hoped that revisions to the tables would provide information from across the United Kingdom's asylums that would bring about better understandings of the aetiology, pathology and treatment of insanity. Although the extra work required to fill in expanded tables was not welcomed by all, the worth of the exercise was ultimately acknowledged by a majority of members of the MPA.[58] The standardised data pooled from all institutions across England and Wales could allow cross-sectional analysis with enormous potentials for the development of psychiatric research.

Growing interest in finding out if recovery rates varied in patients diagnosed with different forms of insanity was part of the reason why calls to revise the statistical tables commenced again in 1880.[59] The hope was that if the tables were revised correctly, they would provide improved data which would lead to useful findings about how long those who suffered from each of the different forms of insanity tended to stay in asylums, and whether they were at any point discharged.[60] Asylum superintendents suspected that a diagnosis of dementia would provide a grim outlook,

[57] Major, 'Dr Major on Statistical Tables of the Causes of Insanity' in *JMS*, vol. 23, no. 104, January 1878, pp. 573–575; P. Maury Deas, 'Five Years of Statistics' in *JMS*, vol. 25, no. 109, April 1879, pp. 8–9.

[58] See Sir John Charles Bucknill, *The Care of the Insane and Their Legal Control*, London, Macmillan, 1880, p. 51.

[59] Daniel Hack Tuke, 'On the Best Mode of Tabulating Recoveries from Insanity in Asylums Reports', vol. 26, no. 115, October 1880, pp. 375–383; Campbell, remarks in 'Report of the Thirty-Fifth Annual Meeting of the Medico-Psychological Association' in *JMS*, vol. 26, no. 115, October 1880, pp. 444–460 (p. 449).

[60] Ibid.

with the patient likely to remain in the asylum until their death. Those diagnosed with a mania would also, in all likelihood, have a very long stay, and perhaps would never be released, yet hope remained for those diagnosed with a form of melancholia, who tended to see the best recovery rates. Those classified as idiots would often find themselves in different institutions entirely, and this would come to be especially marked after the passing of the 1886 Idiots Act, which made different provisions for those diagnosed with forms of insanity that were considered incurable, as either congenital or having existed from birth.[61]

These considerations on prognosis led to another set of debates on classification commencing in July 1880. These would lead to the first major revision to the Table of the Forms being published in 1882 (see Table 4.1). The revisions committee attempted to make a compromise between the disciples of Skae and those who wanted to retain the existing symptom-based concepts of mental disorder. In order to placate those like Crichton-Browne who wanted to retain a tried and tested classification system and who were fearful of the potential damage of Skae's system, the main classes from the old Table of the Forms were retained. To satisfy those who wanted aetiological classification concepts introduced into asylum statistics, sub-classes of each of the main classes of the existing Table of the Forms were introduced. The crucial element of this compromise however was that filling in these sub-classes was deemed optional, and this undermined efforts by figures like Clouston to have Skae's classification introduced into statistical returns. This compromise then would mean that the question of the MPA's standard forms of insanity would not be resolved in any meaningful way at the end of these debates, and although they had led to the publication of the first revision to the Table, the committee's attempts to please both sides had left many issues raised in the debates unresolved.

This revision to the statistical tables commenced with the appointment of a committee in July 1880. Thomas W. McDowell, who had served as a pathologist under Crichton-Browne at the West Riding Pauper Lunatic Asylum, put forward this motion, and it was seconded by Henry Sutherland who had also spent time with Crichton-Browne during his training

[61] Peter Bartlett, The Poor Law of Lunacy: The Administration of Pauper Lunatics in Mid-Nineteenth Century England (with special Emphasis on Leicestershire and Rutland), PhD Thesis, UCL, 1993.

years spent in Wakefield.[62] Unlike Clouston's call in 1876 to appoint a revisions committee, McDowell did not offer any kind of agenda in proposing a motion to revise the statistical tables. Instead, this reappointment was more of a fluke that occured as result of McDowell asking for an update on the progress of the revisions committee appointed in 1876 and which he believed was still working on revisions.[63] Upon hearing that the committee in charge of them had not sat, McDowell called for its reappointment to once again consider how the MPA could improve the quality of the diagnosis data.[64] To achieve this, the committee was given the task of revising the tables to improve the uniformity of the data submitted by asylum superintendents in statistical returns.

A large committee of eighteen members was appointed in response to calls to revise the statistical tables. Daniel Hack Tuke was nominated as chairman of this revisions committee due to his prominent role within the association, and Henry Rayner, due to his previous work and expertise on statistics, was appointed as secretary. Prominent members included John Sibbald, who was at that time the Commissioner in Lunacy for Scotland and who had worked under Skae at the Edinburgh Royal Asylum, where he had been a colleague of Clouston, who was also appointed to serve on the committee.[65] Herbert Major was appointed; he had succeeded Crichton-Browne as medical superintendent at the West Riding Lunatic Asylum. Major had previously expressed hopes in the pages of the *JMS* that carefully compiled statistical tables would yield more reliable details and numbers on the admissions to asylums, which would in turn inform research on the treatment, prognosis and causes of insanity.[66] Other members of the committee included Campbell, due to having previously worked on statistics, including a call for uniformity of statistics

[62] Michael Anthony Finn, The West Riding Lunatic Asylum and the Making of the Modern Brain Sciences in the Nineteenth Century, PhD Thesis, Leeds, September 2012, p. 77 and 'Obituary: Henry Sutherland' in *JMS*, vol. 48, no. 200, January 1902, pp. 208–209.

[63] Dr Blandford, remarks recorded in 'Report of the Thirty-Fifth Annual Meeting of the Medico-Psychological Association' in *JMS*, October 1880, pp. 444–460 (p. 447).

[64] Ibid.

[65] 'Obituary: John Sibbald' in *JMS*, vol. 51, no. 214, July 1905, pp. 636–637.

[66] Hebert C. Major, 'Remarks on the Results of the Collective Record of the Causation of Insanity' in *JMS*, vol. 30, no. 129, pp. 1–7.

published in the *JMS* in 1873, and a defence of the use of Skae's classification as the standard;[67] William Henry Parsey, who served as president of the MPA in 1876 and was London trained;[68] Isaac Ashe, steward to Bethlem, who had published research in the *Journal of Mental Science* on general paralysis;[69] Robert Boyd who, as discussed, had made a number of contributions to the debates concerning statistics that occurred in 1869–1870; Hayes Newington, who would rise to become a prominent member of the society during the early part of the twentieth century, and who was a part of the Newington dynasty that had established the Ticehurst asylum and had trained in London and at Morningside Asylum in Edinburgh under the stewardship of David Skae;[70] James Murray Lindsey, another Edinburgh trained alienist who worked with Sankey at Hanwell County Asylum;[71] William Chapman Begley, who had worked with John Connolly at the Hanwell Asylum;[72] and T.W. McDowall.

The committee presented their proposed revisions to the statistical tables the following year at the 1881 summer annual general meeting.[73] The secretary for the committee, Henry Rayner, took the floor and proposed that the statistical tables be approved without discussion and instead, delegates were instructed to send comments and suggestions by mail directly to the committee. He appealed for power to be granted to the revisions committee to implement the revised statistical tables once any minor adjustments were made in response to these suggestions, and details of the changes would be published in the *JMS*. Rayner's justification was that this would allow the revisions to be implemented sooner, avoiding the lengthy and acrimonious discussions that had accompanied

[67] J.A. Campbell and J. Todd, 'Uniformity in Public Asylum Reports' in *JMS*, vol. 19, no. 85, April 1873, pp. 67–78 (p. 69).

[68] 'Obituary: William Henry Parsey' in JMS, vol. 30, no. 129, April 1884, pp. 166–167.

[69] Isaac Ashe, 'Some Observations on General Paralysis' in *JMS*, vol. 22, no. 97, April 1976, pp. 82–91.

[70] 'Obituary: Herbert Francis Hayes Newington' in *JMS*, vol. 63, no. 263, October 1917, pp. 461–467.

[71] 'Dr James Murray Lindsay' in *JMS*, vol. 58, no. 240, January 1912, p. 197.

[72] 'Obituary: William Chapman Begley' in *JMS*, vol. 33, no. 142, July 1887, pp. 337–339.

[73] Henry Rayner, remarks recorded in 'Report of the Thirty-Sixth Annual General Meeting of the Medico-Psychological Association' in *JMS*, vol. 27, no. 119, October 1881, pp. 434–444 (p. 440).

previous attempts to revise the statistical tables. Whether this was a political move on Rayner's part is difficult to tell: it may be the case that he was sincere in his desire to not take up precious time during the annual meetings to discuss the minutiae of the statistical tables, as this was after all the only opportunity for members from across the British Isles to meet. Rayner may also have wanted to prevent a repeat of the kind of bombastic debates that surrounded previous revisions of the statistical tables: MPA annual general meetings were becoming increasingly prestigious, with increasing membership seeing grander audiences and more attention from other branches of medicine. Mindful that even the learned members of the Association may at times let the occasion go to their heads, Rayner's proposal to switch the discussion to the pages of the Association's journal may have been a strategy to elicit a clearer headed discussion of the revisions to the statistical tables. His motion however was met with disapproval, with prominent members of the Association raising their voices in protest. Clouston argued that the revisions were widely considered to be a matter of paramount importance, which made it necessary for them to be presented for full discussion at an annual meeting.[74] He suggested that the tables be sent for discussion to the regional divisions of the Association for further discussion before the next year's annual meeting, where they would be discussed in light of feedback gathered from members across the British Isles. Either way, Rayner's plan was emphatically rejected by the president of the Association Dr G.W. Mould, superintendent of the Cheadle Royal Asylum, and a motion was passed to present the revisions to the regions before they would be discussed at the next annual general meeting.[75]

Members of the Association reconvened in July 1882 to discuss the revisions and the statistical report that had been penned by Rayner and Daniel Hack Tuke.[76] The Table of the Forms presented in the report retained the separation between the causes of mental disease and the forms of insanity. Aetiological considerations had not been incorporated into the core concepts of this committee's classification. The

[74] Thomas Clouston, remarks recorded in ibid.

[75] G.W. Mould, remarks recorded in ibid.

[76] Daniel Hack Tuke et al., 'Report of Committee on the Statistical Tables of the Medical-Psychological Association' in *JMS*, October 1882, pp. 463–464.

report stated that the causes of psychological disorder can be best understood by cross-referencing the information collected by the Table of the Causes of Insanity with the Table of the Forms. The Table of the Forms would not become an aetiological classification and concepts based on symptomology would continue to be used as main classes. Skae's aspiration for a scientific classification of the insanities was dealt a fatal blow. The concern of the revisions committee instead was to make 'the [recording of the] forms of mental disorder in those admitted in as practical a manner as possible'.[77] In an attempt to resolve the debates and appease Skae's followers, the committee had introduced concepts of aetiology as sub-classes to the main forms. As Table 4.4 demonstrates, these included factors like pregnancy and alcoholism, which could be recorded against a primary diagnosis of melancholia or mania.[78] The committee recommended that these sub-classes be used at the discretion of the superintendent, and that filling them in on statistical returns was then optional. This angered those who had fought a long battle for the classification of the causes to be used as the standard in asylum statistics. The Table of the Forms that was produced by the 1882 committee added 'Acquired Epilepsy' and 'General Paralysis of the Insane' to the symptomatic concepts of melancholia, mania and dementia. A sixth primary category of 'Congenital or Infantile mental deficiency' would introduce to the Table a division between disorders assumed to be hereditary and those believed to be acquired. This move to separate congenital disorder from those believed to be acquired would define all subsequent versions of the Table of the Forms. As mentioned, sub-categories were added by the committee to each of the original four classes of Prichard's symptomology: congenital deficiency was divided into two classes to describe those diagnosed with and without epilepsy; mania was divided into six classes of acute, chronic, recurrent, *a potu*, puerperal and senile forms; melancholia was divided into acute, chronic, recurrent, puerperal and senile types; and, finally, dementia was divided into primary, secondary, senile and 'organic'—the final class describing those suspected to be

[77] Ibid.

[78] For a full treatment of puerperal insanity see Hilary Marland, ''Destined to be a Perfect Recovery': The confinement of Puerperal Insanity in the Nineteenth Century' in *Insanity, Institutions and Society, 1800–1914: A Social History of Madness in Comparative Perspective*, edited by Joseph Melling and Bill Forsythe, Routledge, 1999, pp. 137–156.

linked to tumours or brain disease.[79] The committee did not provide descriptions of any of the disorders, and instead suggested that members consult textbooks for definitions. A desire to expand upon the symptom-based classification then in use in asylum statistics led the committee to differentiate between two sorts of epilepsy in their classification, splitting it into 'acquired' and 'congenital'.

A number of criticisms were aired in response. Opening proceedings, J.A. Campbell complained that the table proposed by the committee divided the forms of insanity into 'curable' and 'incurable' forms:

> Table XI. subdivides the patients in a valueless mode. The first division into curable and incurable is clearly antagonistic to what should be, from a physician's point of view, and some of the other subdivisions are unworkable.[80]

Campbell's concern was that unproven metaphysical assumptions were being made about the future course of a disease, which would have consequences for treatment and the efforts made to cure patients. He feared that curable and incurable as a prominent feature of psychological categories would over-determine the treatment that was provided to a patient at the point of diagnosis. There was limited knowledge about the prognosis of each of the forms of insanity during this period, and Campbell articulated concerns that mistaken assumptions about how to classify patients according to conjectures on their outlook may have a detrimental impact upon the treatment that they receive. Having unproven assumptions on the outlook of a form of insanity feature so prominently within the Table of the Forms also introduced judgements on the prognosis of a patient that were not well-suited to a statistical exercise that was designed to minimise the influence of subjective judgements on the data collected (Table 4.3).

Clouston added to Campbell's criticisms, and complained that the tables were 'like everything else in this country [...] a compromise between the views of a great many members of this Association'.[81] Clouston's comment on the failure of the Association to deliver anything

[79] Anon, 'The Statistical Tables' in *JMS*, vol. 28, no. 124, January 1883, p. 653.

[80] J.A. Campbell, 'Proposed Statistical Tables' in *JMS*, vol. 28, no. 122, July 1882, pp. 318–319.

[81] Ibid.

Table 4.3 Recommended changes to the Table of the Forms of mental disorder presented to the Annual General Meeting of the MPA in 1882[82]

TABLE XI.

Showing the form of Mental Disorder in the Admissions, Recoveries, and Deaths of the Year 18 , and of Inmates on 31st December, 18 .

Form of Mental Disorder.	Admissions.			Recoveries.			Deaths.			Remaining in Asylum.		
	Male.	Female.	Total.	Male.	Female.	Total	Male.	Female.	Total.	Male.	Female.	Total.
Congenital or Infantile Mental Deficiency...												
" α with Epilepsy												
" β without Epilepsy												
Epilepsy acquired												
General Paralysis of the Insane												
Mania—												
" Acute												
" Chronic												
" Recurrent												
" A Potu												
" Puerperal												
" Senile												
Melancholia—												
" Acute												
" Chronic												
" Recurrent												
" Puerperal												
" Senile...												
Dementia—												
" Primary												
" Secondary												
" Senile												
" Organic (*i.e.*, from Tumours, Coarse Brain Disease, &c.)												

[82] 'Report of the Thirty-Seventh Annual General Meeting of the Medico-Psychological Association' in *JMS*, vol. 28, no. 123, October 1882, pp. 437–462 (p. 460).

Table 4.4 Recommended changes to the Aetiological Table of the MPA presented by the Statistical Committee and presented at the 1882 Annual General Meeting of the Association[83]

Causes of Insanity.	Number of Instances in which each Cause was Assigned. Admissions { M. No. of Cases. F. T.											
	As predisposing cause.*			As exciting cause.			As predisposing or exciting (where these could not be distinguished).			Total.†		
	Male.	Female.	Total.	Male.	Female.	Total.	Male.	Female.	Total.	Male.	Female.	Total.
Moral: Domestic trouble (including loss of relatives and friends)												
Adverse circumstances (including business anxieties and pecuniary difficulties) ...												
Mental anxiety and worry (not included under the above two heads), and overwork												
Religious excitement												
Love affairs (including seduction)												
Fright and nervous shock...												
Physical: Intemperance in drink...												
" sexual...												
Venereal disease												
Self-abuse (sexual)												
Over-exertion												
Sunstroke												
Accident or injury												
Pregnancy												
Parturition and the puerperal state												
Lactation												
Uterine and Ovarian disorders												
Puberty...												
Change of life...												
Fevers												
Privation and starvation												
Old age												
Other bodily diseases or disorders												
Previous attacks												
Hereditary influences ascertained (direct and collateral)...												
Congenital defect ascertained												
Other ascertained causes												
Unknown												

Note.—* With reference to the distinction between "predisposing" and "exciting" causes, it must be understood that no single cause is enumerated as both predisposing and exciting in the case of any individual patient.

† The figures in the Total column represent the entire number of instances in which the several causes (either alone or in combination with others) were stated to have produced the mental disorder. The excess of the aggregate of such causes over the number of patients admitted is owing to combinations of causes.

83 'Report of the Thirty-Seventh Annual General Meeting of the Medico-Psychological Association' in *JMS*, vol. 28, no. 123, October 1882, pp. 437–462 (p. 459).

that lived up to his hopes was born out of the frustration that all compromise had seemed to achieve was stasis, with the committee publishing a table that strongly resembled the one that was originally used, albeit with optional sub-classes.[84] Hack Tuke then addressed the meeting and stated that the Table of the Forms was the most contentious out of the statistical tables.[85] He believed the debates over psychological diagnosis showed that the main bone of contention between members of the Association was how to implement the suspected causes of insanity into statistical returns given the then current state of knowledge on pathology and aetiology. He thought that more research and better evidence was needed before the kind of certainties that Skae had offered in his classification system could be confirmed. In other words, implementing speculative causes into the classification used to collect statistics may distort the data returned on psychological diagnosis, and potentially open up false avenues of research. Like Crichton-Browne, Skae's detractors held that knowledge on the physical causes of mental disorder was still crude, and the aetiology presented in his system did not account or explain variations in behaviour and other symptoms observed in patients. Hack Tuke responded to Clouston's criticism over making the categories of aetiology optional by stating that due to the lack of breakthroughs in pathology and anatomy, it was simply not possible to implement Skae's causes as necessary categories of the statistical tables:

> When Dr Clouston proposed the [revisions] Committee, he said that such was the advance of cerebral pathology that he hoped some of our tables could be improved in accordance with it, but he was sorry to say the Committee found that to attempt to construct any tables based upon our advance in cerebral pathology could not be carried out. The Table of the Forms of mental disease agreed upon was, he thought, a workable one. It was not absolutely necessary to fill up the sub classes. The table would be practically complete if any superintendent preferred filling up only the major and omitting the minor or sub-classes.[86]

[84] Thomas Clouston. Remarks recorded in 'Medico-Psychological Association: Quarterly Meeting January 1882' in *JMS*, vol. 28, no. 121, April 1882, pp. 136–146.

[85] Daniel Hack Tuke, remarks recorded in ibid.

[86] Ibid.

Campbell objected that having the sub-classes as optional would mean the statistical tables would fail to collect enough information about the physical condition of the patient upon admission to make the exercise worthwhile, claiming that findings were increasingly suggesting 'physical causes to be more and more the cause of mental disease'.[87] Clouston however relented, and suggested that the revised tables be adopted for one year in a trial form, and that the committee be reappointed so that it could receive feedback from members of the Association. Campbell expressed concern at the disruption caused by the introduction of a flawed system for only one year, but his objections were ignored, and the proposed revisions were given their trial run[88] (Table 4.4).

An announcement of the approval of the Statistical Tables was published in January 1883 in the *JMS*, and it called for members to use the tables in their annual reports; and whilst they were not limited to recording the statistics that were required to fill in the tables, they were requested to fulfil the basic requirements of them. Members of the MPA were also asked to send any problems they had encountered using the tables during the year's trial period to Rayner as the secretary of the committee.[89] The revisions became permanent without much fanfare as members lost interest in the Table of the Forms of Insanity by the time it came to the summer meeting. Rayner went on to present the Table of the Forms on behalf of the MPA in September 1885 to the International Congress of Psychiatry in Antwerp as part of a discussion set to pave the way for an international classification, with national associations from the main centres for psychiatric treatment being asked to submit their official classifications for consideration.[90] Writing in the *JMS* the following year, Rayner stated that the Association had decided to submit the 1882 Revisions as a proposed transnational classification, stating that 'the [MPA] Council felt that a classification intended for international adoption must be extremely simple, while freedom is left to individual alienists to add supplementary sub-divisions to the classification'.[91] Rayner's remarks

[87] J.A. Campbell, remarks recorded in 'Medico-Psychological Association: Quarterly Meeting January 1882' in *JMS*, vol. 28, no. 121, April 1882, pp. 136–146.

[88] Ibid.

[89] Ibid.

[90] Henry Rayner, 'Classification of Insanity' in *JMS*, vol. 32, no. 138, July 1886.

[91] Ibid.

demonstrate that practical efficiency over theoretical complexity had been the deciding consideration of these debates, with pragmatism winning the day over science. There is unfortunately no evidence to suggest the MPA's classification received much of a reception when it was presented at the congress.

Conclusion

By the time it came to the end of nearly two decades of debate over classification, the concepts of Pinel and Esquirol were still being employed in asylum medical statistics, despite attempts to develop a classification of causes for use in statistical returns. Even in the face of Skae's classification, that found a welcome reception amongst physicalists who wanted diagnosis to be made on the foundations of natural science, symptomology proved to be resilient to the criticisms from individuals like Batty Tuke and they continued to be used in medical bureaucracy. Concepts based on symptomology as in the Table of the Forms first drafted by Prichard for the Lunacy Commission and published in 1845 had become 'locked in' to asylum statistics due to a complex set of institutional and administrative factors. Although viewed by sympathisers as flawed but part of the development of scientific knowledge, for critics like Crichton-Browne, Skae's classification failed even the basic tests of scientific rigour, making it more trouble than it was worth to incorporate his categories into asylum statistics on diagnosis. The compromise put forward by those responsible for the 1882 Revision put to rest the debates until the beginning of the twentieth century, but there is no indication that the revisions were particularly well-received or popular. Rather, the main protagonists, including Crichton-Browne and Skae, were no longer practising physicians, with those remaining seemingly having lost the appetite for continuing the debate.[92]

Nevertheless, the debates outlined in this chapter chart an episode in the history of psychiatry that can assist in broadening our understanding of the history of mental health statistics on psychological diagnosis. The discussions surrounding the statistical tables show how medical bureaucracy functioned as a catalyst for discussions on what a standardised

[92] Except Thomas Clouston, since he continued to use Skae's classification in medical statistics published by Morningside Asylum on diagnosis until the early years of the twentieth century.

classification should look like. Growing dissatisfaction with the symptom-based classification that was used in admissions led to a clash between those influenced by Skae, which in turn provoked a reaction from those who did not think his concepts were scientific enough. Attempts to revise the statistical tables along aetiological or pathological grounds, as we saw with Batty Tuke, were unsuccessful because in opposition to these radical attempts to revise the forms of insanity, a number of other alienists favoured sticking with Prichard's diagnostic concepts, despite the growing questioning of their scientific value. These oppositions were fuelled by two concerns: first, those articulated by Crichton-Browne, who thought that Skae's system was conceptually flawed and inconsistent, and would place the future course of research into the causes and treatment of insanity on a misguided path; and second, those who wanted a simple set of diagnostic concepts that would not complicate the completion of statistical returns.

The debates on uniformity in asylum medical statistics also demonstrate how diagnosis became increasingly standardised during the second half of the nineteenth century. As outlined in the previous chapter, recommendations for the terms that ought to be used in statistical tables were published in the first report of the Lunacy Commission published in 1845, but as we will see in Chapter 6, there was still much divergence in the terms used in statistical submissions. This made compiling statistics on diagnosis from asylums for those who used different sets of diagnostic terms a difficult and time-consuming exercise. The publication of the 1882 Revisions therefore was a step towards uniform completion of asylum statistical returns on diagnosis, which contributed to the regular publication of national statistics on diagnosis. This changed the task of the asylum superintendent from that of a skilled practitioner, employing loose diagnostic concepts to make a judgement on the condition suffered by a patient, to that of a professional who must record a diagnosis according to the set of uniform concepts included on statistical returns.

The classification that was produced in 1882 signalled a compromise between Skae's followers and those who wanted to stick with the classification concepts that had been introduced by Pinel and which had been used for around half a century. They had proven to be effective, even if vague and potentially leading to misdiagnosis. The concern with Skae's system were so severe that some thought their adoption could lead to the corruption of asylum statistics, putting into jeopardy the future of psychiatric research. Ultimately, the diagnostic concepts that were established attempted to compromise by including categories that were along the Pinealean lines, yet introduced sub-classes picked from Skae's aetiology, although the use of these sub-classes was optional. This compromise signals wider cracks that were appearing in the aspirations for a scientific psychiatry, one which would provide mechanistic, somatic explanations for the different forms of insanity. The increased importance placed upon statistics during this period and during these discussions reflects the lack of pathological breakthroughs in the study of madness, and statistics garnered from asylum admittances were increasingly being viewed as the horizon on which future discoveries would be made. Indeed, one commentator, in a laudatory comment upon Emil Kraepelin's *Psychologische Arbeiten* and his use of the methods of the emerging field of experimental psychology, wrote in 1897 in the *JMS* that '[i]t is an astonishing and unaccountable fact that in English asylums, where the anatomical study of the dead brain is well established, the exact study of the living brain is often almost ignored'.[93] It is to the reception of Kraepelin's work and the next set of revisions to the Table of the Forms that this volume now turns.

[93] '[Review of] Psychologische Arbeiten. Herausgegeben von Emil Kraepelin' in *JMS*, vol. 43, no. 181, 1897, pp. 363–365.

CHAPTER 5

'A Higgledy Piggledy Conglomeration': The 1907 Revisions to the Table of the Forms of Mental Disorder

In 1905 and whilst sitting on a revisions committee appointed by the MPA to revise and modernise the diagnostic concepts used in asylum admittances, the then president of the Association Robert Armstrong-Jones gave a lengthy address to the Psychological Section of the British Medical Association stressing the importance of making accurate predictions on the course of an illness when diagnosing a patient with insanity.[1] According to Armstrong-Jones, the development of knowledge on the prognosis of insanity and its different forms had been hindered by imprecision in the diagnostic concepts used within medical statistics. To better understand the causes and outlook of its different forms, greater precision was needed:

> Insanity is a generic term, having many species and varieties, some of these differing widely as to prospects of recovery, and also, as to the occurrence in their course, of life and death.[2]

[1] Robert Armstrong-Jones, 'Prognosis in Mental Diseases' in *BMJ*, December 16th, 1905, pp. 1578–1582.

[2] Ibid., p. 1578.

K. M. Jones, *Psychological Classification and Diagnosis in Asylum Statistics, 1800–1948*, Mental Health in Historical Perspective,
https://doi.org/10.1007/978-3-031-46154-5_5

Research on the prognosis of each of the different forms of insanity would allow a diagnosis that would provide a clearer indication of the outcome of a patient. For the patient it could help avoid a lengthy stay in an asylum, with slim prospect for recovery and discharge. If a diagnosis was made as early as possible, Armstrong-Jones thought, it could avoid problems for the family of anyone admitted to an asylum, including financial ruin and the stigma cast upon having a family member admitted. For medical superintendents, it meant fewer patients in crowded and underfunded asylums that were making fewer discharges than hoped for.[3] Making the right diagnosis as soon as possible was vital because the chances of recovery dwindled after the first year of internment within an asylum:

> [It is] absolutely essential to obtain early treatment for insanity and the chances of recovery dwindle out of all proportion by delay. [...] insanity is curable in inverse ratio to its duration, and that if actively and skilfully treated within the first month, more than 70 percent of the recoveries are sent out cured [...] whereas after the first year only about 10 percent recover, after the second year 3 percent, and the third up to the fifth 2.3 percent, and after the fifth recovery is exceptional.[4]

Armstrong-Jones used statistics on psychological diagnosis gathered from his Claybury asylum to back up these claims on the chances of recovery. He also presented recovery-rates for each of the forms of insanity admitted. He observed that melancholic patients had the best prognosis and the highest number of discharges. Patients diagnosed with mania had a less positive outlook, and the worst of all were those diagnosed with delusional insanity, acute forms of mania and monomania: Armstrong-Jones deemed these to be incurable, yet there were still chances for recovery for those diagnosed with even acute forms of melancholia.[5] The cause of insanity could indicate clues about its prognosis: for instance, when alcoholism was present, or any other 'single and powerful cause be operative – such as disappointment in love to a sensitive woman – the prognosis is better than if several causes, such as poverty, anxiety, and

[3] S.W.D. Williams, 'Our Over-Crowded Lunatic Asylums' in *JMS*, vol. 17, no. 80, 1872, pp. 515–518.

[4] Robert Armstrong-Jones, 'Prognosis in Mental Diseases' in *BMJ*, December 16th, 1905, pp. 1578–1582.

[5] Ibid.

domestic bereavement acted in conjunction'.[6] Yet, despite there being some optimism in the outlook for certain cases, Armstrong-Jones warned that even in patients whose recovery lasted long enough for the patient to be discharged, a weakness would always remain that could lead to readmission.[7]

Armstrong-Jones delivered these findings on prognosis as he sat on a committee appointed by the Association in 1902 to revise the concepts used in asylum medical statistics. The debates that accompanied these revisions were characterised by an emphasis upon prognosis because firstly, the large county asylums built in the wake of the 1845 Lunacy Acts were beginning to fill up towards the end of the nineteenth century, and secondly because of the growing popularity of Emil Kraepelin's work on classification. Kraepelin was seen to have developed a set of diagnostic concepts that provided a reasonably accurate prognosis of a disorder. In many ways, Kraepelin had come to be seen as realising the project of using statistical data to develop psychiatric research, eventually providing a classification of insanity that had incorporated considerations on prognosis into concepts of diagnosis.

This chapter details how debates over classification explored in the last chapter would reignite in 1902 thanks to a paper on asylum medical statistics and bureaucracy given to the Medico-Psychological Association (MPA) annual meeting by Poor Law Commissioner Lawrence Brock. They would be resolved with the publication of the second set of revisions to the Table of the Forms of Insanity, published in 1907. They began in the summer of 1902 when, in response to Brock's paper, the MPA appointed a committee to revise the 1882 Revision, and thereby commencing the second major set of revisions to the Table of the Forms. The appointment of a revisions committee reignited debates that had reached some sort of truce in 1882 with the publication of a table that sought to reconcile Skae's classification of aetiology with symptomology. As we will see, Kraepelin's work on classification had some degree of influence upon the committee established to revise the Table of the Forms at the turn of the twentieth century, and they introduced the relatively novel notion of dementia praecox into the statistical tables. Although the

[6] Ibid.

[7] This point was hotly debated by Thomas Clouston in his response to Armstrong-Jones's paper in ibid.

evidence from the discussions suggests that Kraepelin's work had been received well by members of the MPA, the work of the committee came under attack, with the most sustained criticisms coming from the London physician Charles Mercier. The revisions undertaken by the Association also attracted the interest of prominent figures from beyond psychiatry, including Francis Galton and Karl Pearson. Seeing the potential of mental health statistics in furthering eugenic aims, both had advised the revisions committees as statistical experts, with an eye to developing mental health epidemiology from asylum statistics. These revisions to the Table of the Forms led to major changes in the way that information was recorded in logbooks, and this is reflected in the more in-depth statistics that broke down insanity by its forms that was presented in lunacy administration reports from 1907, when the revised Table of the Forms was published, until the outbreak of the First World War.

The 1907 Revisions were part of a set of developments to psychiatric epidemiology and asylum administration between 1890 and 1910 that circulated Kraepelinian concepts of psychopathology, contributing to them becoming common parlance amongst British psychiatrists by the beginning of the First World War.[8] This chapter will therefore explore the debates between 1902 and 1907, and in so doing, understand the ways they shaped psychological diagnosis and asylum medical statistics during the first quarter of the twentieth century. They led to major changes in the ways that data on admissions were collected, with the introduction of a standardised logbook issued to asylums that had been designed to cut down on the time needed to fill in statistical returns. This episode led to a move away from the diagnostic categories used for much of the heyday of the asylum in admissions and the emergence of concepts of mental disorder that would characterise diagnosis during the first half of the twentieth century. The concepts of psychopathology that Kraepelin offered catered to a desire for accurate predictions on the course of an illness that arose from the 1880s onwards as discharges fell, asylums were beginning to fill up, and a therapeutic nihilism came to be directed towards asylum treatment. In outlining the debates and the publication of the MPA's 1907 Revision, this chapter also argues that these revisions were decisive in Kraepelinian concepts of psychopathology

[8] David Healy, F. Farquhar, et al., 'Historical Overview: Kraepelin's Impact on Psychiatry' in *European Archive of Psychiatry and Clinical Neuroscience*, no. 258, 2008, pp. 18–24.

becoming common parlance amongst British psychiatrists within ten years of the publication of the committee's report.

The Lead-Up to the Revisions

A renewed interest in asylum statistics at the beginning of the twentieth century led to new discussions to revise the statistical tables. These discussions involved not only alienists, but also public health officials and figures from the eugenics movement, namely Karl Pearson and Francis Galton. The potential of asylum statistics was changed by the 1890 Lunacy Act, as it had widened the field of those included in the statistics to voluntary patients – before the act only pauper or rate-aided lunatics were included. An increase in the pool of data, so to speak, coupled with the potentials offered by the exciting new fields of psychometrics and mathematical statistics made the potential of asylum medical statistics even more appealing. The desire to revise the tables was also motivated by a recognition that the mental sciences had undergone some change, and there was a general acknowledgement leading up to the revisions that something needed to be done to modernise the classifications used in admissions procedures.

Discussions on prognosis gained momentum from the 1890s onwards, with a number of lectures, papers and addresses to medical societies discussing the problem of prognosis and psychological diagnosis.[9] An ability to make a diagnosis that provided a reasonably accurate indication of the future course of a disorder had so far eluded alienists, but this was becoming ever pressing as the large Victorian asylums were becoming old and overcrowded. Kraepelin's division of insanity on the basis of a differing prognosis of each of its forms had garnered interest partly

[9] See: Robert Armstrong-Jones, 'Prognosis in Mental Diseases' in *BMJ*, December 16th, 1905, pp. 1578–1582; Sir William R. Gowers, 'A Lecture on the Prognosis and Treatment of Syphilitic Disease of the Nervous System' in *JMS*, April 4th, 1903, pp. 773–778; Judson S. Bury, 'Prognosis in Relation to Disease of the Nervous System' in *BMJ*, November 9th, 1901, pp. 1389–1396; W.R. Gowers, 'The Lettsomian Lectures on Syphilis and the Nervous System' in *BMJ*, February 9th, 1889, pp. 283–285; G. Fielding Blandford, 'The Lumleian Lectures on the Diagnosis, Prognosis and Prophylaxis of Insanity' in *BMJ*, April 6th, 1895, pp. 741–747; George Green, 'The Prognosis in Dementia Paralytica' in *JMS*, no. 52, no. 217, pp. 84–305; A.R. Urquhart, 'The Morison Lectures on Insanity, with Special Reference to Heredity and Prognosis' in *JMS*, vol. 52, no. 217, April 1907, pp. 233–321.

because it catered to this desire. As mentioned, Kraepelin's work on classification was characterised by diligent recording and storing of patient data which had allowed the course of the different forms of insanity to be traced. Kraepelin had in essence performed on a smaller scale what the MPA had been attempting to do through standardising national medical statistics. Indeed, Armstrong-Jones's work was the latest in a set of papers penned by asylum medical superintendents that had made attempts to link psychological diagnosis to statistical data on outlook. D.G. Thomson's 1882 paper on 'The Prognosis in Insanity' was the first notable work on prognosis since the 1882 revisions to the Table of the Forms.[10] In it he made the case that medical statistics held the key to prognosis, but in their current state they relied upon imprecise concepts of psychological diagnosis. His findings were based upon data from his own asylum and employed the main forms of Skae and the MPA's classification in addition to the concepts of mania, melancholia and dementia. He focused on melancholia as 'the most frequent and the most hopeful of all forms of insanity', and claimed that 'the consideration of statistics and personal observation fully confirm this observation'.[11] Although factors including age, weight and 'constitution' may affect the outlook of any particular case, along with physical conditions like pregnancy, Thomson claimed that 'in a person without visceral disease and in fair health, simple melancholia should be recovered in [between] six to twelve weeks'.[12] Thomson's work is approvingly cited by H. Hayes Newington in a paper read two years later to a quarterly meeting of the MPA held in Bethlem Hospital, in which he discussed the relationship between individual cases and the sort of general laws that statistical enquiry can yield.[13]

Kraepelin's work on classification and diagnosis was beginning to attract attention from British medical circles because it catered to a desire for accurate prognosis, with some believing he had realised the goal of

[10] D.G. Thomson, 'The Prognosis in Insanity' in *JMS*, vol. 28, no. 122, 1882, pp. 195–210 (p. 206).

[11] Ibid.

[12] Ibid., p. 209.

[13] H. Hayes Newington, 'Unverified Prognosis' in *JMS*, vol. 30, no. 130, 1884, pp. 223–233.

developing diagnostic categories that indicated the outlook of a patient.[14] His work was particularly attractive to some because he had arrived at his findings through statistical analysis. In a paper delivered to the Association in 1896, W.H.R. Rivers sought to convince alienists of the power of methods developed by the emerging experimental psychology movement for medical psychology.[15] He described Kraepelin as 'the chief worker' in the application of psychometrics to study the problems posed by insanity, and to understand the mental pathology of 'the abnormal mind'.[16] His paper recounted the experiences he had had working with Kraepelin in Heidelberg. Rivers described the German's work as 'forming not only the foundation for a systematic plan of measurement of mental capacity, but has also in itself brought out many points of direct importance to mental pathology'.[17] The response to Rivers' account of Kraepelin's research was mixed, with Percy Smith wanting more details on individual cases, and many in attendance voicing concerns about the practicality of introducing similar methods of measurement into the context of British asylums.

Nevertheless, Rivers' lecture on his experience of the methods Kraepelin had borrowed from experimental psychology shows the interest alienists had in applying methods from psychometrics to the study of abnormal pathology. By the time the revisions committee sat, Kraepelin's work was regularly being cited in British medical journals.[18] The sixth edition of Kraepelin's 1899 *Lehrbuch der Psychiatry* had received a relatively positive review in the *Journal of Mental Science* the year it was

[14] The remarks of Edward Mapother, commenting towards the end of Kraepelin's life, are particularly illuminating: 'He had also approximated to the modern view that all type-forms represent syndromes which may be combined in varying measure, and that any syndrome may run every possible course, though a statistical correlation exists between certain forms and courses.': Edward Mapother, 'Emil Kraepelin: Psychiatrist' in *JMS*, vol. 73, no. 302, October 1927, pp. 509–34.

[15] W.H.R. Rivers, 'Experimental Psychology in Relation to Insanity' in *JMS*, no. 41, 1895, pp. 591–599.

[16] Ibid.

[17] Ibid., pp. 592–593.

[18] R.M. Ion and M.D. Beer, 'The British Reaction to Dementia Praecox 1893–1913. Part 1' in *History of Psychiatry*, vol. 13, no. 51, 2002, pp. 285–304.

published, and in 1902 its first English translation appeared.[19] The same year, descriptions of dementia praecox were published in the Association's journal, as well as a report on the Società Freniatrica Italia that characterised the classification used in Italian statistical returns as being Kraepelinian.[20] The attraction of Kraepelin's work was in the methodology, which involved the collection of large amounts of information on the symptoms and the course of illness of asylum patients, both of which were meticulously recorded on *Zählkarten*, or counting cards. Kraepelin's work was regarded as a new direction because his textbooks, as Kendler notes, did not contain the lengthy descriptions of symptoms from individual cases that populated textbooks by figures such as Wernicke and Kraft-Ebbing.[21] They combined what Berrios and Hauser call cross-sectional information, that is to say, details on the presentation of the symptoms at the time of diagnosis, usually when a patient entered the asylum, with longitudinal data on the progression of an illness during a patient's time in the asylum.[22] The *Zählkarten* allowed Kraepelin to cross-reference data on symptoms presented at diagnosis to data on the outcome of a patient, and he sorted these into two groups of incurable and deterioration. Information management of the kind that allowed large amounts of data on the progression of psychological symptoms to be analysed facilitated Kraepelinian's dichotomy of psychosis, with dementia praecox and manic-depressive insanity each having a different prognosis. From the data he collected, Kraepelin concluded that those diagnosed with dementia praecox were incurable, facing a gradual deterioration

[19] "Psychiatrie: Ein Lehrbuch Für Studirende Und Aerzte (Psychiatry: A Manual for Students and Physicians). Von Dr Emil Kraepelin, Professor an Der Universität, Heidelberg. Leipzig: Barth, 1899, 2 Vols. Price, vol. I, 9 Marks; vol. II, 15 Marks." *JMS*, vol. 45, no. 190, 1899, pp. 581–583 (p. 583).

[20] See: W.C. Sullivan 'Report of a Case of Dementia Praecox. (Amer. Journ. Med. Sci.,Jan., 1902.) Dunton, IV. R.' and A.W. Wilcox 'On the Classification of the Psychopathies [Sulla classificazione delle Psichopathie]. (Riv. Sper. di Freniatria, vol. xxviii, fasc. i, 1902.) De Sanctis.' In *JMS*, vol. 48, no. 203, Oct 1902, pp. 778–779.

[21] Kenneth Kendler and Eric J. Engstrom, 'Criticisms of Kraepelin's Psychiatric Nosology: 1896–1927' in *The American Journal of Psychiatry*, vol. 174, no. 4, 2016.

[22] G.F. Berrios and R. Hauser, 'Kraepelin: Clinical Section—Part II' in *A History of Clinical Psychiatry: The Origin and History of Psychiatric Disorders*, the Athlone Press, 1995, pp. 280–301.

in their condition and increasingly intense symptoms of hallucinations, mania or melancholia.[23]

Although Kraepelin's work was, for the most part, cited favourably, there were prominent critics who attacked the work for being vague and devoid of the kind of descriptions of symptoms that had filled the textbooks of the nineteenth century.[24] Some thought his work provided inaccurate prognosis, and others thought that it relied too heavily on the methods of experimental psychology, which were ill-suited to medical psychology.[25] Thomas Clouston, for instance, had criticised primary dementia on the basis that:

> When the mental condition of the cases of confusion and stupor [are] carefully studied, in the attack and afterwards, we find that in about one-half of them there is no consciousness, and the patients do not remember what took place during the attack. Those are called anergic cases by Hayes Newington [*sic*]. Some authors improperly call this 'primary dementia', and popularly it is often called 'trance'. It is a curable disease, and occurs most frequently among persons under thirty years of age, with a neuropathic constitution and a bad mental heredity.[26]

Dementia praecox and manic-depressive insanity were therefore by no means universally accepted by the time it came to the revisions. Statistics and epidemiology were becoming increasingly viewed as the way that discoveries into the course of different forms of insanity would be made, and usurped the work of Victorian anatomists who believed that establishing causal connections between symptoms observed in the forms of insanity, and physical conditions such as lesions and bodily states, was the key to understanding madness.[27] Like Kraepelin's counting cards, the Table of the Forms was viewed as a part of a system collecting

[23] Edward Shorter, 'The History of Nosology and the Rise of the Diagnostic and Statistical Manual of Mental Disorders' in *Dialogues of Neuroscience*, vol. 17, no. 1, March 2015, pp. 59–67.

[24] Kenneth Kendler and Eric J. Engstrom, 'Criticisms of Kraepelin's Psychiatric Nosology: 1896–1927' in *The American Journal of Psychiatry*, vol. 174, no. 4, 2016.

[25] Ibid.

[26] Thomas Clouston, *Unsoundness of Mind*, Methuen, 1911, p. 176.

[27] See Michael Finn's discussion of William Bevan-Lewis's work as pathologist at the West Yorkshire Lunatic Asylum, which is described by as being 'the final flourish' of pathological accounts of mental illness developed within the asylum; Michael Anthony

asylum medical data that could, if executed correctly, provide insights on prognosis. The concepts published in the 1907 Revision signalled an attempt to reconcile symptomology with concepts of diagnosis that could provide some indication of the outlook of a patient. Practical considerations guided these attempts, as concerns were aired over introducing unfamiliar terms in the statistical returns may increase workload and introduce ambiguities to the data. Indeed, and as we will see later on in this chapter, dementia praecox had appeared in a draft revision of the document presented to the society in 1904 but was eventually reformulated as 'primary dementia' in the final version published in 1907.

There is some debate over whether the 1907 Revision introduced Kraepelinian concepts to the United Kingdom or not. Healy et al. claim that they did, pointing towards the inclusion of primary dementia in the revisions.[28] Ion and Beer, however, argue that primary dementia does not equate to dementia praecox since it had a different meaning, and had been included in textbooks published by prominent critics of primary dementia.[29] From the detailed account of the revisions that occurred at the beginning of the twentieth century, I demonstrate that the revisions committee had included dementia praecox in drafts of the classification, but had changed this to primary dementia out of concerns that many using the classification would be unfamiliar with Kraepelin's own term. The inclusion of 'alternating insanity' or circular insanity in the 1907 Revisions, a condition that is historically linked to manic-depressive insanity, further suggests that the committee incorporated Kraepelinian diagnostic categories into the 1907 Revision, but had rephrased them for familiarity's sake.[30]

Finn, *The West Riding Lunatic Asylum and the Making of the Modern Brain Sciences in the Nineteenth Century*, PhD Thesis, University of Leeds, 2012, p. 175.

28 David Healy, F. Farquhar et al., Historical Overview: Kraepelin's Impact on Psychiatry' in *European Archive of Psychiatry and Clinical Neuroscience*, no. 258, 2008, pp. 18–24.

29 R.M. Ion and M.D. Beer, 'The British Reaction to Dementia Praecox 1893–1913. Part 1' in *History of Psychiatry*, vol. 13, no. 51, 2002, 285–304.

30 William Drewry's article on Circular Insanity includes 'Alternating Insanity' as an alternative term: William Drewry, 'Circular Insanity, Report of Three Cases' in *The Journal of Mental and Nervous Disease*, vol. 20, no. 4, April 1895, pp. 223–230; Healy argues for the continuities between circular insanity and manic-depressive insanity in: David Healy, *Mania: A Short History of Bipolar Disorder*, John Hopkins University Press, 2008, pp. 53–88.

Despite attempts going back to 1845 to standardise the tables used to collect statistical data on psychological diagnosis from asylums, the concepts of the Table of the Forms were still considered unacceptably vague for purpose. At the annual meeting of the Association in July 1902, the Poor Law Commissioner Charles Hubert Bond gave a paper voicing these concerns, calling for the revision and modernisation of the statistical tables.[31] Bond raised issues about the time it took for asylum medical superintendents to complete the yearly statistical returns of patient data to the Lunacy Commission. Under the terms of the 1890 Lunacy Act, requirements to log a psychological diagnosis were expanded to include private 'voluntary' patients. This in effect expanded the remit of statutory requirements to provide patient data, which expanded the data set, so to speak, but also increased the demands placed on asylum superintendents to fill in statistical returns. Bond proposed changes that would alleviate the work by simplifying the admissions processes and the paperwork. This would entail a revision of statistical tables and the terms used in psychological diagnosis. The data returned from these revised processes would, it was hoped by Bond, be of higher quality and could be more effectively employed in psychiatric epidemiology. Focusing on the Table of the Forms, Bond argued that revisions needed to be made to the concepts of diagnosis used in the tables since statistics on psychological diagnosis were at the heart of asylum medical data. Bond was articulating a growing appreciation of asylum medical statistics on diagnosis: as one member of the revisions committee appointed to conduct revisions to the statistical tables would later remark, the Table of the Forms was regarded as 'the hub around which the other [tables] revolve'.[32]

Bond thought the statistical tables in use compromised the quality of the data returned from asylums. They had not been revised for twenty years and, as outlined in the previous chapter, were a compromise to placate competing factions engaged in debates over how to standardise concepts of psychological diagnosis. In making this compromise, the

[31] Charles Hubert Bond, 'Medico-Psychological Statistics: The Desirability of Definition and Correlation, with a View to Collective Study' to the Annual General Meeting of the Association in 1902 in Minutes of the Annual Meeting of the Medico-Psychological Association of Great Britain and Ireland, July 1902' in *JMS*, vol. 48, no. 203, October 1902, pp. 795–805.

[32] Henry Rayner, 'The Classification of Insane States in Revised Statistical Tables' in *JMS*, vol. 51, no. 212, January 1905, pp. 140–143.

committee had published a classification system that quickly came to be viewed as confusing, ambiguous and vague. The main cause of dissatisfaction was the mixing of causes, since there was a separate statistical table of the causes, rendering forms such as puerperal insanity largely unnecessary. Bond complained that the sub-types of the 1882 Revisions were a particular problem that a revisions committee should fix, although Bond did not suggest a set of diagnostic categories to replace them, stating:

> Considerable diffidence is felt in approaching this table owing to the wide differences of opinion that exist on the subject of classification. No suggestions as regards nomenclature are going to be offered, but a strong protest is ventured to be lodged against the usual practice of mixing symptomatological and aetiological terms. We cannot serve two masters; one is inevitably neglected, and probably neither is served satisfactorily. It is contended that the inclusion of such terms as 'acute mania' and 'puerperal mania' in the same column is a flagrant breach of statistical laws.[33]

He thought that it had been a mistake to introduce the sub-classes because they were vague, and the decision to make them optional had created unacceptable ambiguity in the data by introducing subjective judgement into the completion of the statistical tables. To remedy the situation, Bond proposed that aetiological factors be removed from the psychological diagnostic concepts included in the Table of the Forms. Keeping the statistics on psychological diagnosis and physiological causes separate would keep the data separate and allow the two data sets to be effective for analysis. Careful analysis may lead to trends to be identified, allowing links between symptoms, causes and outlook of an illness to be charted.

In response to Bond's paper, a motion was passed at the annual general meeting of the Association in July 1902 to appoint a committee to revise the Table of the Forms. The Scottish psychiatrist and former colleague of Skae, David Yellowlees, was appointed Chairman, and Bond was appointed Honorary Secretary. Other prominent members included Henry Rayner, who served as a member of the committee responsible for the 1882 Revisions, and Bedford Pierce, medical superintendent of the

[33] C. Hubert Bond, 'Medico-Psychological Statistics: The Desirability of Definition and Correlation with a View to Collective Study' in *JMS*, vol. 48, no. 203, October 1902, pp. 709–732.

Retreat in York.[34] Although expressing a desire to make radical changes to the Association's classification, the committee sought to alleviate concern of any possible increase in workload caused by the adjustments, emphasising that one of the guiding principles of the proposed revisions was to reduce the time it took members to fill in yearly statistical returns, including those relating to psychological diagnosis.[35] Through a simplification of the processes of statistical returns, as well as the classifications used in psychological diagnosis, it was hoped that separating aetiology from symptomology would increase the quality and accuracy of the data garnered from asylum statistical returns.

In October of the same year, the revisions committee published a manifesto of sorts in the *Journal of Mental Science*, along with a call for suggestions from members across the country.[36] Restating their aim to retain 'simplicity of form as far as is consistent with accuracy' the committee emphasised their aims to balance practical considerations with attempts to improve the quality of the data.[37] The announcement was designed to alleviate concern that the introduction of a new set of statistical returns would increase workload, although the committee did state that the changes were designed to improve the accuracy of the medical data collected through yearly returns. The committee proposed to follow Bond's suggestion of separating aetiology from the diagnosis, and hoped that this move would simplify and improve the statistical tables.

The work of the statistical committee was eagerly anticipated over the next two years. It met four times between February and June 1903, and at the annual general meeting of the Association in July, an interim report was presented that included revisions to the statistical tables, which were described as the 'most important matter that the Association now has on hand'.[38] In it, the committee reiterated their aim to introduce a

[34] 'Minutes of the Annual Meeting of the Medico-Psychological Association of Great Britain and Ireland, July 1902' in *JMS*, vol. 48, no. 203, October 1902, pp. 795–805.

[35] David Yellowlees and Charles Hubert Bond, 'Committee for the Revision of the Statistical Tables of the Medico-Psychological Association', in *JMS*, vol. 48, no. 203, October 1902, pp. 812–813.

[36] Anon., 'Committee for the Revision of the Statistical Tables of the Medico-Psychological Association' in *JMS*, vol. 48, no. 203, October 1902, pp. 812–813.

[37] Ibid., p. 812.

[38] 'Occasional Notes: The Annual Meeting of the Medico-Psychological Association' in *The Journal of Mental Science*, vol. 49, no. 207, October 1903, pp. 703–705 (p. 704).

streamlined set of tables that would 'save an enormous amount of clerical work' and increase their 'value and accuracy'.[39] They also criticised the existing forms as being too complicated for clinical use, despite conceding that they may have some scientific value. The committee stated that any revisions would be applied across the United Kingdom, having had the agreement of the Scottish and Irish Lunacy boards, and that the tables produced by the MPA would be uniform 'across all three kingdoms': up until this point, Scottish asylums used a classification based on Skae's alongside that of the MPA in their statistical returns, and Ireland used a version of the table adopted in 1882.[40] By standardising the admissions diagnostic categories across the British Isles, the committee hoped that their work would lead to a valuable and powerful new epidemiological resource based on simplified and more accurate concepts of psychological diagnosis.

Tensions arose between those who desired change that would increase the scientific credentials of the classification, and those who prioritised the need for a practical and efficient diagnostic framework. David Yellowlees delivered the first full revisions committee report to the annual general meeting of the Association in July 1904. It emphasised the practical implications of the introduction of any new classification:

> we [the committee] felt that an asylum physician had something more important in his life than statistics, that he is already burdened far too greatly with statistical labour.[41]

Yellowlees's lack of enthusiasm for the statistical Table of the Forms could be explained through his use of Skae's aetiological classification in his medical practice in Glasgow.[42] Despite these misgivings, Yellowlees's report followed Bond's proposals to remove ambiguity from the concepts

[39] Charles Hubert Bond, remarks recorded in 'Part IV: Notes and News: Medico-Psychological Association of Great Britain and Ireland: Annual Meeting 1903' in *JMS*, vol. 49, no. 207, October 1903, pp. 749–774 (pp. 770–771).

[40] Ibid.

[41] David Yellowlees, 'Report of the Statistical Committee, Appointed at the Annual Meeting Held at Liverpool in 1902, Presented to the Annual Meeting of the Association, July 21st, 1904' in *JMS*, vol. 51, no. 215, October 1905, pp. 799–826 (p. 800).

[42] Jonathan Andrews, 'A Failure to Flourish? David Yellowlees and the Glasgow School of Psychiatry: Part 2' in *History of Psychiatry*, vol. 8, no. 2, September 1997, p. 338.

used in the statistical tables to reduce as far as possible subjective judgement by eliminating the optional sub-classes of the 1882 Revision, which they regarded as superfluous. The report stated that responses to their call had expressed concern about the possibility of misdiagnosis, with the examples of puerperal mania and puerperal melancholia being confused with one another, and organic dementia being mistakenly identified as general paralysis of the insane.[43] To further assist with efficiency in the completion of the tables, the committee suggested that a new medical register be introduced which would be separate from the civil register used to record legally required admissions data on the social background and legal status of the patient. As Table 5.1 demonstrates, the proposed medical register kept by the asylum would record all the data needed for admittances and discharges in one place.

The medical register was designed to cut down on the work required to fill in the statistical returns by collecting the necessary information in one place, including the form of insanity as well as the main suspected cause. One mark was to be made alongside the relevant diagnosis of the form of insanity, and one primary cause was to be recorded, although superintendents could record as many secondary causes as they wished. This medical register was devised in response to complaints from medical superintendents that they often needed to spend time sifting through case notes to find the medical data required to fill in the returns.[44] The report proposed that if kept accurately throughout the year, the register would speed up the completion of the returns because it would collect all the information needed for them in one place.[45] The report announced that the Commissioners in Lunacy for England and Wales were in favour of the changes, and had granted their approval for the separation of a medical and civil register, something that was undoubtedly helped by Bond and Pierce being appointed to the revisions committee – both were at the same time also serving on the board of the Lunacy Commission. As discussed in the previous chapter, collecting this information at the point of admission was a legal requirement for asylum superintendents, but they were becoming increasingly recognised as a potential source of data that could provide

[43] Ibid.

[44] David Yellowlees, Report of the Statistical Committee, Appointed at the Annual Meeting Held at Liverpool in 1902, Presented to the Annual Meeting of the Association, July 21st, 1904', in *JMS*, vol. 51, no. 215, October 1905, pp. 799–826.

[45] Ibid.

Table 5.1 Proposed Medical Register presented in the report of the Statistical Revisions Committee[46]

MEDICAL REGISTER—DIRECT ADMISSIONS.

Date of Admission.	No. in Civil Register.	Name.	Attack. †				If not First Attack, number of Previous Attacks treated to recovery in an Institution or elsewhere.	Previously Certified as Insane.	Age.			Civil State.				Occupation.				Duration of Present Attack from its commencement until the Present Admission, expressed in years, months and days.	Ætiological Factors.				Instances of Epilepsy in Class "Congenital."	Form of Mental Disorder. (No entry to be made here in respect of Congenital Cases.)												Deemed Suicidal by the Medical Officer.	Bodily State on Admission.		Observations.
																Name of	Index Symbol.				Principal.		Con-tributory.																		
			Congenital.	First Attack.	Not First Attack.	Unknown whether First Attack or not.			On Present Admission.	*At commencement of Present Attack.	*On First Attack (*if a Not First Attack admission*).	Single.	Married.	Widowed.	Unknown.		Of Group (*capital letter*).	Of Sub-group (*small letter*).	Of Subdivision (*numeral*).		*One entry and one only to be made for each case in this column.*	Schedule Symbol.	*As many con-tributory factors as are found to be entered here.*	Schedule Symbol.		Epileptic Insanity.	General Paralysis of the Insane.	Dementia from tumours, coarse brain lesions, etc.	Mania :—Recent (R.), Chronic (C.).	Melancholia :—Recent (R.), Chronic (C.).	Alternating Insanity.	Volitional and Moral Insanities.	Delusional Insanity.	Stupor and States of Confusion.	Primary Dementia.	Senile Dementia.	Secondary Dementia.		General Health.	Name of Bodily Disease (if any).	
		Brought forward																																							
		Totals where possible.																																							

NOTE.—It will probably be convenient to use another book as a Register for Transfers. In small Institutions the use of another portion of the same book, substituting the word *Transfer*, for *Direct Admissions* at the head of the page, would possibly suffice. It is intended that separate Registers for the Sexes shall be used.

* Where the information asked for in columns marked with an asterisk is unknown, U.K. should be entered to signify this. In cases where the age on present admission is not with certainty known, an approximate age should be entered.

† Each case must be entered in only one of these four columns.

46 David Yellowlees, 'Definitions of Terms Used in the Report and the Statistical Tables' in *JMS*, vol. 51, no. 215, October 1905, pp. 834–856 (p. 853).

the kinds of insights into the nature of insanity that had thus far eluded psychiatrists.

The first set of revisions removed aetiology from the psychological diagnostic categories that had been included in the Table of the Forms. The accompanying Table of the Causes remained unchanged from those passed in 1882 because the revisions committee thought that producing a new set of revisions was not part of its remit.[47] They had limited their efforts to retaining the main classes of mania, melancholia, dementia, epileptic insanity and GPI from the 1882 table, and removing the aetiological sub-classes as can be seen from a comparison of the existing table and their proposed revisions (see Tables 4.3 and 5.1).

The committee had decided to retain organic forms of dementia as a disease sub-category because they thought that it was a distinct clinical entity which had symptoms that were distinct from the other sub-types of dementia, and distinct from cases of GPI. As we will see, the committee would be reprimanded for this by members of the society because its proposed revisions had not kept to Bond's aims to fully separate aetiology from symptomology categories. Aside from this, all other terminologies associated with causes were removed from the Table of the Forms of Insanity.

The influence of Kraepelin's work is most clearly seen in this draft of the MPA's classification with the inclusion of dementia praecox as a subclass of dementia. The committee's use of the term was one of the earliest in the United Kingdom, and this proved a decisive moment in the spread in popularity of Kraepelin's ideas throughout the British Isles—although the final version of the classification would use primary dementia as a category and would not include Kraepelin's term. Further resemblances to Kraepelinian psychopathology were seen with the inclusion of alternating insanity, the symptoms of which were described in medical textbooks as being close to those described by manic-depressive insanity.[48] Alternating insanity, sometimes known as circular madness, found its origins in the work of Falret and Baillarger, the symptoms of which were 'the opposite conditions of mania and melancholia or of excitement and depression

[47] Ibid., p. 804.

[48] German Berrios, 'Mood Disorders: Clinical Section' in *A History of Clinical Psychiatry*, edited by Berrios and Porter, Athlone, 1995, p. 396.

[that] succeeded each other with a certain amount of regularity'.[49] Alternating insanity to some extent captured the symptoms of mania and depression that were described by Kraepelin's manic-depressive insanity. The committee did not provide definitions of the terms included in its table, seeking instead to rely upon the judgement of medical superintendents in the application of the diagnostic terms, assuming that they would be familiar with the definitions provided in medical textbooks.

Reception of the 1904 Draft

The report of the committee was eagerly anticipated by members of the MPA, with a *Journal of Mental Science* editorial predicting that the results of the committee 'must stand for the guidance of the profession for many years to come'.[50] The responsibilities placed upon the committee and the revisions that it was tasked to carry out were by no means a mere administrative task: many members viewed the future of research on insanity as resting on the committee producing a cutting-edge classification that would improve the data on diagnosis returned from asylums. It had been over twenty years since a revision to the statistical tables had been carried out, and even then, the 1882 Revisions were viewed as a compromise and not the scientific step forward that had been hoped for. For many, the concepts had not been properly changed or modernised for over fifty years since the passing of the 1845 Lunacy Act, and there were big expectations from members of the association that a new classification would capture the complexities of more recent work on classification offered by Skae, Griesinger and Kahlbaum.[51]

The committee thought that the new classification concepts offered by Kraepelin would be further developed, or that new discoveries were on the horizon which would realise the much-valued classification of mental

[49] Edward B. Lane, 'Some Cases of Alternating Insanity with One Case of Recovery' in *Boston Medical and Surgical Journal*, vol. 116, January 20th, 1887, pp. 52–56.

[50] 'Occasional Notes: The Annual Meeting' in *Journal of Mental Science*, vol. 50, no. 11, October 1904, pp. 750–751 (p. 751).

[51] One striking example of a psychiatrist who attempted to unify anatomical, pathological, psychological and biological models of the mind was William Lloyd Andriezen. His work attempted to draw connections between the fundamental cellular microbiology of the brain through to complex mental phenomena including emotions, language and cognitive development. 'On the Bases and Possibilities of a Scientific Psychology and Classification in Mental Disease' in *JMS*, vol. 45, no. 189, April 1899, pp. 257–290.

diseases according to prognosis. Change was in the air, and the beginning of the century was a transition period between the classifications that were used in Victorian asylums and the beginning of the dominance of Kraepelinian concepts of psychopathology that would come to be enthusiastically received by psychiatrists working across Europe and the United States during the interwar period. Although refraining from suggesting comprehensive revisions, the report hoped that the concepts it proposed would include 'so many cases occurred for whom without them there seems no suitable niche'.[52] One of the members of the committee, Henry Rayner, stated that the forms of insanity that were recommended by the committee represented a move to formulate the 'highest and latest views of insanity that were held in this country'.[53] To some extent, this was reflected in the concepts included in Table 5.2: Kraepelin's dementia praecox, although relatively young, was beginning to gather more and more attention from British psychiatrists.[54]

The weight of expectations from members of the MPA made it almost inevitable that the efforts of the committee were doomed to failure. The reception to their recommendations was far from enthusiastic, with many taking the view that the revisions committee had not made enough in the way of changes to the existing 1882 Revision.[55] Despite the committee's lofty aims, their revisions were considered too conservative by a sizeable proportion of the membership. The committee anticipated these criticisms by announcing that they did not think it was the right time to offer radical changes or a new classification of all mental disorders, nor was it their duty to carry out either of these tasks.[56] As a result, the table they suggested only saw minor changes to the categories that were already in use, and these mainly included the removal of sub-categories relating to

[52] Ibid.

[53] Ibid.

[54] Case studies and research employing Kraepelin's categories were appearing in the *JMS* frequently after 1900: for instance: Henry M. Eustace, 'A Case of "Dementia Praecox"' in *JMS*, vol. 50, no. 210, July 1904, pp. 516–521.

[55] Hubert Bond and Henry Yellowlees, 'Report of the Statistical Committee, Appointed at the Annual Meeting Held at Liverpool in 1902, Presented to the Annual Meeting of the Association, July 21st, 1904', in *JMS*, vol. 51, no. 215, October 1905, pp. 799–826.

[56] Hubert Bond and Henry Yellowlees, 'Report of the Statistical Committee, Appointed at the Annual Meeting Held at Liverpool in 1902, Presented to the Annual Meeting of the Association, July 21st, 1904', in *JMS*, vol. 51, no. 215, October 1905, pp. 799–826.

Table 5.2 Forms of Mental Disorder included in the Report of the Statistical Committee presented to the 1904 AGM of the MPA[57]

ADMISSION GROUP, TABLE IV.—*Showing the Form of Mental Disorder on admission in the Direct Admissions during the year 19... (Voluntary Boarders excluded).*

Forms of mental disorder.	M.	F.	T.
Congenital or infantile mental deficiency:			
(*a*) Without epilepsy			
(*b*) With epilepsy			
Epileptic insanity			
General progressive paralysis			
Mania { Recent*			
Mania { Chronic			
Melancholia { Recent*			
Melancholia { Chronic			
Alternating insanity			
Volitional and moral insanities			
Delusional insanity			
Stupor and states of confusion			
Dementia { Primary (including Dementia præcox)			
Dementia { Senile			
Dementia { Organic and paralytic			
Dementia { Secondary			
Total			

* The period of one year is taken as the limit of the term recent.

causation. Although they acknowledged that these were far from perfect and that members 'would perhaps feel disappointed that more of the terms used in modern classifications have not been used', it anticipated this criticism by stating that it 'did not feel either that the time for this was ripe, or that the suggesting of a new classification really formed part of the task imposed upon them'.[58] Members of the MPA were disappointed with the classification presented by the first revisions committee, and that

[57] Hubert Bond and Henry Yellowlees, 'Report of the Statistical Committee, Appointed at the Annual Meeting Held at Liverpool in 1902, Presented to the Annual Meeting of the Association, July 21st, 1904', in *JMS*, vol. 51, no. 215, October 1905, pp. 799–826.

[58] Ibid.

more work had not been put into realising the opportunities offered by revising the classification.

Amongst the most prominent of critics of the 1904 draft of the Table of the Forms was Charles Mercier, who was by this time an influential elder of the Association. Mercier believed that a precise classification based on principles informed by evolutionary biology would help British medical psychology achieve the goal of providing a world leading, scientific standard of psychiatry that would establish the groundwork for an emerging psychiatric epidemiology. His work was infused with social Darwinism, and in a joking remark made in an article devoted to Herbert Spencer, he described his research on classification as being 'more Spencerian than Mr. Spencer'.[59] He thought that the classifications committee had come nowhere near to realising an opportunity to implement evolutionary science into the statistical tables. On this basis he disputed the claim made by the revisions committee that it had presented embodiments of the most advanced clinical concepts available to psychiatrists. Mercier felt that the committee's table was regressive in its over-reliance on symptomology, and he expressed a concern that if adopted, the version of the table presented in 1904 would be a wasted opportunity for British psychiatry to put asylum statistics on firm conceptual grounds. He also thought the MPA's classification could come to set an example for psychological diagnosis and asylum medical statistics further afield:

> I think we have the chance of getting this scheme adopted generally, not only by the administration of this great country, but by the subordinate and inferior administrations of the Isle of man [*sic*], Berwick-upon-Tweed, Scotland (laughter), and Ireland; and also that we may set such an example by which the statistics of insanity of all countries may be comparable with one another.[60]

This was part of a lengthy address given by Mercier to the Association that criticised the revisions presented in 1904.[61] He contested the committee's

[59] Charles Mercier, 'Mr. H Spencer's Classifications of Cognitions' in *Mind*, vol. 8, no. 30, April 1883, pp. 260–267 (p. 260).

[60] The laughter here might refer to the division at the time between Scottish and English Lunacy Commissions: 'Medico-Psychological Association of Great Britain and Ireland: Annual Meeting July 21st 1904' in *The Journal of Mental Science*, vol. 50, no. 211, October 1904, pp. 784–805 (p. 799).

[61] Ibid., pp. 798–799.

claim that it was not a part of their task to provide a new set of concepts for the purposes of the collection of statistics, and their insistence that the changes they had made were necessary for the effective revision of the statistical tables.[62] He began his attack with a lengthy comment on the Table of the Causes, claiming that the categories of 'inheritance' and 'heredity' were too vague to be used as categories of causation. This was especially the case since a detailed family history was usually unavailable, meaning that statistical information would often be based on guesswork on the behalf of an asylum medical superintendent. He considered 'previous attacks' that had been included in the Table of the Causes by the committee as tautologous when it was listed as a principle of causation, since previous attacks could hardly be called a cause, and instead were a symptom of a condition having a pre-history before the current attack. Mercier also contested the inclusion of 'old age' and 'venereal disease' in the Table of Causes, claiming that whilst they may frequently be present in patients alongside a form of insanity, both were not, strictly speaking, always the cause of a mental disorder.[63]

Shifting his criticisms to the categories of the Table of the Forms, he stated three conditions for a good classification:

> A classification, to be good, must include all the things to be classified and nothing else. In the second place, it should separate things which are different, and associate things which are alike. In the third place, it should not include the same thing under more than one class of the same rank.[64]

Like his criticisms of the Table of Causes, Mercier was calling for greater logical clarity in the concepts used in the Table of the Forms. He stated that the classification needed to have some order and not to confusedly include concepts of different classes. The focus of his criticism was the inclusion of 'organic' as a sub-class of dementia, which he deemed an aetiological category, and the omission of psychological symptoms in the table:

[62] Ibid., p. 799.

[63] Mercier railed against the proposed sterilisation of 'degenerates' in a *BMJ* letter in 1904, asking for those calling for this policy to explain and provide a precise definition of a 'degenerate'; Charles Mercier, 'Correspondence: Proposed Sterilisation of Certain Degenerates', in *BMJ*, April 2nd, 1904, p. 808.

[64] Ibid.

> But I regret to say that all those canons of classification have been violated [by the table]. It does not include all the things which have to be classified. I see in it no place for suspicion, no place for illusion, or hallucination; I see no place in it for suicide, nor for the various phobias and manias; and such very distinct forms or varieties of insanity as acute delirious mania and paranoia have no place in it at all. It associates things which are unlike; it puts together under the heading [melancholia] such diverse things as morbid hesitation and kleptomania; it puts together under the same heading stupor, which is an anomaly of conduct, and confusion, which is an anomaly of thought...[65]

Mercier's view was that the foundations for a useful classification were in logical clarity, and by placing disorders in a coherent hierarchy, a rigorous structure would be achieved. However, he considered the classification offered by the committee to have none of these qualities, and that they had failed to completely remove all talk of causes from the Table of the Forms. To demonstrate the incoherence of the draft table, he claimed it was absurd to make general progressive paralysis (GPP) a main class on the same level as mania and melancholia because both could appear as symptoms of GPP. This was not limited to GPP, with there being many other conditions in the table that had mania and melancholia as symptoms. This called into question the validity of the classification, since two doctors could use different diagnoses for one patient with them both being correct, at least in the case of mania and the conditions in the Table for which it was a symptom. The lack of logical rigour led Mercier to conclude that the draft was an incoherent classification that been hurriedly thrown together. The waspish tone of Mercier's comment provides an insight into the general air of ill feeling exchanged over the revisions to the statistical tables. Mercier appealed for the deliberations on the Table of the Forms to be conducted in the open between the members of the MPA, and not behind closed doors as had been the recent trend with MPA committees.[66] As a man who thrived on intellectual debate and disagreement, he took exception, along with the medical superintendent of Murray Royal Asylum in Perth, Alexander Reid Urquhart, to a motion submitted by Carlyle Johnstone to continue further discussions on the

[65] Ibid.

[66] 'Medico-Psychological Association of Great Britain and Ireland: Annual Meeting July 21st 1904', in *JMS*, vol. 50, no. 211, October 1904, pp. 784–805 (p. 799).

revisions in quarterly regional meetings before the Association reconvened at the next annual meeting. Relenting, the chair gave Mercier additional time to further outline his objections, and he convinced the council to place them on the agenda for the adjourned annual meeting pushed to November 1904, which would be attended by members from across the British Isles. Acknowledging that his attacks on the tables at the July 1904 meeting had been 'purely destructive', Mercier would make attempts to provide constructive steps towards reimagining the Table of the Forms later that year. In October 1904, he published an article in the *JMS* that offered a proposal for outlining his vision of a rigorously structured classification, which he contrasted to the 'higgledy piggledy conglomeration' produced by the revisions committee.[67] However, despite the efforts he put into his own classification, Mercier's classification would attract little attention from either the revisions committee or the wider membership of the Association.[68]

The debates conducted over the next two years continued to be acrimonious and drawn out over a series of adjourned annual and regional meetings: the annual meeting would be held in November 1904, and after lengthy discussions came to an impasse, adjourned again until July 1905, the day before the regular yearly meeting of the association. The revisions were presented to the regional meetings, allowing psychiatrists from across the country to be involved in some way in the discussions surrounding the Table of the Forms. External authorities in biology and statistics were consulted by the committee, as well as experts on data collection and epidemiology from the General Records Office (GRO) at Somerset House. Although the committee went to great lengths to reach compromises, it could not avoid impasse, and the debates would become heated as the process was drawn out. The members of the committee received very little in terms of recompense for the time that they had sacrificed, and many had not envisaged that an apparently simple task of carrying out statistical revisions would take up so much of their time over two years. The committee's reactions to quibbles over details and resistance to their proposals became increasingly bad tempered and irritable

[67] Ibid.

[68] Charles Mercier, 'The Statistical Tables' in *JMS*, vol. 50, no. 211, October 1904, pp. 672–697.

as the discussions went on, with barbs being traded in the association's journal through letters and editorials.

Henry Rayner responded on behalf of the committee to Mercier in a piece published in January 1905, dismissing his criticisms of the revisions.[69] He defended the tables published by the committee in 1904 as representing 'the highest and latest views of insanity held in this country', and accused Mercier of not living up to his own high standards with his classification, describing Mercier's attempt as impractical, unwieldy and conceptually confused.[70] He dismissed accusations that the classification was invalid and that the committee had falsely reified melancholia and mania of insanity, deriding Mercier for not having exacted the kind of precision in his criticisms that he demanded from the committee. He accused Mercier of fundamentally misinterpreting their efforts to classify the forms and not the pathology of insanity: 'a philologist should recognise that "form" refers to contour and outward appearance as distinguished from structure'.[71] Rayner stated the committee had not considered that its task was to describe natural kinds of insanity based upon the structure of an underlying pathology. Instead, their task was to develop concepts for the statistical returns that described the symptoms as they would present themselves during an admissions inspection, and not to provide concepts that would satisfy Mercier's desire for logical rigour and scientific validity.

Rayner thought that ignorance of the causes of insanity meant that the forms could only be just that: a description of the symptoms, of insanity's forms and not its natural kinds. The forms proposed were a temporary measure until advances, which he speculated may not be far away, could provide insights that would allow for either an aetiological or pathological classification of insanity.[72] He emphasised the point that the primary divisions presented by the committee of emotional, volitional, intellectual and general insanities were valid because those were the main appearances that insanity presented within the clinic. He rubbished Mercier's claim that the intensity of the disorder should be the basis of the main classes of

[69] Henry Rayner, 'The Classification of Insane States in Revised Statistical Tables' in *JMS*, vol. 51, no. 212, January 1905, pp. 140–143.

[70] Ibid., p. 140.

[71] Ibid.

[72] Ibid.

the forms, and instead defended the decision to sub-divide based on the temporal considerations of *recent* and *chronic*, which would, he thought, provide clues on the prognosis of the disorder. He repeated Bond and Urquhart's call to split the forms into two parts: the first class to include all conditions where the pathology was not known, and the second for those that were. Rayner considered the changes that had been made temporary and argued that being conservative with changes would have the advantage of allowing the table to be adaptable to new developments in research. Rayner suggested that this provided a much more satisfactory approach than Mercier's, which he deemed to be overly complex and impractical: 'in the face of [Mercier's] table I fear that any sort of alienist would be in the condition of a man finding his way through a maze ending in a morass'.[73]

Formulation of the 1907 Revisions

The issue of the statistical tables was adjourned at the 1904 meeting until the next meeting in July the following year. During a series of tense discussions, both the Table of the Forms and the Table of Causes took centre stage.[74] That same year, the statistician Karl Pearson had met with the revisions committee on a number of occasions on an advisory basis as a statistical expert whilst writing in the *British Medical Journal* that improved asylum statistics could enable a better understanding of the heredity and prognosis of insanity.[75] Pearson argued that asylum medical statistics could provide clues on what was becoming the holy grail for psychiatrists, and which had attracted many to Kraepelin's work—the prognosis of its different forms, which could be understood through the collection of 'reliable family records for the solution of the inheritance of pathological character'.[76] He claimed that admissions data from asylums had a role to play in solving this puzzle, but these needed to be correlated to family records because clinicians often did not know the family history of a patient going back more than one generation. The

[73] Ibid., p. 143.

[74] Percy Smith, 'Adjourned Annual Meeting of 1904' in *JMS*, vol. 51, no. 215, October 1905, pp. 733–772.

[75] Karl Pearson, 'On the Inheritance of Insanity' in *BMJ*, May 7th, 1905, pp. 1175–1176.

[76] Ibid.

committee informed the assembly at the 1905 meeting that Pearson had been consulted, and that Francis Galton had taken an interest in the work undertaken.[77]

As in Rayner's response to Mercier, the committee held that the state of psychiatric knowledge did not allow for a pathological classification to be drawn up at this juncture.[78] Although they felt that the time was not ripe, they thought that breakthroughs that could allow symptomatic forms to be dropped entirely from the statistical tables might be as close as ten years away.[79] Despite the furore caused by the draft revision in 1904, radical changes were not made to the version presented in 1905: one category was added, with the debate at that year's annual meeting of the Association being centred around disagreements over which sub-categories of mania were to be included. On the one hand, there were members of the association who thought that the classification was too conservative: for example, Thomas Drapes, who would later go on to write a seminal introduction to Kraepelin in the *JMS*, rejected the notion that the forms presented by the committee would be a temporary measure, and instead speculated that it might be a hundred years before a scientifically informed classification could be possible, at least if revisions committees kept on producing classifications like the one presented in 1905.[80] Adding to the chorus of criticism was D.G. Thomson, who claimed that the categories of alternating, delusional, volitional and moral insanity were 'new-fangled', fashionable terms for existing forms of insanity.[81] In his view, the committee should have kept with familiar terminology and described them as forms of mania instead of differentiating them as distinct disease entities.[82] In the face of these objections and differences of opinion, members of the revisions

[77] Percy Smith, 'Adjourned Annual Meeting of 1904' in *JMS*, vol. 51, no. 215, October 1905, pp. 733–772.

[78] Ibid.

[79] Ibid.

[80] Ibid.

[81] Ibid.

[82] D.G. Thompson, remarks recorded in Ibid.

committee reiterated its belief that it was not its job to carry out a wholesale revision of the system that was in use, but stated that it also wanted to carefully introduce new concepts to British psychiatry.[83]

Mercier, who had been unable to attend the session devoted to discussing the forms of insanity, attempted to raise problems with the tables at the general session the next day.[84] However, by this point the council's patience was beginning to wane, having the previous day sat through eight hours' worth of deliberation over the tables. Nevertheless, Mercier managed to find a way to express his dissatisfaction with the Table of the Forms, pointing out that despite lengthy exchanges, the Table had undergone no significant changes since the last draft.[85] He then proposed that a new and separate classification committee be set up that was devoted entirely to drawing up a classification of the forms of insanity, and offered to serve on it. The committee eagerly seconded this motion, for it was the troublesome Table of the Forms that had taken up most of their time over the last two years, and they were more than willing to pass on the task to Mercier. The new classification committee, which Mercier was appointed to, would sit for one year and deliver its final version of the classification at the next year's annual meeting in July 1906.[86] This was the point at which the MPA devoted energy specifically to drawing up a classification of the forms of insanity: prior to this it had been a statistical table that had contained forms, or clinical appearances, of insanity in the statistical returns submitted by asylums across the country. This was an important turning point, and the beginning of the process for an official classification of the kinds of insanity to be drawn up by the MPA.

The president of the MPA, Robert Armstrong-Jones, introduced his committee's classification with an address on 'the evolution of insanity'.[87] In an ambitious narrative that spanned four millennia from antiquity to the present, he referred to the work of Alexander Crichton, Thomas Arnold, David Davis, Philippe Pinel and Jean-Étienne Esquirol.

[83] Ibid.

[84] 'Medico-Psychological Association of Great Britain and Ireland: Annual Meeting of the Association, July 20th, 1905' in *JMS*, vol. 51, no. 215, October 1905, pp. 773–789.

[85] Mercier, remarks recorded in ibid.

[86] Ibid.

[87] Robert Armstrong-Jones, 'Medico-Psychological Association of Great Britain and Ireland: Presidential Address on the Evolution of Insanity, Delivered July 26th, 1906' in *JMS*, vol. 51, no. 215, October 1906, pp. 629–661.

Armstrong-Jones projected across cultures and into the past the notion that there had been different forms of insanity, with the 'milder forms of mental disorder [being] treated by pilgrimages to the shrines of certain saints' who were reputed to be skilled at exorcism of evil spirits, and that even in 'the most barbarous and least civilised of races there occur two forms of psychic anomalies, viz., the congenital and the toxic, the latter due to some poison, such as occurs from alcohol in our own country'.[88] He speculated on the prevalence of madness in the past, with 'the spread of venereal disease being responsible for increasing certain forms of insanity', whilst 'the congenital varieties of mental deficiency show but little increase, according to asylum statistics'.[89] This historical framing of the nature of the different forms of insanity, as well as the potentials held for treatment by understanding its various guises, was a fitting way to introduce the presentation of the final version of the Table of the Forms.

The classification committee presented its final report that same day. It had sat five times since July 1905. After lengthy deliberations, it presented what would end up being the final adjustments to the classification during this round of revisions (Table 5.3[90]).

The committee had charged itself primarily with rearranging the classes of insanity that were included in the first draft of Table of the Forms presented in 1904. The classification was separated into two main sections: the first relating to congenital illnesses and the second to 'Insanity occurring later in life' which referred to curable illnesses, and reflected similar distinctions made in lunacy legislation. The classification judged moral insanity to be a congenital disorder that was in the same class as intellectual insanity, but moral dementia was included in the second class of insanities that were considered to develop after birth. Many of the diseases included in this category had appeared on the 1904 table, but some had been rephrased: the committee opted for general paralysis of the insane (GPI) over general progressive paralysis (GPP) as included in previous drafts of the table. In a similar vein, and fearful that dementia praecox would be unfamiliar to psychiatrists practising in the British Isles, it came to be replaced with primary dementia, although the terms were not strictly synonymous. Primary dementia had been used in

[88] Ibid., pp. 644 and 652.

[89] Ibid., p. 652.

[90] Ibid., p. 821.

Table 5.3 Table of the Forms presented to the 1906 Annual General Meeting of the MPA[91]

I. Congenital or infantile mental deficiency (idiocy or imbecility), occurring as early in life as it can be observed –

1. Intellectual
   a. With Epilepsy
   b. Without Epilepsy
2. Moral

II. Insanity occurring later in life

1. Insanity with epilepsy
2. General paralysis of the insane
3. Insanity with the grosser brain lesions
4. Acute delirium (acute delirious mania)
5. Confusional Insanity
6. Stupor
7. Primary Dementia

[the committee placed a note here that 4, 5, 6, and 7 were grouped together by the committee because they constituted a 'natural group']

8. Mania
   a. Recent
   b. Chronic
   c. Recurrent
9. Melancholia
   a. Recent
   b. Chronic
   c. Recurrent
10. Alternating Insanity
11. Delusional Insanity
    a. Systematised
    b. Non-systematised
12. Volitional Insanity
    a. Impulse
    b. Obsession
    c. Doubt
13. Moral Insanity
14. Dementia
    a. Senile
    b. Secondary or Terminal

the United Kingdom before the publication and reception of Kraepelin's work, and it had a variety of meanings. Clouston disliked the term for he judged it 'confusing and incorrect', and instead recommended that the term 'stupor' be used to describe cases where consciousness of environs and memory were severely damaged in a patient.[92] Daniel Hack Tuke's

[91] 'Medico-Psychological Association of Great Britain and Ireland' in *JMS*, October 1906, pp. 809–838 (p. 820).

[92] Thomas Clouston, *Clinical Lectures on Mental Disease*, London, J&A Churchill, 1892, p. 299.

Dictionary of Medicine defined primary dementia as 'a variety of insanity which occurs in young persons although it is very acute and requires much care and skilled treatment'.[93] Unlike dementia praecox however, Hack Tuke's primary dementia 'generally terminates in recovery'.

The use of primary dementia was a compromise made by the committee when seeking to include the relatively new concept of dementia praecox, but it is difficult to say for certain because the committee did not provide definitions of the terms included in the final draft. It is possible that the committee sought to placate members with this reframing of dementia praecox. During regional meetings of the MPA, members had expressed some disfavour with the use of a non-English term in the draft classification, with demands being made to replace it with a term familiar to British medical superintendents. With the modification to primary dementia, as it was now known, it had become a main class, instead of being a sub-class of dementia as in the 1904 draft. It was placed into a 'natural group' of disorders that included confusional insanity, acute delirium and stupor because they presented symptoms that would all be apparent in a case of primary dementia. Acute delirium was introduced to make a distinction between extreme cases of delusional insanity and milder forms which would still be classed as delusional insanity, which itself was split into two sub-classes—systematised and non-systematised. This distinction echoes Pinel's distinction between partial and general insanity, with 'systematised' referring to states of delusion from which the patient did not emerge and which had a poor prognosis, and 'non-systematised' referring to patients who suffered intermittent spells of delusion, which had a better chance of recovery.

This final revision then was marked by two features that sought to answer criticisms aimed at the previous draft. Firstly, the committee sought to answer the criticisms of Mercier on logical inconsistency and secondly to realise Bond's aims articulated in 1902 to remove any terminology that implied causes from the Table of the Forms – they sought to do this through removing organic as a sub-category of dementia. Epileptic insanity was changed to 'insanity with epilepsy' since the committee thought that epileptic insanity inferred that the insanity was caused by epilepsy, and changed the phrasing in the hope that it would be clear to users of the table that it referred to cases of insanity that

[93] Daniel Hack Tuke, *A Dictionary of Psychological Medicine*, Philadelphia, P. Blakiston, 1892, p. 1010.

were accompanied with epilepsy, thereby inferring no causal link. A departure though from earlier versions of the table was that differentiations between the main classes were not based on symptomology alone but had also attempted to incorporate concepts that indicated some outlook for the patient. As mentioned above, delusional insanity was thought by members of the committee, in particular Armstrong-Jones, to have a very poor prognosis.[94] Similarly, alternating insanity, which was characterised by fluctuations between mania and melancholia, was thought to have a particularly bleak progression, with gradual decline spanning over decades.[95] Uncertainty existed over the differences in the prognosis of mania and melancholia because they referred to a broad range of patients, but it was agreed that patients treated during the earliest stages of the illness were thought to have better chances of recovery. Chronic forms typically affected middle-aged patients, with fewer chances of full recovery, whereas hopeful prospects were given to those with recurrent forms of mania and melancholia.[96] Uncertainty surrounded the prognosis of primary dementia, but it was generally viewed as better than that of dementia and melancholia due to it often afflicting younger patients who tended to respond better to treatment.

The classification committee faced resistance to these recommendations. Some perceived the draft to be a backwards step. Lewis Campbell Bruce, who had trained under Clouston at Morningside asylum, remarked that not only would the efforts of the committee fall short of the aspirations for the MPA for its classification to be adopted further afield, but it would actually help to damage the reputation of British psychiatry:

> the speciality had advanced a good deal farther than the proposed classification indicated. The committee was a very strong one, and if they considered that no further progress had been made, it would, he thought, be better to leave it entirely, than to print and publish to the world that

[94] Robert Armstrong-Jones, 'Prognosis in Mental Diseases' in *BMJ*, December 16th, 1905, pp. 1578–1582.

[95] G. Fielding Blandford, 'The Lumleian Lectures on the Diagnosis, Prognosis and Prophylaxis of Insanity: Lecture II' in *BMJ*, April 13th, 1895, pp. 797–800 (p. 799).

[96] John G. Havelock, 'A Case of Recurrent Mania' in *JMS*, vol. 4, no. 179, October 1896, pp. 817–881.

> the present effort was all that the British Medico-Psychological Association could do.[97]

Armstrong-Jones responded to Bruce's criticism that the classification retained some elements of symptomology due to the lack of any major breakthrough in the aetiology or pathology of mental disorders.[98]Clouston chipped in, expressing a desire to keep with the 1882 revision that had incorporated elements of the aetiological classification developed by his mentor Skae, calling the prognostic value of the current classification vague and imprecise.[99] Concerns were raised about the symptom-based approach having been imposed upon British psychiatry from France, and calling for the opportunity to be seized to break free from it and draw up a more 'scientifically' valid aetiological approach.[100]

Despite its poor reception, the 1907 Revision would the following year be adopted by the Commissioners in Lunacy. This move would introduce Kraepelinian diagnostic terms into asylum medical statistics. At the quarterly meeting in November 1906, Dr Hayes Newington announced that statistical tables including the classification had been formally adopted and members would shortly be sent them to use in the 1907 statistical returns.[101] Asylum medical superintendents would also be sent the medical registers that had been devised by the first revisions committee to standardise and streamline the recording of data on admissions, which included the Table of the Forms, and the Table of Causes. The diagnostic concepts published by the MPA would be the official classification of the Association until the product of the next set of revisions was published in 1934. The Board of Control would cease to make it compulsory for asylums to complete the medical registers after the Great War, and the

[97] Lewis Campbell Bruce, remarks recorded in 'Medico-Psychological Association of Great Britain and Ireland' in *JMS*, October 1906, pp. 809–838 (p. 822).

[98] Ibid., p. 823.

[99] Clouston would criticise primary dementia in his lectures, describing it as a form of melancholia, and saying that stupor should replace this term. See: Thomas Clouston, *Clinical Lectures on Mental Diseases*, J&A Churchill, 1892, p. 302.

[100] 'Medico-Psychological Association of Great Britain and Ireland' in *JMS*, October 1906, pp. 809–838.

[101] Dr Hayes Newington, remarks recorded in 'The Medico-Psychological Association of Great Britain and Ireland: Quarterly Meeting November 15th 1906' in *JMS*, vol. 53, no. 220, January 1907, pp. 214–217 (p. 215).

Table of the Causes and the Table of the Forms would cease to be used by many institutions after 1919.[102]

The revisions committee was successful in their original aim of keeping the causes of insanity and the symptom derived concepts of mental disorder separate by removing all mention of aetiology from the classification they published. As a point of comparison, that same year, the Royal College of Physicians (RCP) would publish the third edition of their nomenclature, which included a sub-section on mental diseases.[103] This closely resembled the Table of the Forms presented by the revisions committee, with two of the members of the committee appointed by the MPA, George Savage and Percy Smith, acting as the psychiatric specialists for the RCP's nomenclature committee.[104] Like the MPA's classification, the RCP's mental diseases sub-section was split into two, including a section on 'Errors of Development' and a section titled 'Disorders of Function' which corresponded to the MPA's distinction between 'Congenital and Infant Deficiency' and 'Insanity Occurring Later in Life'.[105] These two sections contained disease concepts that bore resemblance to the ones included in the Table of the Forms, though the latter included aetiological sub-categories to the main disorders. Melancholia and mania for instance both had puerperal sub-classes, with the former having climacteric forms and the latter having alcoholic and epileptic forms.[106] Crucially, there were two additional classes which had not found their way into the MPA's classification: these were insanities which were the 'Result of Infective, Toxic, and Other General Conditions' and, most importantly, a section on the 'Degenerations'.[107] Degenerations included general paralysis of the insane and dementia with six different forms: developmental; senile; epileptic; syphilitic; organic; and those 'from other

[102] This was mainly because the Board of Control saw the task of collecting asylum statistics as dispensable in the face of the disruption caused by many asylums being repurposed as war hospitals during the conflict; Anon, 'Statistical Intermission' in *JMS*, vol. 6, no. 56, January 1916, pp. 182–183.

[103] William S. Church, E. Liveing et al., *The Nomenclature of Diseases: Drawn up by a Joint Committee Appointed by the Royal College of Physicians of London*, 4th edition, HMSO, 1906.

[104] Ibid., p. vii.

[105] Ibid., p. 35.

[106] Ibid., p. 36.

[107] Ibid., pp. 37–39.

acute or chronic disease, or from injury'.[108] The college's nomenclature attempted to combine functional mental disorders with their suspected causes, be they in the form of bodily conditions such as pregnancy, habits such as alcoholism, lesions, degenerative disorders that had an observable impact on brain physiology, or were hereditary. This is in stark contrast to the MPA's classification, which attempted to provide a descriptive classification with little in the way of aetiology.

Although some viewed the move away from aetiology as a strength of the latest revisions, others thought this to be a shortfall. John Turner, the medical superintendent of Essex County Mental Hospital in Brentwood, offered an ambitious classification of insanity drawn along an anatomical basis.[109] Like the 1907 Revision, this was divided into two sections: the first dealing with 'the idiopathic or those hereditarily predisposed, embracing by far the larger number of individuals' and the second 'the traumatic or accidental'.[110] Turner also stated that the 'relative interdependence of intrinsic and extrinsic factors is a fundamental point' to his classification system—the intrinsic referred to the hereditarily predisposed, the extrinsic to the traumatic or accidental. The first section was divided 'into three classes according to the degree of anatomical change or developmental defect in the cortex'.[111] The first class were 'imbeciles' whose 'structural defect' was to such a degree 'that the nervous system is incapable, at the outset of life, of performing its functions in an efficient or normal manner'.[112] The second class is based upon a similar principle of structural defect, though it was accompanied by efficient function and was 'incapable of withstanding the physiological and inevitable stresses of life'. The third class comprised those who can withstand 'the ordinary physiological stresses, but break down when exposed to the influence of adventitious unfavourable circumstances, or with advanced age'.[113] Turner's system was presented to a meeting of the South Division of the MPA in 1912, but it drew criticism: its most prominent critic was none other

[108] Ibid.

[109] John Turner, 'The Classification of Insanity' in *JMS*, vol. 58, no. 40, January 1912, pp. 9–25.

[110] Ibid., p. 14.

[111] Ibid.

[112] Ibid.

[113] Ibid., p. 15.

than Charles Mercier, who attacked it on the basis that Turner had not separated aetiological, pathological and symptomatic concepts, and that his work again provided a 'complicated compendium' of the insanities.

Commenting on the 1907 Revision, a review in 1923 expressed sympathy towards the committee, and some degree of respect for implementing the relatively new and untested diagnostic category of primary dementia.[114] The report speculated that it may have not been the right time for a completely new classification, and expressed regret that 'some definition of the scheduled forms of mental disorder was not attempted', commenting that the statistics on psychological diagnosis collected since 1907 were essentially useless since 'names are immaterial so long as we have some idea of the type of case they refer to'.[115] Had definitions been provided, this 're-classification [of cases recorded in statistics] in accordance with advancing knowledge of cases now recorded in our statistics would not have been impossible'.[116] According to the review, authorities in the United Kingdom and Ireland should try to emulate the American Psychiatric Association's success in providing 'workable definitions of the main types of mental disorder in its statistical manual' because these had given some indication of the future course of each form of insanity.[117] The report emphasised that the absence of definitions was an important oversight that hindered communication between psychiatrists, and that whilst there 'was disagreement on whether they work well or not, at least [definitions] functioned well enough to allow communication to occur amongst the community'.[118]

[114] M. Hamblin Smith, 'Review: The Seventh and Eighth Annual Report of the Board of Control for the years 1920 and 1921' in *JMS*, January 1923, pp. 99–108.

[115] Ibid.

[116] Ibid.

[117] Ibid., p. 103.

[118] Ibid.

Conclusion

Writing in 1942 and whilst conducting a review of classifications used in medical statistics, the psychologist and eugenicist Carlos Patton Blacker would label the 1907 Revisions as 'Mesozoic'.[119] In adopting a geological term, Blacker judged the classification to be a bridge between Victorian asylum classification and the Kraepelinian classifications of early twentieth-century medical science. Primary dementia, which had replaced the dementia praecox of an early draft of the 1907 Revision, simultaneously referred to a concept of psychopathology familiar to asylum medical superintendents in primary dementia, and Kraepelin's novel concept of dementia praecox that itself had been developed through statistical methods. The inclusion of alternating insanity completed the picture since it bore a close resemblance to Kraepelin's manic-depressive insanity. Once again the MPA revisions committee had sought compromise between different groups in the Association, but in so doing published a classification that appeared dated once Kraepelinian terminology became widely used after the Great War. Whilst the classification was flawed, and did not live up to the aspirations of many, the MPA's Table of the Forms had anticipated the popularity of Kraepelinian psychopathology.

The revisions to the standard classification of the MPA at the beginning of the twentieth century coincided with pressures placed upon the profession to improve the accuracy of prognosis at the point of diagnosis. Increased emphasis on outlook was in response to the state of the Victorian asylum system, a therapeutic nihilism descending on the profession, and the lasting influence of degeneration theory. The attention to heredity as a causing factor, and the development of a section devoted to congenital disorders in the Table of the Forms, also anticipated the rise of eugenics. Hopes for a breakthrough in the pathology of insanity and its different forms had not materialised by the time it came to the revisions, and this also goes some way to explaining the preoccupation with outlook and heredity in these discussions. As we will see in the next chapter, around the same time there was a strong movement concerned with the borderland of insanity, which thought that improved prognosis was required so as to admit people who ought to be placed

119 Carlos Patton Blacker, 'Redhill Hospital—Notes on Visit Paid by Dr Harris and Dr Blacker on Monday, 16th December 1946 in Papers by Carlos Paton Blacker on Mental Health Records, Carlos Paton Blacker Collected Papers, held by The Wellcome Collection.

in an asylum, but could easily find themselves outside of one for most of their life: this was either because of violent conduct associated with psychopathy, or because of the public health risk degenerationists and eugenicists believed were posed by hereditary illnesses and constitutional weaknesses. The move to establish a committee in 1902 to revise the tables for use in asylum medical statistics was influenced by these broader concerns. Central to their efforts were the standard concepts of diagnosis and aetiology that were used in tables to record admissions data, including the forms of insanity diagnosed. The diagnostic concepts incorporated into the final version of the table were designed to provide a more precise outlook on the course of the illness than those previously used.

In presenting these debates, I hope not only to have told a chapter in the story of the Table of the Forms, but also to have shed new light on the links between asylum medical statistics and the development of psychological diagnosis during the first years of the twentieth century. The role the MPA's classification played in the widespread transmission and application of Kraepelinian concepts of psychopathology across the British Isles was partly down to their use in the medical registers introduced with the 1907 Revisions. The debates outlined in this chapter help to deepen understandings of the circumstances that led to shifts from diagnostic concepts used during the age of the Victorian asylum, to a classification of mental disorder informed by Kraepelin's work. I have suggested that this desire was heightened not only because of admiration for his methods in tracking patient data, which it was hoped would be emulated to some degree through asylum statistics, but also due to changing legal and practical considerations that made prognosis at the point of diagnosis a pressing concern for Victorian psychiatrists. The discussions presented further suggest the tandem development of psychiatric nosology and psychiatric epidemiology, spurred by hopes that efforts undertaken by asylum superintendents to devise a standard classification could be applied to research beyond the asylum. As we will see in the next chapter, asylum medical statistics were drawn upon by lunacy administration and the eugenics movement during the early years of the twentieth century to understand the public health risks posed by insanity.

The classification would not be treated well by history, principally due to the reformulation of Kraepelin's dementia praecox as primary dementia and the lack of definitions accompanying the terms in the table. The practical pressures placed upon the committee shaped the course of the discussions. Members that partook in statistical and classification committees carried out their work on a voluntary basis and had to spend many hours in meetings and consultations with members of the association, having to draft reports, papers and announcements. This all took time, and as we have seen, the grand visions of a figure like Mercier were soon reined in by everyday realities. Bureaucratic procedures and record-keeping are often overlooked in favour of the grand work of psychiatrists recorded in textbooks, but from these debates it becomes clear that this is only part of the story. The retention of symptomatic concepts was partly because symptom-based concepts were familiar and practical. Along with the reparsing of dementia praecox to primary dementia in the final revision, we have seen in this chapter how practical considerations proved to be the decisive factor in shaping the Table of the Forms. The terms included within the 1907 Revision drew upon the experience of the medical superintendent and their familiarity with textbooks and research that described the symptoms associated with each of the disorders that were included in the table. Put simply: symptom-based concepts worked and were familiar, and in the light of the practicalities of the Revisions committee, they were resorted to in lieu of pathological classifications that would allow diagnosis to be made according to causal, physical and mechanistic divisions.

CHAPTER 6

Psychological Classification and Asylum Medical Statistics

In August 1888, Daniel Hack Tuke engaged in correspondence with the editors of *The Times* disputing a pair of claims that had been made in a recent review of the year's *Report of the Commissioners of Lunacy*. The first was that insanity was on the increase and the second was that insanity was more frequently diagnosed in women than in men.[1] The reviewer had come to these conclusions by comparing the numbers published that year to ones that were published in the 1859 report. The conclusion of the review was that insanity had risen, with there being 'one known lunatic to every 535 of the population [whereas] on the 1st January in the present year there was one known lunatic to every 346 of the population, or a total of 82,643'.[2] It claimed that 'male lunatics were one to every 370 of the population, while female lunatics were one to every 326'.[3] Tuke, who at that time was serving as medical superintendent of one of the largest asylums in the country, wrote in his response that the reviewer's conclusions were incorrect. He dismissed as a fallacy the claim that there

[1] Daniel Hack Tuke, 'Lunacy Statistics: To the Editor of the Times' in *JMS*, vol. 34, no. 147, October 1888; *The Times* (London, England), August 30, 1888, no. 32478, p. 6.

[2] Ibid.

[3] Ibid.

K. M. Jones, *Psychological Classification and Diagnosis in Asylum Statistics, 1800–1948*, Mental Health in Historical Perspective,
https://doi.org/10.1007/978-3-031-46154-5_6

was an increase in the rate of insanity, accusing them of conflating an increase in rates of diagnosis with prevalence, or the actual rate of insanity amongst the population. Instead, he claimed that the rate of insanity had in fact remained constant over the years, and the increase in numbers could be accounted for by the expansion of asylum treatment, making an increase in the diagnoses of insanity inevitable.[4] He dismissed as unworthy of comment the possibility that there could be any differences in the rate of diagnosis of insanity between genders.

By the late 1880s, concerns over psychological classification, mental health statistics and diagnosis were no longer limited to those directly involved in running and overseeing asylums. Public fears grew over the rise of insanity and the possibility of being wrongly confined in an asylum.[5] Trust in the judgement of psychiatrists was questioned and the best available statistics to help understand broader questions such as the spread and increase of insanity were viewed as not being of sufficient quality to provide answers. Whilst there had long been criticisms of asylums and their management, alienists now increasingly felt the need to defend their practice and their status. As Andrew Scull notes, the 'institution was, of course, the almost exclusive arena in which the new profession plied its trade' observing that the 'asylum was itself a major weapon [...] in the struggle to cure the insane'.[6] Although Akhito Suzuki has

[4] The historiography on the debate over the increase in insanity during this period is extensive and whether there was an actual increase in the rate of insanity is debatable. Hare gives an assessment of the historical debate, claiming that there was in fact an increase in the rate of insanity, which he interprets as being a schizophrenia-like disorder, and points towards dietary and viral factors as explanations. Social historians like Andrew Scull take the view that the rise in the rate of insanity can be explained as part of a wider political project of 'social control' of the mad, and their removal to asylums was linked to the potential they had to disrupt the means of production: it was therefore in the interests of workhouse owners, and mad doctors to some extent in cahoots with them as employees of the state protecting private interests. Others such as Kathleen Jones also take the view that the increase was artificial, though a humanitarian desire to care for the insane was behind the increase in admittances. See: Edward Hare, 'Was Insanity on the Increase?' in *BJP*, vol. 142, no. 5, May 1983, pp. 439–455 (p. 451); Andrew Scull, 'Was Insanity Increasing? A Response to Edward Hare' in *BJP*, vol. 144, no. 4, April 1984, pp. 432–436; 'The Rise of the Asylum' in *The Most Solitary of Afflictions: Madness and Society in Britain 1700–1900*, Yale University Press, 1993, pp. 3–45; Kathleen Jones, *Mental Health and Social Policy, 1845–1959*, Routledge, 1960 (p. 22).

[5] P. McCandless, 'Liberty and Lunacy: The Victorians and Wrongful Confinement' in *Madhouses, Mad-Doctors, and Madmen*, edited by Andrew Scull, pp. 339–362.

[6] Andrew Scull, 'The Social History of Psychiatry in the Victorian Era' in *Madhouses, Mad-Doctors and Madmen*, edited by Andrew Scull, pp. 5–33 (p. 9).

questioned this view by looking at home care during this same period, it remains the case that mental health statistics for the most part only represented asylum populations.[7]

In the summer of 1905, another set of barbs were traded in the pages of *The Times* over asylum medical statistics, this time between the statistician and eugenicist Karl Pearson and James Crichton-Browne. Crichton-Browne, who had by then retired as asylum medical superintendent of the West Riding Lunatic Asylum, had questioned a set of claims Pearson had made in his 1903 Huxley Memorial lecture. He had criticised Pearson's warnings of a decline in the 'national ability', an assessment of the overall mental aptitude and prowess of the nation. Pearson thought that measuring and maintaining the national ability was key to avoiding a mental and physical deterioration of the British people. Reminiscent of his clash with David Skae explored earlier in this volume, Crichton-Browne thought Pearson's claims were conjecture dressed up as science, and he did not think asylum medical statistics could prove the strong conclusions on heredity Pearson was presenting. Crichton-Browne disagreed on the source of the national decline, with Pearson attributing it to the 'unintellectual' classes outbreeding the intellectual, whereas Crichton-Browne believed the more likely causes were environmental factors:

> His own view was that any dearth of ability from which we might be suffering was to be ascribed not so much to the infertility of the cultivated classes as to the artificial production of stupidity in various ways, and to the incessant draining from the country – which was the fit and proper breeding place and rearing ground of intellect – of the best elements of our people to be swallowed up or deteriorated in our big towns.[8]

[7] Akhito Suzuki's work on the social history of madness from the perspective of the family is important to mention here, because although insanity was mainly treated in the asylum, there was some sort of home care tradition. Suzuki also highlights the importance expressed by Bucknill on the importance of families in the diagnostic procedure. Yet the provisions by 1903 were still opined by psychiatrists as being almost very limited in England, yet more progress had been made in Scotland: Akhito Suzuki, *Madness at Home: The Psychiatrists, the Patient and the Family in England 1820–1860*, University of California Press, 2006 (p. 62); Editorial, 'The Home Care of the Insane Poor in England' in *JMS*, vol. 49, no. 207, pp. 708–711.

[8] 'Sir J. Crichton Browne on Sanitary Reforms' in *The Times*, no. 37789, Friday, August 18th, 1905, p. 9.

These concerns were informed by the eugenic conception of society and the nation as an organism that could suffer a collective mental deterioration.[9] Although a committed eugenicist, Crichton-Browne did not agree with Pearson's deterministic view that intelligence was inherited, and that unless the intellectual classes were encouraged to breed, a deterioration of the overall national abilities would ensue. Instead, he believed that 'unfulfilled intellects' resided in the labouring classes, and that it was the job of public health and education to prevent a decline by maintaining environmental standards that allowed those with potential to realise it.[10]

Pearson responded furiously to these criticisms in a letter published the following week, accusing Crichton-Browne of not even bothering to engage with the statistical evidence he had presented to bolster his claims on genetic inheritance.[11] He clarified his position by describing an insane diathesis, that is to say a mark of insanity, that was carried by those who had inherited a susceptibility to insanity.[12] The diathesis was a suitably loose concept that made no commitments about the nature of madness, but Pearson stressed that the best available evidence poined to its existence, and expected statistical research to discover a congenital mental weakness that was reflected in a person's physical constitution. Pearson believed that the best available data pointed towards insanity being a characteristic mark of a constitutional vulnerability that could be passed on to offspring:

> the statistics at present available suggest – I will not at present assert they do more – that we may ultimately find the insane diathesis, or, more roughly, 'want of mental balance', is inherited with precisely the same intensity as the physical characters in man.[13]

[9] Frank W. Stahnisch, 'The Early Eugenics Movement and Emerging Professional Psychiatry: Conceptual Transfers and Personal Relationships Between Germany and North America, 1880s to 1930s' in *The Canadian Bulletin of Medical History*, vol. 31, no. 1, 2014, pp. 17–40 (p. 23).

[10] Ibid.

[11] Karl Pearson, 'National Deterioration: To the Editor' in *The Times*, no. 37795, Friday, August 25th, 1905, p. 6.

[12] Karl Pearson, 'On the Inheritance of Insanity' in *BMJ*, vol. 1, no. 2317, pp. 1175–1177.

[13] Ibid., p. 1176.

Pearson engaged in studies of phthisis around the same time in an attempt to discover the insane diathesis, which he thought could be traced by studying those who seemed to have a constitutional vulnerability to developing the condition.[14] A number of studies of the Galton laboratories sought to trace parallels between physical and psychological constitution, with the links between tuberculosis and insanity attracting particular interest.[15] Furthering this exchange in another letter published four days later, Crichton-Browne considered the insane diathesis to be unacceptably vague and should not be used to make predictions about the inheritance of insanity.[16] For a medical profession accustomed to proving aetiology through anatomy and pathology, population studies that made strong claims on the causes of insanity were viewed with some degree of suspicion. Crichton-Browne was particularly cautious, and although responding amicably to Pearson, he gently criticised him for having made stronger claims about the potentials of mental health statistics than their current state warranted.

Tensions between mathematical statistics developed by Galton and Pearson and the crude vital statistics that were the norm for asylum medical statistics would come to a head at the turn of the century. This signalled a clash between differing approaches to the investigation of insanity that occurred around the time of the correspondence between Pearson and Crichton-Browne. Since the establishment of lunacy administration, national statistics had been collected in England and Wales, and Scotland and Ireland from the mid-nineteenth century onwards. Medical statistics for much of this time were presented as vital statistics that took the forms of averages and ratios published in lunacy reports. The development of asylum medical statistics followed this trend, with progress

[14] Pearson had developed a number of heat maps of Liverpool to trace the rate of phthisis in an attempt to map rates of insanity to contract of the disease, and had contacted Frederick Mott to explore the possibility of linking the two through statistical records. See Karl Pearson, Correspondence about Schedules on the Hereditary Transmission of Diseases, UCL Special Collections, 1906-07, PEARSON/3/10/2 and Work on the inheritance of Diseases and Insanity, UCL Special Collections, 1906-07, PEARSON/3/10/1-6.

[15] Pearson's own interest in the links between tuberculosis and insanity are documented in his personal papers on insanity: 'Pearson's Work on the Inheritance of Diseases and Insanity' PEARSON/3/10/2, 1906–1907, UCL Special Collections.

[16] James Crichton Browne, 'National Deterioration: To the Editor of the Times' in *The Times*, no. 37798 Tuesday, August 29th, 1905.

being slow. As explored in Chapter 4, the lack of standardisation of terms used in statistical returns had hampered efforts to develop statistics on psychological diagnosis. The development of asylum statistics on psychological diagnosis between 1845 and 1940 was disrupted by what Eileen Magnello calls an epistemic rupture between the Victorian preoccupation with vital statistics, and the development of mathematical statistics that occurred towards the end of the nineteenth century, principally through the work of Francis Galton, W.F.R Weldon and Karl Pearson.[17] Magnello describes how Galton's development of methods including median, correlation and regression analysis served as a bridge between vital statistics and mathematical statistical methods.[18] In his study of statistics in nineteenth century Britain, Donald Mackenzie puts the lack of advances in statistical theory prior to Galton down to the instrumental use of vital statistics, which were invoked by authorities to push through preconceived policy agendas.[19] Although Mackenzie's broad judgement is debatable in the case of asylum statistics, since the Commissioners in Lunacy were an oversight body and were interested in arriving as near as they could to the facts of the matter as opposed to employing statistics instrumentally to achieve a policy goal, he is correct in noting the relatively crude statistical methods available to public health authorities before the advent of mathematical statistics.

This chapter sketches the development of asylum statistics from their introduction in 1845 until the 1920s to show that there were two phases in the presentation of statistics on psychological diagnosis, and that developments in statistical theory played a role in defining these periods. The first phase saw a slow but gradual development of asylum statistics from 1845 until the handing over of powers from the Commissioners in Lunacy to the Board of Control under the terms of the 1913 Mental Deficiency Act. Despite the developments in previous chapters, asylum statistics on diagnosis stalled under the watch of the Board of Control upon its

[17] Eileen Magnello, 'The Introduction of Mathematical Statistics into Medical Research: The Roles of Karl Pearson, Major Greenwood and Austin Bradford Hill' in *The Road to Medical Statistics*, edited by Eileen Magnello and Ann Hardy, Rodopi, 2002, pp. 95–123.

[18] Eileen Magnello, 'The Introduction of Mathematical Statistics into Medical Research: The Roles of Karl Pearson, Major Greenwood and Austin Bradford Hill' in *The Road to Medical Statistics*, edited by Eileen Magnello and Ann Hardy, Rodopi, 2002, pp. 95–123.

[19] Donald A. Mackenzie, *Statistics in Britain, 1865–1930: The Social Construction of Scientific Knowledge*, Edinburgh University Press, 1981.

appointment, and after 1913, statistics on diagnosis appeared infrequently in their annual reports. Furthermore, after 1920, statistics on psychological diagnosis disappeared altogether and would seldom appear during the inter-war period, with regular statistics only emerging again after the end of the Second World War. The second half of this chapter charts the work of statisticians on insanity that drew on asylum records and who were involved in reforming public health statistics. The influence of figures in the eugenics movement over the Board of Control brought an abrupt end to interest in statistics on psychological diagnosis in 1913. The chapter will end by charting statistical studies on madness did not break it down into its different forms and instead employed broad definitions of insanity in their research. In an aim to identify those whose procreation should be regulated in pursuit of improving the national ability, broad definitions of insanity were deemed to be satisfactory.

The Development of Medical Statistics in Lunacy Commission Reports: 1845–1900

In the wake of the passing of the 1845 Lunacy Acts, attention came to be directed towards the significance of the findings gathered from data collected as a part of routine admissions procedures. Looking for clues from across the Channel, an assessment of French asylum data from the earliest years of the nineteenth century was published the spring of 1854 in *The Asylum Journal*.[20] The report reviewed admissions statistics from asylums in Paris and the wider Seine region. The total number of lunatics in Parisian asylums for that year stood at 3,182, which amounted to just under 20% of the total number of asylum inhabitants in the whole of the country. French authorities had worked this out to make this one asylum patient for every 2,128 of the population, and one in every 474 for the Seine region. The report accounted for regional and national differences because 'idiots' were more frequently admitted to asylums in urban areas because of a greater risk of ill-treatment, often becoming spectacles to the masses.[21] In contrast, those in the countryside 'are allowed to be at

[20] Anon., 'Statistics of the Insane in France' in *The Asylum Journal*, vol. 1, no. 4, 1854, pp. 63–64.

[21] Ibid.

large, and are generally treated kindly'.[22] The report went on to describe the occupations of those admitted, with traders and the liberal professions composing the greatest number, and to break down the statistics according to voluntary and official admissions, the former being 'non-dangerous lunatics on the demand of their facilities', with the latter being those deemed a danger to the public by the authorities. Official admissions had increased sharply since the introduction of legislation in 1838 that granted the police powers to admit people to asylums: 1833 had seen a weighting of 2,821 official to 4,242 voluntary admissions, but during the fifteen-year period between 1838 and 1852, the numbers had tipped massively towards official admissions, with 13,664 to 45,961 voluntary.

At this time, asylum medical statistics from the French system were some of the most well-established in Europe and were appealed to as the model of how to make sense of the data collected from large, state-run asylums.[23] France's lunacy statute of 1838 had established state-run lunatic asylums and the administrative procedures that recorded the patient information.[24] Lunacy reports issued by authorities in the United Kingdom were not quite as advanced as those in France, with medical statistics not being compiled for all asylums. Rather, in the two decades immediately following the 1845 Lunacy Acts, information for each asylum was presented as part of an appendix to the Annual Report of the Commissioners in Lunacy. This was partly because of the lack of standardisation of statistical returns, which made compiling them a difficult and time-consuming task, prompting the debates on standardisation outlined in the fourth chapter of this study.[25] The information published in the first Lunacy Commission reports pertained to the number of asylum inmates, broken down into numbers of admissions, deaths and discharges, and classes of patients, beds available, financial information on the running of the institution and information on staffing. By 1855, national findings on mortality and recovery rates were published in reports for England and Wales, and these were based on an analysis of

[22] Ibid.

[23] Terrence D. Murphy, 'Medical Knowledge and Statistical Methods in Early Nineteenth-Century France' in *Medical History*, vol. 25, 1981, pp. 301–319.

[24] Jacques Postel and Claude Quetel, 'Le vote de la loi de 1838' in *Une nouvelle histoire de la psychiatrie*, Dunod, 2004, pp. 180–192.

[25] Ian Dowbiggin, *Inheriting Madness: Professionalization and Psychiatric Knowledge in Nineteenth-Century France*, University of California Press, 1991.

reported deaths and discharges compared to admissions numbers.[26] As in the French system, patients were divided into categories of pauper and voluntary classes, and numbers were also broken down into gender, at least in reports for England and Wales. Combined medical statistics for all asylums were largely absent from these early reports of the Lunacy Commission, but information such as the suspected cause of insanity and psychological diagnosis were included in statistical reports of each individual asylum, although the quality of the information and its level of detail varied between institutions.

Asylum medical statistics remained crude up until the 1860s. Admissions were usually, but not always, divided according to whether the patient was classified as a lunatic or idiot, according to gender and according to whether they had been admitted as a private or pauper patient. During his study on reforms to the admissions data collection procedures of the 1940s, Carlos Patton Blacker concluded that the poor-quality of the data in these early reports was partially because of its incompleteness, with many asylums not returning statistics on diagnosis, and also because of inefficient methods that made compiling the data a time-consuming task.[27] The non-submission of returns and asylums not using standard diagnostic terms contributed to the commission not publishing data on diagnosis until the 1870s. Medical statistics on psychological diagnosis were also not a priority for asylum oversight, with statistics on mortality, breakdowns of institutional finances and information pointing to conditions within the asylum being more essential for the purposes of asylum regulation.

Statistics on psychological diagnosis in the reports of individual asylums varied in detail, with there being some variance in the diagnostic categories used. Some asylums combined main psychological categories with physical symptoms thought to be associated with the form of insanity, such as epilepsy and general paralysis, or 'softening of the brain' as in the report of the *Manchester Royal Lunatic Hospital* (see Tables 6.1, 6.2, 6.3, 6.4, 6.5, and 6.6).

[26] W. Parsey, 'On the Statistics of County Asylums' in *The Asylum Journal*, vol. 1, no. 10, 1855, pp. 149–150.

[27] Carlos Patton Blacker 'Mental Health Records: What We Can Learn From Them?', 27th February 1947, in Papers by Carlos Paton Blacker on Mental Health Records, Carlos Paton Blacker Collected Papers, held by The Wellcome Collection.

Table 6.1 'Table VIII Showing the Probable Causes of Disorder' from the report of the Somerset County Asylum for Insane Paupers, 1848[28]

TABLE VIII Showing the probable causes of disorder					
Moral	Males	Females	Physical	Males	Females
Ambition	3	3	Accidental Injury	5	1
Destitution	2	1	Critical period	0	3
Disappointment	0	1	Disease of the Brain	4	5
Dissipation	1	0	Affection of the organs of hearing	1	0
Dread of poverty	2	0			
Fright	1	5	Fatuity	1	0
Grief	5	13	Fever	4	1
Loss of property	6	5	Hereditary Disposition	23	24
Love	4	3	Intemperance	12	2
Religious Excitement	2	2	Puerperal disease	0	2
Bad education	1	0	Want of rest	2	0

Table 6.2 'Table IX Showing the Forms of Disorder' from the report of the Somerset County Asylum for Insane Paupers, 1848[29]

TABLE IX: Showing the forms of disorder			
Forms of Disorder	Males	Females	Total
Mania			
Acute Mania	6	6	12
Ordinary Mania	20	44	64
Periodical Mania	13	12	25
Dementia or Incoherence	28	30	58
Melancholia	15	16	31
Monomania	13	6	19
Moral Insanity	5	1	6
Congenital Idiocy	6	1	7
Congenital Imbecility	9	3	12
Epilepsy	17	22	39
General Paralysis	6	0	6
Delirium Tremens	2	0	2
Delirium	2	1	3

[28] First Report of the Somerset County Asylum for Insane Paupers, From the 1st March When It Was Opened for Patients To the End of the Year 1848, Samuel Backhouse, 1849, p. 41.

[29] First Report of the Somerset County Asylum for Insane Paupers, From the 1st March When It Was Opened for Patients To the End of the Year 1848, Samuel Backhouse, 1849, p. 41.

Table 6.3 'Table of the Forms of Disease' from the fourth annual report of the Committee of Visitors of the County Lunatic Asylum at Colney Hatch, 1855[30]

The forms assumed by, and the complications of the diseases in the 219 admitted cases, were as follows:	
Mania	46
Melancholia	35
Monomania	25
Dementia	26
Mania, with General Paralysis	7
Mania, with Epilepsy	9
Dementia, with General Paralysis	33
Dementia, with Partial Paralysis	3
Dementia, with Epilepsy	26
Idiocy (associated in one case with Epilepsy	9
Total	219

By the 1860s the situation had begun to change, with greater complexity in medical statistics beginning to occur and the limited inclusion of statistics on psychological diagnostic categories. From 1861, detailed breakdowns of causes of death that included information on psychological diagnoses were being published in annual reports of the Commissioners in Lunacy as some asylums had included causes of death that mentioned a psychological diagnosis. For instance, the Leicester County Asylum reported that six of its patients had died of 'maniacal exhaustion', five of general paralysis and six of apoplexy,[31] whereas the West Riding Pauper Lunatic Asylum reported that thirteen had died from senile decay, ten from exhaustion after mania and ten from exhaustion after melancholia.[32] The 1865 report of the Commissioners in Lunacy contained a note emphasising the need for uniform statistical returns. It described how:

> The Superintendents of most County Asylums publish in their Annual Reports Tables more or less elaborate, and containing a large amount of valuable information. While, however, the facts recorded may be identical in many if not most of the reports, the form in which they are recorded varies so greatly that it becomes impossible to tabulate them for the purpose of showing general results.[33]

[30] *The Fourth Annual Report of the Committee of Visitors of the County Lunatic Asylum at Colney Hatch, January Quarter Session, 1855*, John Thomas Norris, p. 41.

[31] *The Sixteenth Annual Report of the Commissioners in Lunacy*, HMSO, 1862, p. 135.

[32] Ibid., p. 179.

[33] *The Twentieth Annual Report of the Commissioners in Lunacy*, HMSO 1866, p. 45.

Table 6.4 Tables of the Statistical Returns published in the Report of the *Manchester Royal Lunatic Hospital*, 1861[34]

12

TABLE VIII.—FORM OF DISEASE IN THOSE ADMITTED.

	Males.	Females.	Total.
Mania	8	7	15
" with softening of brain	1	0	1
" with acute inflammation of membranes	0	1	1
Melancholia	4	8	12
Moral Insanity	0	2	2
Dementia	1	0	1
" with acute softening of brain	1	0	1
" with chronic softening of brain and cord	0	1	1
General Paralysis	1	0	1
	16	19	35

TABLE IX.—SUPPOSED CAUSE OF INSANITY.

	Males.	Females.	Total.
Hereditary tendency	1	3	4
Intemperance and other excess	5	2	7
Overwork	1	1	2
Loss of money	1	0	1
Religion	1	0	1
Jealousy	0	1	1
Fright	0	1	1
Speculation	1	0	1
Business anxieties	2	0	2
Softening of brain	1	1	2
Miscarriage	0	2	2
Not known	3	8	11
	16	19	35

TABLE X.—OCCUPATION OF THOSE ADMITTED.

Gentleman	1	Carpenters	2
Ladies	3	Housekeepers	2
Merchant	1	Farmer's Wife	1
Manufacturer	1	Tradesmen's Wives	7
Governess	1	Vocalist	1
Reporter	1	Waste Dealer	1
Clerks	2	Provision Dealer	1
Merchant's Wife	1	Warehouseman	1
Schoolmistress	1	Cashier	1
Shopkeeper	1	Cook	1
Retired Tradesmen	2		
Bookseller	1		35
Watch Dealer	1		

[34] *Report of the Manchester Royal Lunatic Hospital*, Thos. Sowler and Sons, 1861, p. 12.

Table 6.5 Table of the Forms of Diseases in Admissions in the *Twentieth Report of the Committee of Visitors of the County Lunatic Asylum at Hanwell, 1865*[35]

TABLE I.

Form of the Disease in the 354 Patients admitted during the Year ending December 31st, 1864.

Form of Disease.	M.	F.	Total.
Mania	72	82	154
" Suicidal	3	—	3
" with General Paralysis	8	4	12
" " " Suicidal..	—	—	—
" Epilepsy	3	—	3
" " Suicidal	2	—	2
" General Paralysis and Epilepsy	1	—	1
" Puerperal	—	5	5
Monomania	—	2	2
Melancholia	14	50	64
" Suicidal..............	14	8	22
" with Mania	—	3	3
" withGeneralParalysis, Suicidal	3	—	3
". Puerperal	—	1	1
Imbecility....................	16	12	28
" with General Paralysis	20	—	20
" withGeneralParalysis, Suicidal..........	3	—	3
" with Epilepsy	7	1	8
" with Epilepsy, Suicidal	1	—	1
Dementia	—	8	8
" with General Paralysis	—	2	2
Idiotcy	1	3	4
" with Epilepsy	1	—	1
Convalescent on admission......	—	4	4
Total......	169	185	354

[35] *Twentieth Report of the Committee of Visitors of the County Lunatic Asylum at Hanwell*, Harrison and Sons, 1865, p. 88.

Table 6.6 Tables from the first annual report of the North Wales Lunatic Asylum, Denbigh, 1849[36]

12

TABLE II.

Showing the form of disease in the 142 patients admitted.

	Males.	Females.	Total.
Mania acute . .	11	13	24
" " attempted suicide	1	1	2
" " chronic .	33	39	72
" " with general paralysis .	2	..	2
Dementia . . .	11	10	21
Melancholia . .	1	4	5
Epilepsy . . .	3	2	5
Idiots . . .	4	2	6
Moral insanity . .	..	4	4
Mania puerperal . .	..	1	1
Total . .	66	76	142

TABLE III.

Showing form of disease in 18 cases discharged cured.

	Males.	Females.	Total.
Mania acute	6	5	11
" chronic	2	1	3
" puerperal	..	1	1
Melancholia	1	..	1
Moral insanity	..	2	2
Total	9	9	18

TABLE IV.

Showing the duration of disease upon the 18 cases on admission.

	Males.	Females.	Total.
Under one month . . .	4	4	8
" three ditto . . .	3	2	5
" six ditto . . .	1	1	2
" ten ditto . . .	1	2	3
Total . . .	9	9	18

TABLE V.

Showing the duration of treatment in the Institution of those cases discharged cured.

	Males.	Females.	Total.
Under three months	2	2	4
" six ditto	6	2	8
" ten ditto	1	5	6
Total	9	9	18

Average—21½ weeks.

[36] The First Annual Report of the North Wales Lunatic Asylum, Denbigh, for the Year MDCCC.XLIX, Thomas Gee Clwydian Office, 1849, p. 12.

As we have seen earlier in this study, attempts to bring uniformity to asylum medical statistics triggered debates that waged throughout the 1860s and 1870s, and which would reach their conclusion in 1881. Whilst waiting for the work of the revisions committee, the Commissioners expressed hope in the 1866 report for the swift publication of the revised statistical tables, but in the meantime offered their own provisional set of tables to allow some degree of standardisation, of which Table 6.7 is an example. The Commissioners expressed enthusiasm about the possibilities offered by standardised information on 'the form of mental disorder under which [patients] labour', and 'hoped that the Medical Officers of Asylums may see the great importance of coming to some agreement' over the terms to use in psychological diagnosis, at least for the purposes of filling in statistical returns.[37] The report also contained a series of recommendations for revision of the statistical tables that emphasised the need for standardised tables to help provide data that would settle the 'vexed question of the increase of insanity' (Table 6.8).[38]

Table I. gives the numbers of admissions, readmissions, discharges, and deaths, with the average numbers resident during the year; the sexes being distinguished under each head.
Table II. gives the same results for the entire period the Asylum has been in operation.
The Table also embraces a column for the mean population, or average numbers resident in each year. In other columns are shown for each year the proportion of recoveries calculated on the admissions; and the mean annual mortality, or the proportion of deaths, calculated on the average numbers resident. It is of the first importance that these two principle results under asylum treatment, when given, should be calculated on a uniform plan, and according to the methods here pointed out.
Table III. furnishes a history of the yearly results of treatment since the opening of the Asylum.
Table IV. gives a history of each year's admissions; how many, for example, of the patients admitted, say in 1855, have been discharged as cured, how many have died, and how many remain in the Asylum in 1865.

[37] Ibid., p. 46.

[38] 'Suggestions for Revised Medical Statistical Tables Drafted by the Commissioners in Lunacy' in ibid., pp. 43–44.

> The value of this table in regard to the vexed question of the increase of insanity is evident. The table is adopted from the Somerset Asylum Reports.
> Table V. shows the causes of classified under appropriate heads. This form is adopted from the Reports of the Commissioners in Lunacy for Scotland, with some addition and modification. It appears sufficiently detailed for statistical purposes.
> Table VI. gives the length of residence in the Asylum of those discharged recovered, and of those who have died during the year.
> Uniformity in recording the ages of Patients on admission, the duration of the existing attack, and the form of mental disorder under which they labour, is also very desirable; and it is to be hoped that the Medical Officers of Asylums may see the great importance of coming to some agreement upon these points. How far the table of the causes of death may require modification or extension will be a matter for subsequent consideration.[39]

The report of 1866 published a table that included a crude breakdown of the patients residing in asylums who had been categorised as 'Probably Incurable Pauper Cases'.[40] Further breakdowns by gender and two tables with further breakdowns of admissions were included: one for patients classified as 'Violent' and one for 'Harmless'. The following year in 1867, the Commissioners reported that tables using standard terms of diagnosis had been returned by more than half of the County and Borough asylums in England and Wales.[41] It proposed an additional three tables that captured the duration of the disorder, ages and causes of mental disorder for all admissions, discharges and deaths (Table 6.9). Repeated attempts were made by the commission, working with the MPA, to bring about standardisation that would enable more detailed medical statistics to be published. Basic data on admissions, discharges and deaths were simpler to compile than clinical data such as those on psychological diagnosis because what defined a pauper or private lunatic was outlined by law, whereas there were no standard definitions of psychological disorders. The task of compiling more in-depth medical data was also made harder because of the different methods asylum superintendents had developed

[39] 'Suggestions for Revised Medical Statistical Tables Drafted by the Commissioners in Lunacy' in ibid., pp. 43–44.

[40] Ibid.

[41] *Twenty Second Report of the Commissioners in Lunacy*, HMSO, 1868, p. 81.

Table 6.7 'Abstract of Returns of Probably Incurable Pauper Cases' broken down according to Form of Mental Disorder, Twenty First Report of the Commissioners in Lunacy, 1867[42]

64 *Twenty-first Report of the*

ABSTRACT of RETURNS (*see* Appendix J.) of PROBABLY INCURABLE PAUPER CASES in COUNTY and BOROUGH ASYLUMS and REGISTERED HOSPITALS, 1st January 1867.

ASYLUM.	Total Number of Incurables.	Form of Mental Disorder.			Condition.			
		Idiot or Imbecile from Birth or Infancy.	Imbecile or Demented, but not from Birth or Infancy.	Other Forms of Mental Unsoundness.	Excited, Violent or Dangerous.	Quiet and Harmless.	Epileptics.	Affected with General Paralysis.
Beds, Herts, and Hunts	477	57	211	209	203	274	80	109
Bucks	302	45	62	195	292	10	41	7
Cambridge and Isle of Ely	261	22	22	217	63	198	45	10
Carmarthen, Cardigan, Pembroke, and Haverfordwest	156	4	27	125	40	116	17	6
Chester	468	27	118	323	368	100	65	32
Cornwall	329	14	123	192	287	42	43	9
Cumberland and Westmoreland	249	12	113	124	181	68	33	10
Denbigh, Anglesey, Carnarvon, Flint, and Merioneth.	321	21	48	252	74	247	23	11
Derby	300	57	75	168	217	83	52	7
Devon	610	54	374	182	482	128	78	34
Dorset	425	21	101	303	167	258	48	17
Durham	378	15	288	75	279	99	27	51
Essex	484	52	237	195	329	155	78	28
Glamorgan	260	22	174	64	100	160	31	26
Gloucester	571	54	276	241	323	248	87	19
Hants	540	103	115	322	393	147	90	20
Kent	679	28	409	242	610	69	85	27
Lancaster, at Lancaster	778	28	597	153	669	109	116	23
" Rainhill	586	26	262	298	330	256	60	31
" Prestwich	843	18	575	250	700	143	98	78
Leicester and Rutland	330	81	84	165	244	86	57	6
Lincoln	499	72	76	351	458	41	58	13
Middlesex, Colney Hatch	1,953	111	1,140	702	1,483	470	357	90
" Hanwell	1,667	66	655	946	1,038	629	176	70
Monmouth, Hereford, Brecon, and Radnor	393	46	28	319	368	25	53	26
Norfolk	300	45	117	138	163	137	52	10
Northumberland	132	10	73	49	69	63	22	13
Notts	306	18	30	258	277	29	44	14
Oxford and Berks	463	56	197	210	160	303	94	23
Salop and Montgomery	371	43	192	136	253	118	62	28
Somerset	388	50	174	164	177	211	78	10
Stafford, at Stafford	434	43	64	327	410	24	95	17
" Burntwood	222	24	43	155	97	125	36	17
Suffolk	330	26	21	283	286	44	25	2
Surrey	893	28	794	71	422	471	138	30
Sussex	495	40	218	237	467	28	58	6
Warwick	389	54	190	145	157	232	64	9
Wilts	379	39	114	226	304	75	69	8
Worcester	503	75	155	273	475	28	110	20
York, North Riding	407	41	120	246	81	326	26	15
" West Riding	916	19	461	436	380	536	144	53
Birmingham	442	30	237	175	107	335	141	37
Bristol	197	24	82	91	170	27	50	8
Hull	117	3	53	61	47	70	20	7
City of London	185	2	70	113	66	119	31	10
Norwich	84	8	19	57	19	65	24	9
Newcastle-on-Tyne	106	4	102	–	59	47	16	6
Northampton Hospital	300	37	70	193	243	57	47	10
York Hospital	39	–	17	22	33	6	10	4
TOTAL	22,257	1,775	9,803	10,679	14,620	7,637	3,354	1,126

[42] *Twenty First Report of the Commissioners in Lunacy, HMSO*, 1867, p. 64.

of collecting, collating and submitting their data to the Lunacy Commission, with there being some resistance to the adoption of standard tables from certain recalcitrant medical superintendents: the Commissioners' report of 1869 announced that some of the largest asylums, including Hanwell, Lancaster and Stafford, had no plans to use statistical tables drafted and issued by the Lunacy Commission, and although thirty-seven asylums including Broadmoor had pledged to take up the tables, only Manchester Royal Lunatic Asylum and Northampton General Lunatic

Table 6.8 '[Proposed] Table V – Showing the Causes of Death during the Year' from 'Appendix I' including Proposed Standardised Returns for Medical Statistics[43]

Table V – Showing the Cause of Death during the Year			
Cause of Death	Male	Female	Total
CEREBRAL OR SPINAL DISEASE:			
Apoplexy and Paralysis			
Epilepsy and Convulsions			
General Paralysis			
Maniacal and melancholic exhaustion or decay			
INFLAMMATION AND OTHER DISEASES OF THE BRAIN, SOFTENING, TUMOURS &C.			
Thoracic Disease			
Inflammation of the Lungs, Pleurae and Bronchi			
Pulmonary Consumption			
Disease of the Heart, &c.			
ABDOMINAL DISEASE:			
Inflammation of the Stomach, Intestines, or Peritoneum			
Dysentery and Diarrhoea			
Fever			
Erysipelas			
Cancer			
General Debility and Old Age			
Suicide and Accidents			
Total			

[43] Ibid., p. 117.

Asylum had actually put the recommendations into practice.[44] By the following year, the report stated that although there had been near-universal uptake, with most asylums at least pledging to use the standard returns in the near future, there still remained a handful of asylums and hospitals that had not used the standard forms in their yearly statistical returns.[45]

By the 1870s, asylum statistics became a focus for public health bodies because they not only could enable asylum oversight and administration but could also be used to make sense of broader questions on insanity. Lunacy Commission reports would regularly be reviewed in newspapers and periodicals, accompanied with commentary on the rates of insanity amongst the population to illuminate matters of national importance, public health requirements and the impact of new technologies upon the human mind. Common approaches used in these reviews included comparisons of admissions rates across asylums in urban and rural areas, assessments of admissions and discharge rates over decades and voicing concerns over mortality rates. The occupation, religion and family background of those admitted was also a common area of discussion. Interest in medical statistics was prompted to some degree by the 1871 and 1881 censuses, which included questions on insanity amongst family members.[46] The Commissioners themselves used this information to make estimations on insane populations beyond the asylum walls, and to make forecasts over asylum admissions.[47]

In answering questions that were attracting wider attention from the press and the public, interest in medical statistics ceased to be limited to asylum administration and the clinic. Understanding the causes behind the increase in admittances to asylums in the larger cities became a matter of growing social importance as urban populations expanded, and public health movements sought to improve living conditions in cities. Developing asylum data was not only a concern for those with an interest in managing and maintaining conditions within the asylum, but also for the wider public as interest grew amongst alienists in how urban living, as

[44] *Twenty-Fourth Report of the Commissioners in Lunacy*, HMSO, 1869, p. 71.

[45] *Twenty-Fifth Report of the Commissioners in Lunacy*, HMSO, 1970, p. 5.

[46] E. Hare, 'Was Insanity on the Increase?' in *British Journal of Psychiatry*, vol. 142, no. 5, May 1983, pp. 439–455 (p. 442).

[47] *Twenty-Fifth Report of the Commissioners in Lunacy*, HMSO, 1970, p. 5.

Table 6.9 Table II: Showing the Ratio of Lunatics, Idiots and Persons of Unsound Mind to the Population 1859–1878 from the Thirty-Second Report of the Commissioners of Lunacy, 1878[48]

10 *Thirty-second Report of the* *Commissioners in Lunacy.* 11

TABLE II.—Showing the Ratio of Lunatics, Idiots, and Persons of Unsound Mind, to the Population on the 1st January in each of the Years 1859–1878, inclusive.

YEAR.	POPULATION (estimated for the middle of each Year). Males.	Females.	Total.	NUMBER OF LUNATICS, &c., on 1st January. Private. Males.	Private. Females.	Private. Total.	Pauper. Males.	Pauper. Females.	Pauper. Total.	Total. Males.	Total. Females.	Total. Total.
1859	9,606,982	10,079,719	19,686,701	2,701	2,279	4,980	14,065	17,727	31,792	16,766	20,006	36,772
1860	9,704,394	10,198,319	19,902,713	2,771	2,294	5,065	14,561	18,432	32,993	17,332	20,726	38,058
1861	9,801,152	10,318,162	20,119,314	2,909	2,357	5,266	15,090	19,291	34,381	17,999	21,648	39,647
1862	9,923,272	10,447,741	20,371,013	3,046	2,374	5,420	15,627	20,082	35,709	18,673	22,456	41,129
1863	10,046,909	10,578,946	20,625,855	3,126	2,381	5,507	16,485	21,126	37,611	19,611	23,507	43,118
1864	10,172,080	10,711,809	20,883,889	3,158	2,418	5,576	17,260	21,959	39,219	20,418	24,377	44,795
1865	10,298,826	10,846,325	21,145,151	3,255	2,535	5,790	17,621	22,539	40,160	20,876	25,074	45,950
1866	10,427,146	10,982,538	21,409,684	3,367	2,647	6,014	18,317	23,317	41,634	21,684	25,964	47,648
1867	10,557,066	11,120,459	21,677,525	3,411	2,644	6,055	18,956	24,075	43,031	22,367	26,719	49,086
1868	10,688,600	11,260,113	21,948,713	3,404	2,636	6,040	19,923	25,037	44,960	23,327	27,673	51,000
1869	10,821,775	11,401,524	22,223,299	3,414	2,761	6,175	20,950	26,052	47,002	24,364	28,813	53,177
1870	10,956,608	11,544,708	22,501,316	3,442	2,838	6,280	21,690	26,743	48,433	25,132	29,581	54,713
1871	11,093,123	11,669,689	22,762,812	3,575	2,879	6,454	22,434	27,867	50,301	26,009	30,746	56,755
1872	11,231,339	11,836,496	23,067,835	3,682	2,960	6,642	23,136	28,862	51,998	26,818	31,822	58,640
1873	11,371,273	11,985,141	23,356,414	3,895	3,128	7,023	23,577	29,696	53,273	27,472	32,824	60,296
1874	11,512,956	12,135,653	23,648,609	4,023	3,269	7,292	24,101	30,634	54,735	28,124	33,903	62,027
1875	11,656,400	12,288,059	23,944,459	4,043	3,347	7,390	24,948	31,455	56,403	28,991	34,802	63,793
1876	11,801,633	12,442,377	24,244,010	4,062	3,447	7,509	25,280	32,127	57,407	29,342	35,574	64,916
1877	11,948,677	12,398,632	24,347,309	4,087	3,510	7,597	26,078	32,961	59,039	30,165	36,471	66,636
1878	12,007,547	12,756,850	24,764,397	4,172	3,520	7,692	26,852	33,994	60,846	31,024	37,514	68,538

RATIO (per 10,000). Private Lunatics to Population. Males.	Females.	Total.	Pauper Lunatics to Population. Males.	Females.	Total.	Total Lunatics to Population. Males.	Females.	Total.	YEAR.
2·81	2·26	2·53	14·64	17·59	16·14	17·45	19·85	18·67	1859
2·86	2·25	2·54	15·00	18·07	16·58	17·86	20·32	19·12	1860
2·97	2·28	2·62	15·39	18·70	17·09	18·36	20·98	19·71	1861
3·07	2·27	2·66	15·75	19·22	17·53	18·82	21·49	20·19	1862
3·11	2·25	2·67	16·41	19·97	18·23	19·52	22·22	20·90	1863
3·10	2·25	2·67	16·97	20·50	18·78	20·07	22·75	21·45	1864
3·16	2·34	2·74	17·11	20·78	18·99	20·27	23·12	21·73	1865
3·23	2·41	2·81	17·57	21·23	19·45	20·80	23·64	22·26	1866
3·23	2·38	2·79	17·96	21·65	19·85	21·19	24·03	22·64	1867
3·18	2·34	2·75	18·64	22·23	20·48	21·82	24·57	23·23	1868
3·15	2·42	2·78	19·36	22·85	21·15	22·51	25·27	23·93	1869
3·14	2·46	2·79	19·80	23·16	21·52	22·94	25·62	24·31	1870
3·22	2·46	2·83	20·22	23·88	22·08	23·44	26·34	24·93	1871
3·28	2·50	2·88	20·60	24·38	22·54	23·88	26·88	25·42	1872
3·43	2·61	3·01	20·72	24·78	22·81	24·16	27·39	25·82	1873
3·49	2·69	3·08	20·93	25·24	23·15	24·42	27·93	26·23	1874
3·47	2·72	3·09	21·40	25·60	23·55	24·87	28·32	26·64	1875
3·44	2·77	3·10	21·42	25·82	23·68	24·86	28·59	26·78	1876
3·42	2·83	3·12	21·82	26·58	24·25	25·24	29·41	27·37	1877
3·47	2·76	3·11	22·36	26·65	24·57	25·84	29·41	27·68	1878

48 Ibid.

well as the particular social circumstances of an individual, could help to explain their admittance to the asylum. Questions like whether there were significant differences in the rate and kinds of diagnoses of insanity in admissions to rural and urban asylums proved as divisive as those over the rate of insanity that opened this chapter. The development of germ theory gave further impetus to improve public health towards the end of the nineteenth century, and statistics indicating trends in mental hygiene were seen as particularly desirable during the first decades of the twentieth century. Asylum medical statistics did come under scrutiny however, and as the exchanges that opened this chapter show, much ink was spilled fuelling debates over the true significance of trends identified in statistics (Table 6.10).[49]

By 1877, combined medical statistics for all English and Welsh asylums were being regularly published in Lunacy Commission annual reports.[50] Despite apparent progress, the report emphasised the need for further standardisation, noting that it 'would be of the greatest utility in statistical comparison, and supply the chief requisites for a scientific application of the results of medical statistics'.[51] The 1877 *Report of the Commissioners of Lunacy* provided the first set of standardised tables that classified patients according to the suspected cause of insanity. It introduced tables that compared causes in pauper and private patients, making distinctions in the data between admissions to county and borough asylums, and those admitted to Hospitals and Licensed Houses.[52] The 1877 report's Table of the Causes (see Table 6.11) was divided into moral and physical sections, with 'moral' roughly meaning social or cultural since the disorders included in the moral part were influenced by social change. It included 'domestic troubles' and 'disappointment in love' as categories of moral causes, and 'hereditary taint' and 'onanism' in the physical section.[53] The categories devoted to hereditary and congenital disorders were considered less susceptible to social influences, but the distinction

49 P. Maury Deas, 'Five Years of Statistics' in *JMS*, vol. 25, no. 109, April 1879, pp. 8–19.

50 *Thirty-First Report of the Commissioners in Lunacy*, HMSO, 1877.

51 Ibid., p. 3.

52 Ibid., pp. 6–7.

53 Ibid., pp. 32–33.

Table 6.10 Showing the assigned causes of insanity in the general paralytics from the Report of the Commissioners in Lunacy for the year 1877[54]

TABLE XVIII.—Showing the assigned CAUSES OF INSANITY in the GENERAL PARALYTICS ADMITTED into County and Borough Asylums, Registered Hospitals, Naval and Military Hospitals, State Asylums, and Licensed Houses in England and Wales, during the Year **1876**.*

(The Total Number of these Admissions was 1,221, being 987 Males and 234 Females.)

CAUSES OF INSANITY.	Total Number of Instances in which each Cause was Assigned.			Proportion per Cent. to the Total Number of General Paralytics Admitted.		
	M.	F.	T.	M.	F.	T.
MORAL:						
Domestic Trouble (including loss of relatives and friends).	31	18	49	3·1	7·6	4·0
Religious Excitement - - - - -	8	1	9	·8	·4	·7
Adverse Circumstances (including business anxieties and pecuniary difficulties).	72	4	76	7·2	1·7	6·2
Love Affairs (including Seduction) - -	–	1	1	–	·4	·0
Mental Anxiety: "Worry" - - -	49	9	58	4·9	3·8	4·7
Fright and Nervous Shock - - - -	4	2	6	·4	·8	·4
PHYSICAL:						
Intemperance, in Drink - - - -	248	24	272	25·1	10·2	22·2
" Sexual - - - -	33	8	41	3·3	3·4	3·3
Venereal Disease - - - - - -	4	2	6	·4	·8	·4
Self-Abuse (Sexual) - - - - -	5	–	5	·5	–	·4
Overwork - - - - - - -	41	1	42	4·1	·4	3·4
Sunstroke - - - - - - -	33	5	38	3·3	2·1	3·1
Accident or Injury - - - - -	56	1	57	5·6	·4	4·6
Pregnancy - - - - - -	–	1	1	–	·4	·0
Puerperal - - - - - - -	–	4	4	–	1·7	·3
Lactation - - - - - - -	–	1	1	–	·4	·0
Puberty, and Change of Life - - -	–	10	10	–	4·2	·8
Uterine Disorders - - - - -	1	1	2	·1	·4	·1
Fevers - - - - - - - -	2	–	2	·2	–	·1
Other Bodily Diseases or Disorders, including Old Age.	14	5	19	1·4	2·1	1·5
Hereditary, with other ascertained cause in combination.	64	6	70	6·4	2·5	5·7
Hereditary, other combined cause not ascertained.	25	8	33	2·5	3·4	2·7
Congenital, with other ascertained cause in combination.	2	–	2	·2	–	·1
Congenital, other combined cause not ascertained.	2	2	4	·2	·8	·3
Other ascertained causes - - - -	4	2	6	·4	·8	·4

In the cases of 178 General Paralytics (142 males and 36 females) the cause of insanity was stated to be unknown.

* This table may be compared with Table XIV. in last year's Report, which shows the Causes of Insanity in the cases of *all* the patients admitted during 1876.

54 *Thirty-First Report of the Commissioners in Lunacy*, HMSO, 1877, p. 34.

between social and natural was not so clear cut at this time, as categories such as 'intemperance of drinking' and 'intemperance – sexual' were included in the physical section of the tables. Stages of life such as 'old age' and 'puberty' were included in the Table of the Causes, as were categories related to reproduction as in Skae's classification, including 'pregnancy', 'lactation' and 'puerperal' states.[55] Physical problems like 'uterine disorders' and 'venereal disease' sat alongside categories like 'sunstroke', 'accident or injury' and 'sexual self-abuse'.[56]

Crude early demographic exercises in the form of proportions of asylum inmates to the general population were published during the Victorian period. They were construed by the Lunacy Commission as studies that attempted to make sense of the proportion of lunatics to the rest of the population. Although broader social questions such as increases in insanity were of interest to the Lunacy Commission in an abstract sense, practical considerations were the determining factor in working towards collating national data on asylum numbers. For example, the commission wanted to develop means to predict 'the probable prospective requirements of each county in the way of future accommodation of the insane poor'.[57] The following year, the tables for medical statistics were expanded upon to include national statistics on psychological diagnosis (see Table 6.12). The 1878 report showed statistics on diagnosis for people deemed to be displaying 'suicidal tendencies', and these were broken down into the diagnostic categories that were recommended in the first report of 1845.

The statistics on diagnosis amongst patients with suicidal propensities were some of the earliest statistical tables published in the Lunacy Reports that broke down national patient data according to psychological diagnosis. It set the template for subsequent reports, and in 1879 a table displaying the rate of diagnosis for all patients in asylums in England and Wales was published (see Table 6.13). Between 1879 and 1900, information on diagnosis would be presented in yearly reports of the Lunacy Commission of England and Wales.[58] During these years, statistics on diagnosis were broken down into the categories of mania, melancholia,

55 *Thirty-First Report of the Commissioners in Lunacy*, HMSO, 1877, p. 34.

56 Ibid.

57 Ibid.

58 For detailed information on these tables, see: 'General Statistics' in *Thirty-Seventh Report of the Commissioners in Lunacy*, 1883, pp. 3–5.

Table 6.11 Forms of mental disorder and suicidal propensity: from the Report of the Commissioners in Lunacy for the year 1878[59]

Table XXVII – Showing the Number of Patients with Suicidal Propensity who were admitted to County and Borough Asylums, Registered Hospitals, Naval and Military Hospitals, State Asylums and Licensed Houses for the Year 1878, arranged according to their Forms of Mental Disorder									
Form of Mental Disorder	Total Number of Patients Admitted During 1878			Number with Suicidal Propensity			Proportion per Cent. of the Number with Suicidal Propensity to the Total Number.		
	M	F	T	M	F	T	M	F	T
Mania	3,491	3,674	7,165	740	847	1,587	21.1	23	22.1
Melancholia	1,224	1,649	2,873	757	974	1,731	61.8	59	60.2
Dementia									
Ordinary	1,192	697	1,889	194	118	312	16.2	16.9	16.5
Senile	222	286	508	38	51	89	17.1	17.8	17.5
Congenital Insanity (including idiocy and other mental defects from birth or infancy)	452	275	727	33	23	56	7.3	8.3	7.7
Other Forms of Insanity	85	62	147	20	14	34	23.5	22.5	23.1
Total	6,666	6,643	13,309	1,782	2,027	3,800	26.7	30.5	28.6

59 *Thirty-Second Report of the Commissioners in Lunacy*, *HMSO*, 1878, pp. 46–47.

Table 6.12 Table XVII: Showing the FORMS of MENTAL DISORDER in the Patients admitted into County and Borough Asylums, Registered Hospitals, Naval and Military Hospitals, State Asylums and Licensed Houses during the year 1879; arranged according to CLASS of the Patient[60]

Table XVII: Showing the FORMS of MENTAL DISORDER in the Patients admitted into County and Borough Asylums, Registered Hospitals, Naval and Military Hospitals, State Asylums, and Licensed Houses during the year 1879; arranged according to CLASS of the Patients.																		
Year	Number of Patients Admitted									Proportion per cent. to the Total Number Admitted								
	Private			Pauper			Total			Private			Pauper			Total		
	M	F	T	M	F	T	M	F	T	M	F	T	M	F	T	M	F	T
Mania	576	485	1,061	2,777	3,146	5,923	3,353	3,631	6,984	51.7	50.3	51.1	52.8	54.6	53.7	52.6	54.0	53.3
Melancholia	244	333	577	964	1,482	2,446	1,208	1,15	3,023	21.9	34.5	27.8	18.3	25.7	22.2	28.9	27.0	23.1
Dementia (ordinary)	125	59	184	924	611	1,535	1,049	670	1,719	11.2	6.1	8.8	17.6	10.6	13.9	16.4	10.0	13.1
Dementia (senile)	18	17	35	228	276	504	246	293	539	1.6	1.8	1.7	4.3	4.8	4.6	3.9	4.3	4.1
Congenital Insanity (including Idiocy, and other mental defects from Birth or Infancy)	130	56	186	256	192	448	386	248	634	11.7	5.8	8.9	4.9	3.3	4.1	6.1	3.7	4.8
Other Forms of Insanity	21	14	35	113	54	167	134	68	202	1.9	1.5	1.7	2.1	1.0	1.5	2.1	1.0	1.6
Total	1,114	964	2,078	5,262	5,761	11,023	6,376	6,725	13,101	100	100	100	100	100	100	100	100	100

60 *Thirty-Fourth report of the Commissioners in Lunacy*, HMSO, 1879.

congenital insanity and dementia which had two forms: ordinary and senile. The sub-categories of aetiology introduced by the MPA in their 1882 Revisions were not used in Lunacy Commission reports and do not appear to have been put into practice as intended. The classification that was used in Lunacy Commission reports included what Susan Leigh Star terms a residual category of 'Other Forms of Insanity', and it is a sign perhaps of the effectiveness of the classification that between 10 and 25% of cases were consistently included in this residual category.[61] In 1899, the tables would be slightly modified to show breakdowns in the diagnosis of admissions by month with averages for the year 1897 being presented, and in the 1900 report these displayed the figures across three years (Table 6.14).[62]

The 1901 report presented yearly statistics from 1899, with a slightly revised table that had split dementia into four forms instead of two, with primary and secondary added, and ordinary dementia replaced by organic dementia. Statistics on diagnosis would be broken down according to these categories until the 1907 Revision to the Table of the Forms, detailed in the previous chapter. In the three years from 1899 to 1901, melancholia and mania had accounted for 70% of cases alone, and both had higher rates of diagnosis in women.[63] The following year, the report noted that 'there would appear to have been a certain decrease in maniacal and an increase in melancholic types' and reiterated the claim from the 1902 report that diagnosis for mania and melancholia had been higher amongst women, whilst general paralysis and dementia had higher rates of diagnosis amongst men.[64] The report published two tables, one showing the admissions diagnosis average between the years 1899 and 1902, and the second showing the diagnosis data for 1903 alone. The report for 1903 provided considerations on the rate of insanity compared to the rest of the population, with charts that depicted ratios of the insane within an asylum as a proportion of the general population.[65] These were accompanied by lengthy passages on the relative worth of the expansion of the

[61] Susan Leigh Star, 'Residual Categories: Silence, Absence and Being an Other' in *Zeitschrift für Medien- und Kulturforschung*, 2010, no. 1.

[62] *Fifty-Third Report of the Commissioners in Lunacy*, HMSO, 1899, p. 122.

[63] *Fifty-Sixth Report of the Commissioners in Lunacy*, HMSO, p. 10.

[64] *Fifty-Seventh Report of the Commissioners in Lunacy*, HMSO, p. 15.

[65] *Fifty-Eighth Report of the Commissioners in Lunacy*, HMSO, 1904, pp. 1–10.

asylum system: the Commissioners expressed concern about the ability of expanding institutions to take care of the pauper insane which was motivated by the cost of maintaining an asylum population in an expanded system (Fig. 6.1, Table 6.15, and Fig. 6.2).

Despite these advances in asylum medical statistics, insanity was still being used as a catch-all term in statistical investigation. The identification of the dividing line between sanity and insanity for the most part informs statistical enquiry, with investigations from beyond medicine and lunacy administration rarely utilising breakdowns of insanity into different forms. The assistant to William Farr at the General Registry Office (GRO), Noel Humphreys, in his 1890 paper on statistics in England, articulated

Table 6.13 Forms of Mental Disorder in Admissions, Fifty-fifth Report of the Commissioners in Lunacy[66]

Table XXV – Showing the FORMS of MENTAL DISORDER in the Patients admitted to County and Borough Asylums, Registered Hospitals, State Asylums, and Licensed House during the YEAR **1899**						
Forms of Mental Disorder	Number of Patients Admitted					
	Private			Pauper		
	M	T	F	M	T	F
Congenital, or infantile mental deficiency	37	16	53	517	410	957
Mania, either acute, chronic, or recurrent	345	511	856	3,452	3,843	7,205
Melancholia	280	416	702	1,787	2,907	4,694
Delusional Insanity	82	104	186	290	291	581
General Insanity of the Insane	120	11	131	897	200	1,097
Primary Dementia	97	17	114	219	276	495
Secondary Dementia	34	18	52	460	257	717
Senile Dementia	35	27	62	435	438	873
Organic Dementia	7	6	13	126	64	190
Total	1,043	1,126	2,169	8,213	8,086	16,899

66 *Fifty-Fifth Report of the Commissioners in Lunacy*, HMSO, 1901.

Table 6.14 'Appendix A to the Fifty-fourth Report of the Commissioners in Lunacy for the year 1900 – Table XVI' (Admissions broken down by psychological diagnosis)[67]

122 *Appendix A. to Fifty-fourth Report of the Commissioners in Lunacy.*

TABLE XVI.—Showing the Annual Average of the NUMBER of PATIENTS admitted into INSTITUTIONS for the INSANE in England and Wales

Forms of Mental Disorder.	January.			February.			March.			April.			May.			June		
	M.	F.	T.	M.	F.	T.	M.	F.	T.	M.	F.	T.	M.	F.	T.	M.	F.	T.
Mania - - - - - - -	384	375	759	307	340	647	386	372	758	354	411	765	393	438	831	413	382	795
Melancholia - - - - - -	184	251	435	159	214	373	194	249	443	193	209	402	199	308	507	189	282	471
Ordinary Dementia - - -	112	65	177	92	59	151	117	64	181	101	70	171	114	75	189	103	67	170
Senile Dementia - - - -	40	47	87	34	36	70	39	39	78	38	44	82	44	47	91	35	38	73
Congenital Insanity - - -	Omitted.		–	–	–	–	–	–	–	–	–	–	–	–	–	–	–	–
Other Forms - - - - -	34	22	56	27	22	49	26	24	50	25	24	49	27	21	48	22	24	46
TOTAL (excluding Congenital Insanity) - - -	754	760	1,514	619	671	1,290	762	748	1,510	711	818	1,529	777	889	1,666	762	793	1,555

Daily Average of the Number admitted in each Month (calculated upon the Average Number of Days in each Month, excluding Sundays). The Monthly

Forms of Mental Disorder.	January, 27 Days.			February, 24 Days.			March, 26 Days.			April, 26 Days.			May, 26 Days.			June, 26 Days.		
	M.	F.	T.	M.	F.	T.	M.	F.	T.	M.	F.	T.	M.	F.	T.	M.	F.	T.
Mania - - - - - - -	14·2	13·9	28·1	12·8	14·2	27·0	14·8	14·5	29·2	13·6	15·8	29·4	15·1	16·8	32·0	15·9	14·7	30·6
Melancholia - - - - - -	6·8	9·3	16·1	6·6	8·9	15·5	7·5	9·6	17·0	7·4	10·3	17·8	7·7	11·8	19·5	7·3	10·8	18·1
Ordinary Dementia - - -	4·1	2·4	6·6	3·8	2·5	6·3	4·5	2·5	7·0	3·9	2·6	6·6	4·4	2·9	7·3	4·0	2·6	6·5
Senile Dementia - - - -	1·5	1·7	3·2	1·6	1·3	2·9	1·5	1·5	3·0	1·5	1·7	3·2	1·7	1·8	3·5	1·3	1·5	2·8
Congenital Insanity - - -	Omitted.		–	–	–	–	–	–	–	–	–	–	–	–	–	–	–	–
Other Forms - - - - -	1·3	·8	2·1	1·1	·9	2·0	1·0	·9	1·9	1·0	·9	1·9	1·0	·8	1·8	·8	·9	1·8
TOTAL (excluding Congenital Insanity) - - -	27·9	28·1	56·1	25·8	28·0	53·8	29·3	28·8	58·1	27·3	31·5	58·8	29·9	34·2	64·1	29·3	30·5	59·8

67 *Fifty-Fourth Report of the Commissioners in Lunacy*, HMSO, 1900, p. 122.

in each Month during the Years **1895, 1896,** and **1897,** and suffering from the following assigned Forms of MENTAL DISORDER.

July.			August.			September.			October.			November.			December.			TOTAL.			Forms of Mental Disorder.
M.	F.	T.	M.	F.	T.	M.	F.	T.	M.	F.	T.	M.	F.	T.	M.	F.	T.	M.	F.	T.	
397	402	799	356	335	691	332	352	684	358	345	703	344	351	695	342	378	720	4,366	4,481	8,347	Mania.
192	316	508	170	257	427	152	240	392	174	227	401	163	248	411	167	249	416	2,136	3,110	5,246	Melancholia.
118	64	182	96	66	162	93	60	153	96	58	154	94	59	153	104	66	170	1,240	773	2,013	Ordinary Dementia.
39	44	83	35	32	67	36	31	67	38	39	77	32	44	76	43	40	83	453	481	934	Senile Dementia.
–	–	–	–	–	–	–	–	–	–	–	–	–	–	–	–	–	–	–	–	–	Congenital Insanity.
29	20	49	24	20	44	26	15	41	25	27	52	19	22	41	25	23	48	309	264	573	Other Forms.
775	846	1,621	681	710	1,391	639	698	1,337	691	696	1,387	652	724	1,376	681	756	1,437	8,504	9,109	17,613	TOTAL (excluding Congenital Insanity).

Averages which are above the Yearly Average are printed in thick type, and those not above the Yearly Average in thin type.

July, 27 Days.			August, 26 Days.			September, 26 Days.			October, 27 Days.			November, 26 Days.			December, 27 Days.			Daily Average for the whole Year (excluding Sundays), i.e., 313 Days.			Forms of Mental Disorder.
M.	F.	T.	M.	F.	T.	M.	F.	T.	M.	F.	T.	M.	F.	T.	M.	F.	T.	M.	F.	T.	
14·7	**14·9**	**29·6**	13·7	12·9	26·6	12·8	13·5	26·3	13·3	12·8	26·0	13·2	13·5	26·7	12·7	14·0	26·7	13·9	14·3	28·3	Mania.
7·1	**11·7**	**18·8**	6·5	9·9	16·4	5·8	9·2	15·1	6·4	8·4	14·9	6·3	9·5	15·8	6·2	9·2	15·4	6·8	9·9	16·8	Melancholia.
4·4	2·4	**6·7**	3·7	2·5	6·2	3·6	2·3	5·9	3·6	2·1	5·7	3·6	2·3	5·9	3·9	2·4	6·3	4·0	2·5	6·4	Ordinary Dementia.
1·4	**·6**	**3·1**	1·3	1·2	2·6	1·4	1·2	2·6	1·4	1·4	2·9	1·2	**1·7**	2·9	**1·6**	1·5	**3·1**	1·4	1·5	3·0	Senile Dementia.
–	–	–	–	–	–	–	–	–	–	–	–	–	–	–	–	–	–	–	–	–	Congenital Insanity.
1	7	1·8	·9	·8	1·7	1·0	·6	1·6	·9	**1·0**	**1·9**	·7	·8	1·6	·9	**·9**	1·8	1·0	·8	1·8	Other Forms.
28·7	**31·3**	**60·0**	26·2	27·3	53·5	24·6	26·8	51·4	25·6	25·8	51·4	25·1	27·8	52·9	25·2	25·0	53·2	27·2	29·1	56·3	TOTAL (excluding Congenital Insanity).

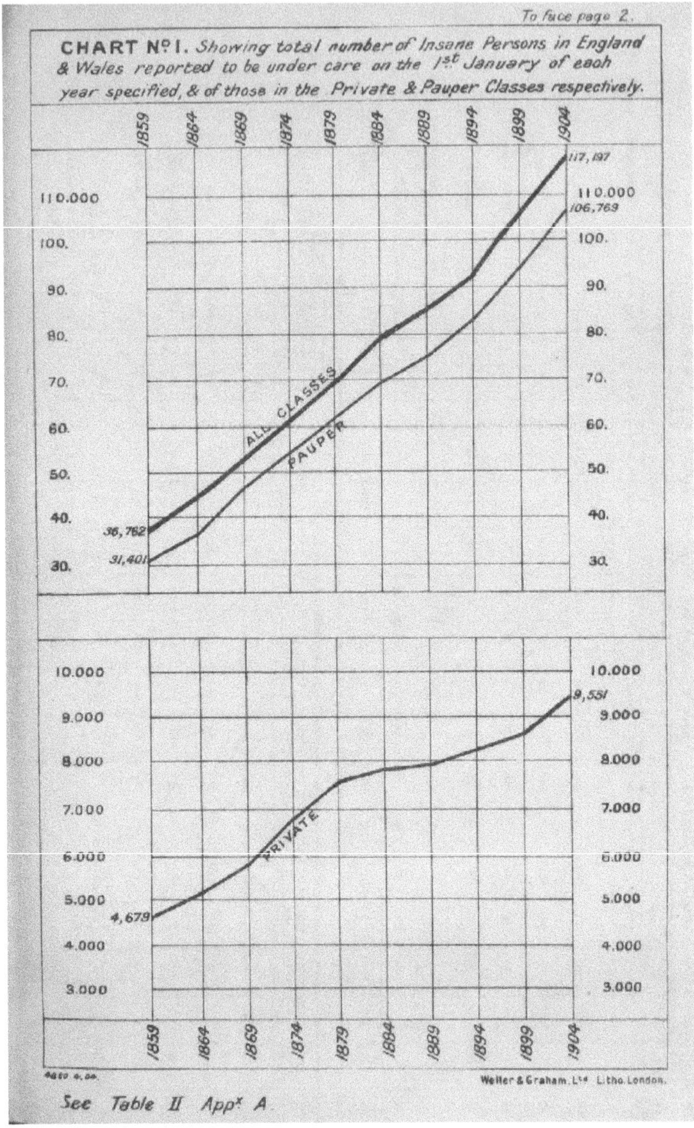

Fig. 6.1 Showing total number of insane persons, from the Report of the *Commissioners in Lunacy*, 1904[68]

[68] *Fifty Eighth Report of the Commissioners in Lunacy*, HMSO, 1904, p. 3.

Table 6.15 Forms of mental disorder from the Report of the Commissioners in Lunacy for 1881[69]

Table XVII: Showing the FORMS of MENTAL DISORDER in the Patients admitted into County and Borough Asylums, Registered Hospitals, Naval and Military Hospitals, State Asylums, and Licensed Houses during the year 1879; arranged according to CLASS of the Patients.

Forms of Mental Disorder	Number of Patients Admitted									Proportion per cent. to the Total Number Admitted								
	Private			Pauper			Total			Private			Pauper			Total		
	M	F	T	M	F	T	M	F	T	M	F	T	M	F	T	M	F	T
Mania	576	485	1,061	2,777	3,146	5,923	3,353	3,631	6,984	51.7	50.3	51.1	52.8	54.6	53.7	52.6	54.0	53.3
Melancholia	244	333	577	964	1,482	2,446	1,208	1,15	3,023	21.9	34.5	27.8	18.3	25.7	22.2	28.9	27.0	23.1
Dementia (ordinary)	125	59	184	924	611	1,535	1,049	670	1,719	11.2	6.1	8.8	17.6	10.6	13.9	16.4	10.0	13.1
Dementia (senile)	18	17	35	228	276	504	246	293	539	1.6	1.8	1.7	4.3	4.8	4.6	3.9	4.3	4.1
Congenital Insanity (including Idiocy, and other mental defects from Birth or Infancy)	130	56	186	256	192	448	386	248	634	11.7	5.8	8.9	4.9	3.3	4.1	6.1	3.7	4.8
Other Forms of Insanity	21	14	35	113	54	167	134	68	202	1.9	1.5	1.7	2.1	1.0	1.5	2.1	1.0	1.6
Total	1,114	964	2,078	5,262	5,761	11,023	6,376	6,725	13,101	100	100	100	100	100	100	100	100	100

69 Thirty-Fourth Report of the Commissioners in Lunacy, HMSO, 1881, p. 36.

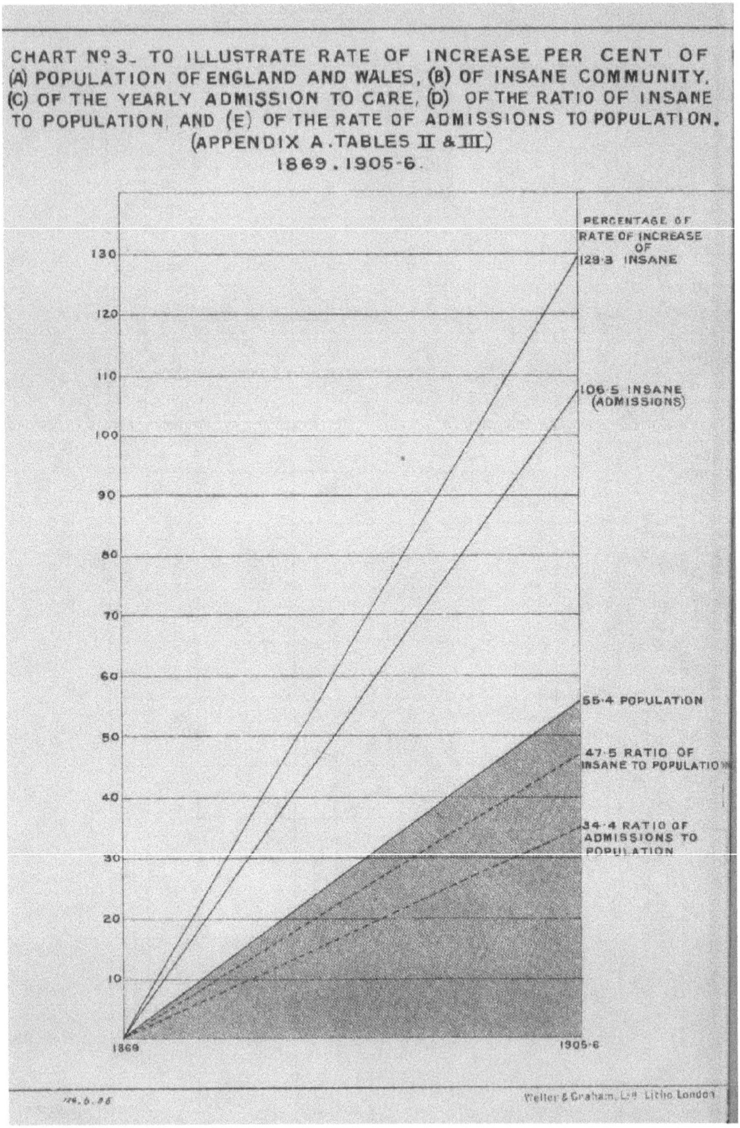

Fig. 6.2 Rate of increase of insanity from the Report of the Commissioners in Lunacy for the year 1906[70]

[70] *Sixtieth Report of the Commissioners in Lunacy*, HMSO, 1906, p. 6.

the rationale for using a unitary concept of insanity in his study on its increase:[71]

> It should moreover be explained that the word insanity is used in this paper as a generic term, signifying all forms of mental unsoundness, and includes all degrees and all varieties of mental unsoundness, which is classed, by the various authorities called upon to deal with the insane, as lunacy, idiocy, or imbecility. In the Census Report for 1881, it was pointed out that no accurate line of demarcation can be drawn between the general conditions indicated by the terms lunatic, idiot and imbecile; although generally speaking, the term lunatic is used to describe persons suffering from the more acute forms of mental disease; idiot to describe those suffering from congenital mental deficiency; and imbecile, to describe persons suffering later in life from chronic dementia.[72]

In response to Humphreys, the asylum medical superintendent George Savage observed that the lack of any kind of differentiation of the forms of insanity risked making any findings from studies using a unitary concept of insanity misleading and erroneous:

> he felt the futility of collecting statistics, for it might be that though there was no great increase of insanity as [qua] insanity, the form of mental disorder was changing for the worse. Insanity being, as Dr Tuke had said, a relative term, there are a large number of persons who are on the borderland, who are or are not lunatics according to the convenience or affluence of their friends. The statistics with regards to the persons found lunatics and recognised as such by the Commissioners' report are of importance; but it is of still greater importance to remember that the forms of insanity differed greatly in their gravity. If, for instance, there were no increase in the number of the insane, but if the form of insanity was getting worse, then there would be cause for very much greater alarm than if the numbers were not increased and the form of insanity was worse, but unfortunately

[71] Simon Szreter, *Fertility, Class and Gender in Britain, 1860–1940*, Cambridge, 1996, p. 79.

[72] Noel A. Humphreys, 'Statistics of Insanity in England, with Special Reference to Its Alleged Increasing Prevalence' in *Journal of the Royal Statistical Society*, vol. 53, no. 2, June 1890, pp. 201–252.

> he was not in a position to back it up with statistics. The addition of new statistical tables was endless, and each new one suggested others.[73]

The 'borderland' Savage referred to was the realm that existed between sanity and insanity, and may include people who have fared well enough outside an asylum, but may have been admitted to an asylum had they actually been inspected by a clinician. Given this, these individuals would therefore would not be represented in statistics that relied on asylum admissions data and statistical returns.[74] The danger posed by the borderland was bound up in Victorian anxieties over degeneration, both in the immediate-future because of the problem of criminal behaviour that many thought was linked to the borderland of insanity, and in the long-term due to the possibility that such individuals would pass on their faulty constitution to their offspring. The need to identify the early signs of insanity in order to recognise 'peculiar' lineages and identify individuals who 'do sometimes inherit a positive tendency to a particular nervous disease' was emphasised by Henry Maudsley in 1895.[75] The borderland proved an obstacle to this task because there were no means available to identify the many individuals who inhabited it.

Before we move on to discuss the developments linked to the definitions and categories of insanity used in asylum medical statistics during the first decades of the twentieth century, it is important to note that much of the assessment of lunacy reports presented in this chapter is related to those for England and Wales. This is principally for concision's sake, since there are many divergences between those of Scotland and Ireland; as Farquarson's detailed account of the Scottish system shows, there are significant differences between the history of asylums in Scotland and in England and Wales, with Scotland having a separate Poor Law system and a distinct Lunacy Commission.[76] The diagnostic categories used in

[73] George Savage, remarks recorded in discussion in response to Noel A. Humphreys, 'Statistics of Insanity in England, with Special Reference to its Alleged Increasing Prevalence' in *Journal of the Royal Statistical Society*, vol. 53, no. 2, June 1890, pp. 201–252 (p. 248).

[74] Mark Jackson, *The Borderland of Imbecility: Medicine, Society and the Fabrication of the Feeble Mind in Late Victorian England*, Manchester University Press, 2000, pp. 10–15.

[75] Henry Maudsley, *Responsibility in Mental Disease*, D. Appleton & Company, 1895, pp. 34–40.

[76] Lauren Farquharson, 'A 'Scottish Poor Law of Lunacy'? Poor Law, Lunacy Law and Scotland's Parochial Asylums' in *History of Psychiatry*, vol. 28, no. 11, 2017, pp. 15–28.

Scottish asylums are linked to the ones developed by the MPA, but there were attempts to implement Skae's classification of aetiology as the standard for medical statistics, despite it never being formally adopted by the Association: at Skae's former asylum in Edinburgh run by Clouston, the classification of causes was used to diagnose admissions until the beginning of the twentieth century. As we have seen, Clouston was adamant that Skae's aetiology was the best available and insisted on using his classification, with the statistics on psychological diagnosis according to both his own and the MPA 1882 Revision being published in reports of the Morningside asylum (Tables 6.16 and 6.17). Indeed, it was only when Clouston retired in 1909 and was replaced by George Robertson that admissions were no longer classified under Skae's classification and solely according to a classification that resembled that published by the MPA in 1907 (Table 6.18). Finally, the Scottish Lunacy Reports also did not use the 1907 Revisions of the MPA Tables and instead kept to a simpler classification as late as their 1909 Report (Table 6.19).

Peak and Decline: Psychological Diagnosis and Asylum Statistics 1900–1928

The turn of the century saw a transition between the classifications used in Victorian asylums and the beginning of the dominance of Kraepelinian concepts of psychopathology. Dementia praecox and manic depressive insanity promised an insight into the outlook of a patient and had been arrived at by statistical investigation. They would be enthusiastically received in the United Kingdom, with diagnosis based on prediction being prominent in the Association's 1907 Revision, seen most starkly with the inclusion of Kraepelin's primary dementia and alternating insanity. The introduction of a medical register in 1907 to further improve standardisation in statistical returns marked a turning point, albeit brief, in asylum statistics and mental health records. As a result of the introduction of the medical register, statistics presented in Lunacy Commission reports up until the outbreak of war in 1914 saw a greater level of detail and sophistication than had previously been seen, with more sophisticated forecasts and projections of patient numbers beginning to appear. The Association's classification would be adopted by the Commissioners in Lunacy at the quarterly meeting in November 1906, with Hayes Newington announcing that the statistical tables had been formally adopted by the association and would be published in

Table 6.16 Forms of Insanity in those Admitted [diagnosed according to] Skae's Classification in the *Seventy Sixth Annual Report of the Royal Edinburgh Asylum for the Insane, 1888*[77]

Table XIII

Forms of Insanity in those Admitted – Skae's Classification

	Males	Females	Total
Congenital Insanity	4	2	6
Epileptic Insanity	9	4	13
Insanity of Puberty	1	0	1
Insanity of Adolescence	15	16	31
Climacteric Insanity	0	21	21
Senile Insanity	5	15	20
Insanity of Pregnancy	0	2	2
Puerperal Insanity	0	8	8
Insanity of Lactation	0	7	7
Ovarian Insanity	0	1	1
Anaemic Insanity	0	2	2
Insanity of Masturbation	2	0	2
General Paralysis	19	2	21
Insanity from Brian Disease	6	10	16
Traumatic Insanity	0	1	1
Phthistical Insanity	6	2	8
Insanity of Cocaine Habit	1	0	1
Insanity of Alcoholism	25	15	40
Post-febrile Insanity	1	1	2
Idiopathic Insanity	18	22	40
Insanity after Surgical Operations	2	1	3
Insanity of Heart Disease	1	0	1
Insanity of Deprivation of the Senses	0	1	1
Insanity of Bright's Disease	0	1	1
Unknown	56	42	98
Total	171*	176	347*
*One male not insane			

[77] *The Seventy Sixth Annual Report of the Royal Edinburgh Asylum for the Insane, Morningside*, 1889, p. 47.

Table 6.17 Forms of Insanity in those Admitted [diagnosed according to] the MPA's Classification in the *Seventy-Sixth Annual Report of the Royal Edinburgh Asylum for the Insane, 1888*[78]

TABLE XI – Showing the Form of Mental Disorder on Admission in the Admission, Recoveries and Deaths of the Year 1888, and the Form of Mental Disorder of the Inmates on 31st December 1888.

Forms of Mental Disorder	Admissions			Recoveries			Deaths			Remaining in Asylums |[diagnosis as of] Dec. 31 1888		
	M	F	T	M	F	T	M	F	T	M	F	T
Congenital or Infantile Mental Deficiency												
a) with epilepsy	2	1	3	0	0	0	0	0	0	4	0	4
b) without epilepsy	2	1	3	0	0	0	1	0	1	7	4	11
Epilepsy acquired	9	4	13	3	0	3	0	1	1	28	22	50
General Paralysis of the Insane	19	2	21	0	0	0	11	2	13	28	5	33
Mania												
Simple	49	46	95	23	14	37	7	15	22	62	50	112
Acute	5	31	36	1	15	16	0	7	7	4	12	16
Delusional	8	11	19	3	5	8	1	1	2	52	52	104
Chronic	0	5	5	0	0	0	0	2	2	16	84	100
Homicidal	1	1	2	0	0	0	0	0	0	3	1	4
Melancholia												
Simple	33	23	56	8	14	22	6	3	9	30	22	52
Hypochondriacal	4	3	7	1	0	1	1	0	1	11	3	14
Delusional	7	15	22	1	2	3	0	0	0	25	30	55
Excited	3	8	11	1	2	3	1	3	4	2	6	8
Suicidal	21	12	33	10	5	15	2	3	5	12	9	21
Resistive	2	9	11	1	2	3	1	2	3	3	13	16
Organic	1	0	1	1	1	2	2	0	2	0	0	0
Dementia												
Secondary	5	4	9	0	0	0	3	4	7	128	98	226
Organic	0	0	0	0	0	0	0	0	0	0	0	0
Total	171*	176	347*	53	60	113	36	43	79	415	411	826

*One Male not Insane

78 *The Seventy Sixth Annual Report of the Royal Edinburgh Asylum for the Insane, Morningside*, 1889, p. 45.

Table 6.18 Showing the form of Mental Disorder amongst on Admission in the Admissions, Recoveries and Deaths to the Royal Edinburgh Asylum, Morningside, 1913[79]

TABLE XI – Showing the form of the Mental Disorder on Admission, in the Admissions, Recoveries and Deaths of the Year 1913										
Form of Mental Disorder		Admissions			Recoveries			Deaths		
		M	F	T	M	F	T	M	F	T
Melancholia	Manic Depressive Insanity	16	53	49	5	14	19	3	5	8
Mania		8	13	21	6	7	13	4	12	16
Infective Exhaustive Insanity		18	26	44	11	9	20	3	9	12
Dementia Praecox		25	7	32	2	0	2	1	0	1
Systematised Delusional Insanity		13	17	30	2	0	2	6	2	8
General Paralysis of the Insane		18	4	22	0	0	0	19	3	22
Epileptic Insanity		4	3	7	0	0	0	1	0	1
Korsakoff's Psychosis		3	0	3	1	0	1	0	0	0
Insanity of Gross Brain Disease		1	0	1	0	0	0	1	0	1
Morphiomania		2	1	3	2	0	2	0	0	0
Senile Insanity		15	9	24	0	0	0	7	5	12
Congenital Defect		2	0	2	0	0	0	0	1	1
Total		125	113	238	29	30	59	45	37	82

Table 6.19 Mental defects and disorders[80]

Table III | Mental Defects and Disorders			From which 108 Patients entered upon the Register in 1908, suffered.					
COUNTIES	Imbecility, congenital or acquired in early life	Dementia	Senile or Organic	Mania or Melancholia	Delusional	Other Forms | Ill defined	Total	Percentage of Imbecility
Perth	8	12	1	0	2	0	23	34
Banff	6	4	2	1	1	0	14	43
Western Isles	7	1	1	2	1	0	12	58
Inverness	6	2	1	0	2	0	11	54
Ross	4	1	1	1	0	0	7	57
Aberdeen	6	2	2	1	0	1	12	50
Forfar	4	2	0	0	1	1	8	50
Caithness	5	3	0	0	1	0	9	55
Kinross	0	4	0	0	1	1	6	0
Other 5 Counties*	5	1	0	0	0	0	6	99
Totals	51	32	8	5	9	3	198	47
* Elgin, Sutherland, Nairn, Clackmannan and Kincardine								

79 *The One-Hundred and First Report of the Royal Edinburgh Asylum, Morningside*, 1913.

80 *Fifty-First report of the General Board of Commissioners of Lunacy for Scotland*, Neil and Co. for HMSO 1909, p. 150.

1907.[81] The new medical registers that had been devised by the revisions committee to standardise and improve the recording of medical data would be distributed to asylum medical superintendents as part of the annual statistical returns. This would include the revised Table of the Forms, and the Schedule of Causes and Associated Factors of Mental Disorder, both of which would be used in returns until the outbreak of war.

From 1908 until 1914 then, the 1907 Revision would structure admissions diagnosis figures, with three tables being published including national figures on psychological diagnosis amongst pauper and private patients. *The Report of the Commissioners* for the year 1908 contained a lengthy analysis of the forms of mental disorder admitted to asylums. This would be repeated each year until the powers of lunacy administration were handed over to the Board of Control in 1914. In a move away from the language of forms and towards the language of different types or kinds of insanity, the 1908 report stated that 'in the case of so complex a condition as insanity, the tendency must be towards increasing differentiation of types'.[82] It also described the 1907 Revision as a work in symptomology and acknowledged the difficulty of arriving at one classification given that 'there have been almost as many different classifications of the forms of insanity as there have been writers on the subject'.[83] The 1908 report states that the 1907 Revision was adopted principally for practical reasons because 'any alternative would have only resulted in difficulty and confusion'.[84] Seeking to allay fears that the expanded classification would itself cause confusion with its additional categories and sub-categories, the report justified the additions by describing them as 'well defined and recognisable', with it singling out moral insanity for special mention (Table 6.20):

> The need for such an expansion and separation of recognisable conditions from hitherto established forms must have been obviously due to a desire for more accurate definition and record; whilst the introduction into the list

[81] Dr Hayes Newington, remarks recorded in 'The Medico-Psychological Association of Great Britain and Ireland: Quarterly Meeting November 15th 1906' in *JMS*, vol. 53, no. 220, January 1907, pp. 214–217 (p. 215).

[82] *The Sixty-Third Annual Report of the Commissioners in Lunacy*, HMSO, 1909, p. 24.

[83] Ibid.

[84] Ibid.

> of moral imbecility and moral insanity is significant of prevailing scientific opinion upon a much-debated question of far-reaching importance.[85]

The new tables on psychological diagnosis were divided into classes of patient and gender, and into separate tables showing admissions for those who had suffered their first and not-first attack.[86] Another table displaying percentage distribution in each age-group of first attacks was included that was broken down according to diagnostic category. In an analysis of the figures, the report arrived at the finding that 'in both classes the proportion of males was higher than that of females in the congenital forms', whilst of the forms occurring later in life, there were greater numbers of female patients diagnosed with mania and melancholia both amongst the private and pauper classes.[87] Amongst private voluntary patients there were higher proportions of cases of delusional insanity and primary dementia in males than in females, but no marked differences in pauper patients. The analysis goes on when presenting percentage distribution in each period:

> It will be seen that in each age-period cases of mania and melancholia were, with two exceptions, by far the most numerous of any of the forms of insanity. These exceptions were in the age-periods 35 to 44, and 45 to 54, where in the male sex general paralysis predominated, especially in the former of these two periods. In the age-period — 'under 25' — apart from mania and melancholia, the chief incidence was in cases of insanity with epilepsy, primary dementia, and stupor for each sex; in the period — 25 to 34 — general paralysis, delusional insanity, and insanity with epilepsy in males, delusional insanity, insanity with epilepsy, and stupor in females; from 35 to 44 there is the same relative prevalence in the male cases, whilst in females delusional insanity was about twice as frequent as either general paralysis, insanity with epilepsy, or confusional insanity. In the next age-period — 45 to 54 — we find cases of secondary dementia, as well as of confusional insanity, approximating or exceeding those of primary dementia and epileptic insanity; whilst in the final period (55 and upwards), when general paralysis is comparatively rare, and mania and melancholia below the mean, the chief place is taken by senile dementia, which accounts

[85] Ibid.

[86] Ibid.

[87] Ibid., p. 26.

Table 6.20 The Forms of Insanity in all Direct Admissions from the year 1907 [The First Statistical Tables on Psychological Diagnosis Using the 1907 Revision] in *The Sixty-Third Annual report of the Commissioners in Lunacy* [for the year 1909][88]

TABLE XIX: Showing the Forms of Insanity in the cases of ALL DIRECT Hospitals, Naval and Military Hospitals, State Asylums, County and Borough Asylums and Licenced Houses: arranged according to age																					
Forms of Insanity	Ages																				
	Under 15			15 – 19			21 – 24			35 – 44			45 – 54			55 – 64			+65		
	M	F	T	M	F	T	M	F	T	M	F	T	M	F	T	M	F	T	M	F	T
I. CONGENITAL OR INFANTILE MENTAL DEFICIENCY (IDIOCY OR IMBECILITY) OCCURRING AS EARLY IN LIFE AS IT CAN BE OBSERVED :-																					
Intellectual																					
With Epilepsy																					
Without Epilepsy																					
Moral																					
II. INSANITY OCCURRING LATER IN LIFE:-																					
Insanity with Epilepsy																					
General Paralysis of the Insane																					
Insanity with the grosser Brain Lesion s																					
Acute Delirium (Acute Delirious Mania)																					
Confusional Insanity																					
Stupor																					
Primary Dementia																					
Mania																					
Recent																					
Chronic																					
Recurrent																					
Melancholia																					
Recent																					
Chronic																					
Recurrent																					
Alternating Insanity																					
Delusional Insanity																					
Systematised																					
Non-systematised																					
Volitional Insanity																					
Impulse																					
Obsession																					
Doubt																					
Moral Insanity																					
Dementia																					
Senile																					
Secondary or Terminal																					
Total																					

[88] Ibid, pp. 184–185.

> for nearly one-third of the total admissions at this age. [At 65 years and upwards the numbers admitted under this head were more than one-half of the total.] Another analysis shows that in each sex the age at which the largest number of cases of mania were met with was between 25 and 34, whilst as regards melancholia there were more cases at 55 and upwards in the male sex than at any other period, but for females the largest number of cases of this type occurred in the same early period as those of mania. General paralysis in both sexes was most abundant from 35 to 44, the age at which in males there were most cases of delusional insanity, a type of mental disorder which, in females prevailed almost equally at all ages from 35 onwards. There were more cases of insanity with epilepsy in either sex between 25 and 34, and of primary dementia and stupor below 25 years of age than at any other period of life. Secondary dementia, confusional insanity, insanity associated with gross lesions of the brain, and senile dementia, were mostly to be found in later life.[89]

The 1909 Report published for the first-time breakdowns on diagnosis for urban and rural populations, with the qualifier that the majority of asylums were in urban areas and had mixed populations, with thirty-one years old being the average age of a patient upon admittance to an asylum in 'urban counties' and eighteen years old in asylums in 'the rural counties' (Tables 6.21 and 6.22).[90]

The report concluded that primary and senile dementia, along with mania, were more frequently diagnosed in the countryside, with melancholia, delusional insanity and general paralysis being diagnosed more frequently in urban asylums. It also provided breakdowns on the occupation of a patient which had been cross-referenced to diagnostic data, albeit this was gendered, with only statistics for male patients presented—there is no explanation for why statistics on the employment of female patients were not published. Data on diagnosis for 'Town and factory workers' came from Prestwich, Whittingham, Lancaster, Stafford, Winston Green and Leicester Borough. For miners, the data came from Durham, Northumberland and Glamorgan. For agricultural workers, the data came from Cambridgeshire, Dorset, Hereford, Norfolk, Suffolk and Wiltshire (Tables 6.23 and 6.24).

[89] Ibid., pp. 26–27.

[90] *The Sixty-Fourth Annual Report of the Commissioners in Lunacy*, HMSO, 1910, p. 15.

Table 6.21 Forms of insanity, percentage distribution in each age-period—first attacks only[91]

Forms of Insanity: Percentage Distribution in each Age-Period – First Attacks only										
	Males					Females				
	Under 25	-34	-44	-54	55 and over	Under 25	-34	-44	-54	55 and over
Mania (all forms)	40.4	33.5	27.4	25.0	18.8	48.3	38.0	33.0	27.0	21.1
Melancholia (all forms)	24.9	25.3	19.5	25.3	26.7	27.7	37.8	37.9	42.1	27.7
General paralysis	1.0	11.9	31.6	26.2	4.3	0.9	2.8	4.5	4.6	0.6
Delusional insanity	6.0	11.1	8.3	6.2	4.8	2.1	5.5	9.3	10.7	7.4
Insanity with epilepsy	13.0	7.9	5.8	4.3	2.3	7.6	6.3	4.3	2.4	1.6
Primary dementia	7.4	2.4	1.0	2.0	1.3	4.8	1.7	2.0	2.6	0.6
Secondary dementia	1.2	1.6	1.4	3.5	4.7	0.6	0.9	1.8	3.7	5.3
Senile dementia	0	0	0	0.6	28.8	0	0	0	0.4	29.6
Confusional insanity	1.6	2.5	2.7	3.9	3.0	3.0	3.1	4.3	3.4	2.4
Stupor	3.0	1.3	0.6	0.3	0.1	3.7	1.3	1.3	0.8	0.5
All other forms	1.5	2.5	1.7	2.7	5.2	1.3	2.6	1.6	2.3	3.2

Table 6.22 Psychological diagnosis in urban and rural counties[92]

	General Paralysis	Mania (all forms)	Melancholia (all forms)	Delusional Insanity	Primary Dementia	Senile Dementia	All forms
Males							
Urban	1,267	2,688	2,358	655	124	347	9,184
Rural	163	918	504	87	62	237	2,357
Females							
Urban	239	3,194	3,780	643	143	374	9,495
Rural	23	1,041	831	111	54	218	2,718
Percentage Distribution							
Males							
Urban	13.7	29.2	23.5	7.1	1.3	3.8	100
Rural	6.9	38.8	21.3	3.7	2.6	10.0	100
Females							
Urban	2.3	33.6	34.5	6.7	1.5	3.9	100
Rural	0.8	38.8	30.6	4.1	2.0	8.0	100

[91] *The Sixty-Third Annual Report of the Commissioners in Lunacy*, HMSO, 1909, p. 26.

[92] *The Sixty-Fourth Annual Report of the Commissioners in Lunacy*, HMSO, 1910, p. 15.

The following year in 1910, diagnosis rates for 1907–1909 were published breaking down rates of diagnosis by age (Tables 6.25 and 6.26):

> From this it would appear that the age-periods 25-34, and 35-44, yield the largest proportion of cases of insanity, that of 45-54 being next, whilst the proportion at ages under 25 is almost the same as that of the period 55-64; and the fewest occur after 65 years of age, although this period includes the great majority of all the cases of senile dementia. In the above selected types a comparison shows that cases of epileptic insanity and mania occur largely at ages below 45 years; melancholia and delusional insanity

Table 6.23 Nature of employment and form of insanity (males only)[93]

Nature of Employment and Form of Insanity (Males only)								
Nature of Employment	General paralysis	Mania (all forms)	Melancholia (all forms)	Delusional Insanity	Primary Dementia	Senile Dementia	Other Forms	Total
Towns and Factory	402	904	881	230	9	61	576	3,063
Mines	219	446	280	137	23	66	293	1,464
Agriculture	60	431	237	34	20	114	221	1,117
Percentage Distribution								
Towns and Factory	13.1	29.5	28.8	7.5	0.3	2.0	18.8	100
Mines	15.0	30.4	19.1	9.4	1.6	4.5	20.0	100
Agriculture	5.4	38.6	21.2	3.0	1.8	10.2	19.8	100

Table 6.24 Distribution of congenital cases [by district], 1907–1909[94]

Distribution of Congenital Cases 1907 – 1909						
In Asylums in	Males	Females	Both Sexes	Proportion per cent. in Total Admissions		Both Sexes
				Males	Females	
Urban Districts	203	98	301	6.6	3.4	5.0
Mining Districts	94	70	164	6.4	5.5	6.0
Rural Districts	96	86	182	8.6	6.1	7.2

93 *The Sixty-Fifth Annual Report of the Commissioners in Lunacy*, HMSO, 1911, p. 17.

94 Ibid.

Table 6.25 Forms of insanity—age distribution[95]

Forms of Insanity Age Distribution						
	Insanity with epilepsy	General Paralysis	Mania	Melancholia	Delusional Insanity	All Forms
Under 25	26.1	1.5	19.5	11.4	7.0	13.1
25 – 34	27.3	17.5	26.6	23.0	23.5	21.7
35 – 44	21.9	43.6	21.1	21.3	25.9	21.7
45 – 54	12.3	30.1	15.8	21.0	22.7	18.5
55 – 64	8.2	6.7	10.3	16.2	13.6	13.0
65 and over	4.2	0.6	6.7	7.1	7.3	12.0
Total	100	100	100	100	100	100

Table 6.26 *The Sixty-Fifth Annual report of the Commissioners in Lunacy*, HMSO, 1911[96]

Forms of Insanity at Various Ages										
	Males					Females				
	Under 25	25 – 44	45 – 64	65 and over	**All ages**	Under 25	26 – 44	45 - 64	65 and over	**All ages**
Insanity with Epilepsy	13.5	7	3.7	2.4	**6.2**	8.0	5.0	3.1	1.4	**4.4**
General Paralysis	1.2	23.4	18.7	0.8	**16.4**	0.9	3.7	3.4	0.1	**2.8**
Confusional Insanity	2.5	2.7	4.0	1.9	**3.0**	2.9	4.0	4.4	1.5	**3.7**
Primary Dementia	7.8	2.0	1.7	0.2	**2.4**	5.9	2.0	1.7	0.4	**2.2**
Mania (acute and chronic)	38.3	27.8	22.1	15.5	**23.8**	46.3	34.5	25.0	16.6	**31.0**
Melancholia (acute and chronic)	24.2	22.2	28.8	16.8	**24.0**	27.2	38.0	40.8	18.4	**35.0**
Delusional Insanity	6.8	10.4	7.9	3.9	**8.4**	2.4	8.5	11.2	6.1	**8.2**
Senile Dementia	0	0	4.1	52.0	**7.5**	0	0	2.7	49.8	**6.9**
Secondary Dementia	1.2	1.8	4.9	3.2	**2.9**	0.5	1.3	4.3	3.7	**2.4**
Other Forms	4.5	2.7	4.1	3.3	**3.4**	5.9	3.0	3.4	2.6	**3.4**

95 Ibid.

96 Ibid., p. 18.

> prevail most between 25 and 55, whilst cases of general paralysis fall chiefly between 35 and 55, and especially between 35 and 45.
> Further analysis of Table XX. may be made by dealing with the cases assigned to each sex, and distributing the forms of insanity from which they suffered into age-periods, so as to ascertain which of these forms were most frequently met with in the particular age-period. This scheme is necessary to supplement the results obtained above, where the converse method was adopted, viz.: — the distribution of all the cases suffering from a particular form of insanity into their respective age-periods.[97]

In reports published for the years 1908–1912, analysis of admissions by sex was provided. The reports showed increased attempts to understand the statistics on psychological diagnosis amongst admissions. The report included analysis that attempted to make sense of statistics on gender, age and geography, and these were in many ways the high point of the project to develop asylum statistics that had been undertaken since the 1860s to standardise data on psychological diagnosis. Despite these developments, subsequent reports published from 1913 by the Board of Control do not provide analysis for the figures on diagnosis. The 1913 report provides an extensive analysis of the causes of insanity, concluding that heredity is the prevailing causing factor of all its forms.[98] Ascribing a common cause for all forms of insanity under heredity reflects the prevailing tendency in statistical investigations to treat insanity as one concept and to break it down into different forms. A further clue for reasons behind the abrupt end of analysis of figures on the diagnosis of the forms of insanity comes from the 1908 Commission on the Feeble Minded, which was pivotal in setting up the Board of Control, and recommended that the legal and medical categories of idiots and lunatics be collapsed into a single legal classification of mental defectives (Fig. 6.3).[99]

Further clues can be find by looking towards the research undertaken by statisticians of the time who took an interest in insanity and mental health data. Karl Pearson and his Galton laboratory colleague David Heron were interested in linking mental health to population studies, but their use of asylum medical data was by no means universally supported. As Crichton-Browne's reaction and Pearson's ill-tempered

[97] Ibid.

[98] *The Sixty-Eighth Report of the Royal Commission on Lunacy*, HMSO, 1914.

[99] *The Royal Commission on the Feeble-Minded*, HMSO, 1908.

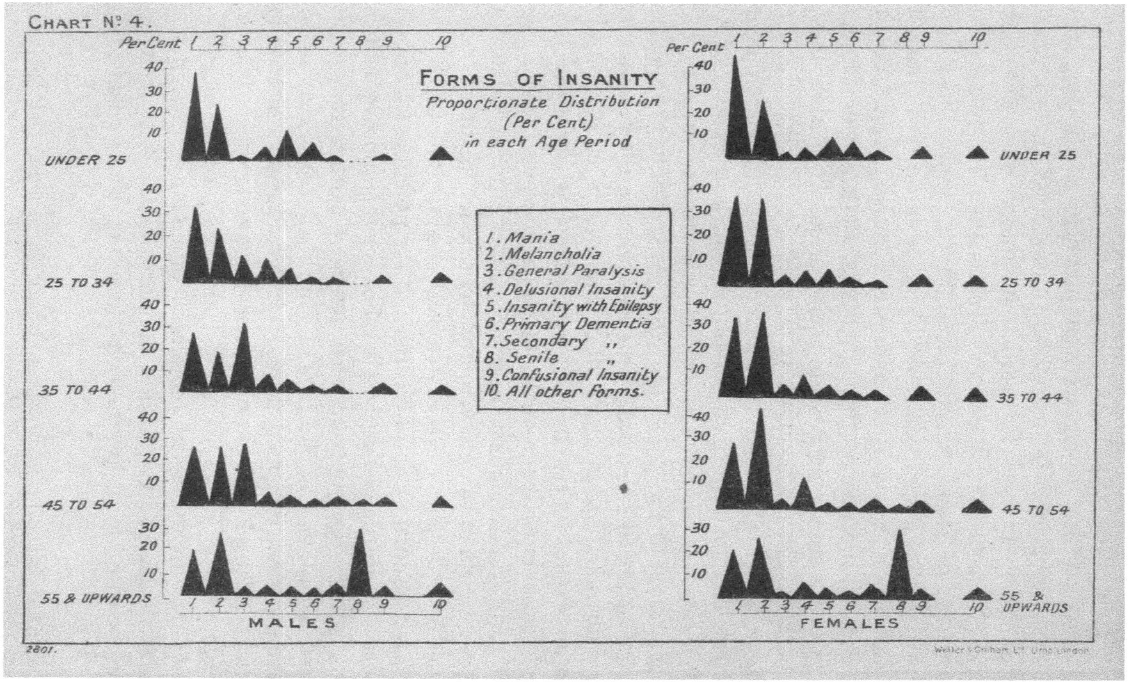

Fig. 6.3 Visualisation of proportionate distribution of forms of insanity in each age group[100]

100 *The Sixty-Fifth Annual report of the Commissioners in Lunacy*, HMSO, 1911, p. 17.

response that opened this chapter suggest, opinion differed on what constituted a proper scientific method on insanity and population studies, even amongst committed eugenicists; despite having been a strong supporter of eugenics, and having acted as president of the Eugenics Society in 1908, Crichton-Browne publicly questioned the statistical evidence presented by Pearson to justify state intervention to realise eugenic aims. As Michael Neve and Trevor Turner note, the pair shared a common interest in eugenics, but had different approaches, with Crichton-Browne having adopted a more liberal position on individual freedoms to procreation than the state-socialism of Pearson, which sought to influence and regulate births through policy, especially of families that had traces of the insane diathesis in their lineage.[101] Despite these differences, there were strong alignments between psychiatrists and the eugenics movement by the beginning of the twentieth century. Prominent members such as Frederick Mott enthusiastically engaged in correspondence with Pearson and Galton, and he had become a member of the Eugenics Society upon its formulation in 1907. As mentioned in the last chapter, Pearson had been consulted by the MPA during the revisions to the statistical returns and had taken an interest in asylum records, mostly in relation to his studies on phthisis and tuberculosis, which themselves were designed to understand the fitness of the nation and the national ability. Galton had also taken interest in asylum records and mental health statistics, although his motivations were not identical to Pearson's.

During the first decade of the twentieth century, Pearson had frequently written on insanity and heredity, and the potential for reform in public records to aid eugenic goals. He called for the improvement of family records, and co-operation between general practitioners, psychiatrists and statisticians to compile patient information in an effort to understand the inheritance of mental instability.[102] Pearson's interest in asylum statistics is relatively straightforward: as a committed hereditarian, he was interested in the use of asylum statistics as a possible means to extrapolate findings on the wider prevalence of insanity amongst the general population. He had emphasised the need for the state to intervene and prevent those from lower stocks, including those detained in

[101] Michael Neve and Trevor Turner, 'What the Doctor Thought and Did: Sir James Crichton-Browne (1840–1938)' in *Medical History*, no. 39, 1995, pp. 399–432.

[102] Karl Pearson, 'On the Inheritance of Insanity' in *British Medical Journal*, vol. 1, no. 2317, May 27, 1905, pp. 1175–1177.

asylums, from procreating. This was to be done mostly through incentives bestowed upon the more gifted through policy, but in the case of the 'feeble-minded', he agreed with Crichton-Browne that internment in an asylum was the best eugenic solution.

Galton's interest in asylum statistics however is a bit harder to assess. He had wanted to avoid the label of a crude hereditarian and was as interested in the role of the environment in the development of character and intelligence as much as in the influence of hereditary constitution. Indeed, Galton had approached asylum medical superintendents for information on twins as a part of his twins study, although it is unclear whether he received any responses.[103] Nevertheless, clues to Galton's interest in statistics are included in a 1905 address to the British Sociological Society that outlined some of the broader goals of the eugenics project.[104] A key component was reliable information on the composition and condition of the population, or what he termed 'the national stock', which he divided into three sets: gifted, above average and below average families. He proposed drawing upon public and private records to map the population, with asylum records to be used to determine which families were below the average level:

> Biographies of families, who are distinctly below the average in health, mind, or physique, are to be collected. These include the families of persons in asylums of all kinds, hospitals, and prisons. To be kept for statistical use only.[105]

The implication was that any family who has had a relation interned in an asylum would be considered sub-normal stock within any eugenic bureaucracy, at least according to Galton's plans. Although British eugenicists proposed measures to control and regulate the transmission of the insane diathesis, considerations on the form of insanity were absent: Galton's vision was crude in its attempts to identify and regulate the dividing line between insanity and sanity. Galton envisaged the introduction of stock

[103] John C. Waller, 'Commentary: The Birth of the Twin Study—A Commentary on Francis Galton's 'The History of Twins'' in *International Journal of Epidemiology*, vol. 41, no. 4, August 2012, pp. 913–917.

[104] Francis Galton, 'Studies in National Eugenics' in *Essays on Eugenics*, Macmillan, 1909, pp. 60–67.

[105] Ibid.

honour certificates to those clear of insanity in their backgrounds, which would grant benefits and perks. During the discussions that followed the delivery of the paper, he acknowledged that in the short term, it was not possible to realise these ambitions because the data were simply not available. Despite the current condition of mental health statistics preventing these goals from being realised in the immediate future, it was possible with existing records from schools, local authorities and asylums to identify the most problematic sections of society. Indeed, he approvingly referenced remarks made earlier in the same discussion by Frederick Mott, who with A.R. Urquhart of the Perth asylum, was perhaps one of the most committed of MPA eugenic psychiatrists, and had testified to seeing signs of 'the effect of heredity markedly on the people admitted into the Asylums' within the jurisdiction of the London County Council.[106] Mott had attempted to emulate Kraepelin's *Zahlkarten* system by introducing an index card system that recorded 'the date of admission, age of onset, and type of psychosis of both relatives'.[107] In approvingly citing Mott's remarks, Galton stated that the data were already there in public records to conduct a crude but necessary segregation of the lowest stock, with further refinements of the eugenic programme being made possible by developing systems of medical data collection.

The paucity of data and the state of public records did not prevent psychiatrists like Mott from actively promoting segregation of the mentally unwell. An extraordinarily cruel paper he penned on the inheritance of the forms of insanity offered some of the starkest conclusions reached by a psychiatrist writing at the time, adopting racist stereotypes to claim that 'it has always struck me that the Jews were, on account of their neurotic temperament, more liable to insanity than Christians'.[108] In the same paper Mott invoked statistics to argue that forms of insanity barring alcoholic insanitywere caused by hereditary predisposition:

[106] Frederick Mott, remarks recorded in Discussion, *The Sociological Review*, vol. 2, no. 1, 1905, pp. 18–25 (p. 19). Urquhart had penned the 'Insanity' section to the Galton Laboratory's *Treasury of Human Intelligence*, edited by Karl Pearson, Vol. 1, Dulau and Co., 1912, pp. 61–66.

[107] Arthur S. Paterson, 'The So-Called Law of Anticipation in Mental Disease' in *The Journal of Neurology and Psychopathology*, vol. 13, no. 51, January 1933, pp. 193–210 (p. 195).

[108] Frederick Mott, 'Heredity and Insanity' in *Eugenic Review*, no. 4, 1911, pp. 257–281.

> One in particular is so instructive that I will show it, for it illustrates the truth of the law that 'like tends to beget like,' not 'like begets like'; it is not necessarily insanity that is inherited, but a neuropathic tendency in the stock which manifests itself in many *forms*, e.g., epilepsy, asthma, migraine, diabetes, exophthalmic goitre, insanity, eccentricity, criminality, neurasthenia, hysteria, etc.[109]

From these strong hereditarian views of Mott, to the disagreement between Crichton-Browne and Pearson, the complex relationship between asylum medical superintendents and eugenicists often comes to the surface in debates over mental health statistics. Pearson could see a huge potential resource in asylum statistics, but they were inadequate as they were and needed to be revised in a way that broke with the tradition of asylum data collection, it being a product of medico-legal and administrative developments: a record of diagnosis provided legal justification for admission, although as this study has outlined, there was recognition of the scientific potential of the data.[110]

An influential monograph on the insane diathesis by Heron, then the Galton Research Fellow in National Eugenics, demonstrates that statisticians at the forefront of the discipline did not concern themselves with the nuances of psychological diagnoses.[111] The grounding assumption to Pearson and Heron's statistical work on insanity was the notion of unitary insanity, that is to say, an understanding of insanity to be one kind with different forms. They also ignored the borderland and instead based their work on the assumption that there was a clear dividing line between the sane and insane. As Heron's wrote in 1907:

> Some forms of insanity may be of singular distinctness and capable of differentiation from the mass of others practical unanimity of the experts.

[109] Ibid.

[110] Francis Galton, 'Studies in National Eugenics' in *Essays on Eugenics*, Macmillan, 1909, p. 64.

[111] There has lately been some resurgence in interest in Heron's statistical work on insanity. Kendler considers Heron's work as historically significant because it helped to 'set the stage for all biometrical modelling work done in psychiatric genetics based on the liability threshold model which formed the core of Pearson's concept of the tetrachoric correlation'. See: K.S. Kendler, 'The Beginnings of Biometrical Psychiatric Genetics: Studies of the Insane Diathesis 1905–1909' in *American Journal of Medical Genetics Part B: Neuropsychiatric Genetics*, vol. 189, no. 1–2, pp. 6–15 (p. 30).

> But can we say that the experts will themselves agree to a general classification of types, or admit that some of these types may not be manifestations at different stages of the same original constitutional defect? It would seem that already there is more than a tendency among experts to revert to Dr Sankey's position 'that insanity is but the process, and that the so-called varieties are merely differentiated by non-essential phenomena; that all insanities begin with melancholia, and tend to pass through a succession of stages in the order – melancholia, mania and dementia, a succession liable at any time to interruption by recovery.' In short, to take Dr Urquhart's position that 'Insanity is a unity, not a fortuitous collection of kaleidoscopic systems each requiring a proper name'. It is not for a layman to express an opinion on this point, but while there is diversity of expert views, and while many hold the possible transition from one type to another, and treat insanity as a unity, the popular statement that John Smith had an 'insane' ancestor may not be of such small scientific value as it appears at first sight. Initially this compulsory limitation of the method by which we may hope to reach conclusions may not result in such a heterogeneous and loose classification as some mental experts would suggest.[112]

For Heron, recent disputes over classification went some way to proving that dividing insanity into separate forms was a futile task, as were attempts to classify a disease according to its stages or degrees of intensity. At the very least they showed that a simple definition of insanity was sufficient for the purposes of statistical research. Although dated, Heron's views on unitary insanity were by no means those of a complete outlier or crank for they were informed by the work of Urquhart and Sankey, then prominent alienists who had participated in the debates surrounding the 1907 revisions covered in the last chapter. Heron though did not shut the door entirely to the possibility that there could be different forms, but as we see from the extract below, given the state of public records and the work that needed to be carried out in the short term, this ought to very much be a goal for the distant future:

> When the classification of the types of insanity shall have proceeded further, when above all the family records shall have given us information as to these types in ascendant, descendent and collateral, then our insight will be deeper and we shall be able to test statistically the inheritance of each

[112] David Heron, *A First Study on the Statistics of Insanity and the Inheritance of the Insane Diathesis*, Dulan and Co., 1907, p. 5.

> type and the correlation in heredity between types. In the opinion of the present writer this correlation should always be kept in view as a goal, even if a distant one, in dealing with family histories under the present difficulties.[113]

Despite these qualifiers, Heron went on to describe the diathesis, or predisposition to insanity:

> Theoretically we suppose that there exists a quantitative scale of this insane diathesis. In some individuals the extent or intensity of this constitutional condition is so low, that under no physical or mental strain would they be in the least likely to become insane. In others the intensity so great, that they are unlikely under any circumstances to escape the slight pressure which will suffice to send the balance down on the wrong side. In others again an absolutely easy and physically well-regulated life will preserve them, as similar conditions will preserve the well-to-do who come of tuberculosis stock. But the possibility of such conditions lies only with the well-to-do, not with the struggling and often exceedingly ignorant mass of humanity which provides the bulk of the population of our public asylums [...] Is the intensity of the insane diathesis sufficient in such cases to lead to temporary or permanent conferment in an asylum? Theoretically we want a mark on the scale of the insane diathesis, and then we shall say that under the normal environment of the present age, all who fall below this escape the asylum, all who exceed it will sooner or later be certified. Now it is quite clear that this is practically unattainable; A and B may be sensibly in equal possession of the insane diathesis, but A's environment or habit of life may preserve his sanity and B's destroy his. But the question is not whether any theoretical mark can be exact, but whether it can be drawn sufficiently close to the actual state of affairs to be useful in describing that state in the mass. We believe that the classification into the sane and insane is probably as close as any made in vital statistics. There are undoubtedly a considerable number of neurotics, eccentrics and 'cranks' who under a modified environment would need to be classed as insane. The time may actually come when we shall be able to recognise other marks on the scale of insane diathesis beside the division which under the normal environment of modern life leads to a certificated insanity.[114]

113 Ibid.

114 Ibid. [italics added for emphasis].

Heron's definition of insanity according to the unitary model was enough for quantitative studies that sought to identify the diathesis and develop a quantitative scale for it. Nevertheless, this was a view that was growing in popularity and is part of a trend of treating insanity as a single concept that was reflected in mental health statistics of the time.

In 1921, analysis of the statistics on psychological diagnosis returned from asylums briefly reappeared in lunacy reports.[115] The Board of Control's report took its cue from the reports published before the war by analysing age and gender, but also for the first-time cross-referenced data on the causes of insanity to those of diagnosis of the forms—this had been allowed in part due to the introduction of the medical registers in 1907. When comparing the figures on assigned causes for all disorders for the year 1920 to those that had appeared in 1909–1913, the recording of 'insane heredity' as a causing factor had fallen by 4.9% for males and 3.5% for female admissions. In analysis of the causing factor for the forms of insanity, insane heredity was still one of the most frequent causal factors recorded, being the second or third most popular in most cases. Insane heredity was used more frequently for female than male admissions, and for confusional insanity, primary dementia, mania, melancholia and delusional insanity in both men and women.

Conclusion

Initially established by legal requirements to keep accurate records on patients under the terms of the 1845 Lunacy Act, the subsequent development of asylum statistics was motivated by attempts to provide data that would help to develop them for use in the mental sciences. They would also help in lunacy administration, including anticipating increases in the rate of insanity, identifying asylums with higher-than-average mortality rates, understanding common causes of death amongst inmates and assessing the impact of outbreaks of diseases such as dysentery and phthisis. Reports of the Commissioners in Lunacy frequently mentioned the cost of asylums and the need to understand the conditions in asylums as well as their capacity. As we have seen from our assessment, administrative data that allowed oversight of institutions comprised asylum statistics in early reports: this included finances, staffing and the numbers of beds.

[115] *The Eighth Annual Report of the Board of Control*, HMSO, 1922, p. 16.

Admissions data divided by gender and the legal classes of pauper lunatics and voluntary patients was also included, and, later on, medical statistics that further assisted in asylum oversight on mortality and causes of death statistics were presented in reports. Medical statistics on the causes of insanity and forms of insanity became some of the last additions to asylum statistics. This is principally because they were of less direct use for asylum administration, but also because their standardisation was a more complicated matter.

The drive to bring about standardisation had culminated in a series of reports by the early 1900s that provided some of the most in-depth analysis of asylum statistics on psychological diagnosis that were seen in a Lunacy Commission report. The progress ended abruptly because of notions of insanity that informed enquiry into it in the works of statisticians, but also partly because of the disruption caused by the Great War.[116] Attitudes to asylum medical statistics changed as the Board of Control assumed the responsibility of asylum oversight. As per the recommendations of the 1908 Commission, all classes of asylum patients were reclassified as mental defects under the terms of the 1913 Mental Deficiency Act, and this, along with statistical investigations into the hereditary causation of insanity, led to waning interest in analysing statistics returned on the forms of insanity.

This chapter can be read as providing additional framing of the debates covered in the first part of this study by showing the application of the Table of the Forms of Insanity in the publication of asylum statistics. Admissions statistics were used by the Lunacy Commission in attempts to draw up findings that largely conformed to the Victorian trend of compiling vital statistics for public health. These included attempts to map the prevalence of certain disorders according to gender, class of patient and geographical region, and these largely conform to the Victorian preoccupation with vital statistics. Detailed data on psychological diagnosis came relatively late because of the complications in standardising the terms used in admissions diagnosis, and the difficulty of compiling data from asylums across England and Wales. During the last quarter of the nineteenth century, a set of changes linked to the MPA revisions of the

[116] The Board of Control saw the task of collecting asylum statistics as dispensable in the face of the disruption caused by asylums being repurposed as war hospitals during the conflict; Anon, 'Statistical Intermission' in *JMS*, vol. 6, no. 56, January 1916, pp. 182–183.

statistical tables had led to new stage in the development of medical statistics on diagnosis, but these were still descriptive vital statistics. Although there had been attempts to use asylum returns to understand the rate of insanity amongst the general population, from the beginning of the twentieth century a number of studies attempted to develop new statistical approaches to make predictions on the rates of insanity amongst the general population. These approaches were not interested in understanding different forms of insanity, or building on the work undertaken to realise national statistics on psychological diagnosis.

This chapter has traced this long process of development, that commenced in the 1860s and coincided with the statistical work undertaken by the MPA. Once a degree of standardisation was introduced at the end of the 1870s, the Lunacy Commission of England and Wales began to publish yearly medical statistics on psychological diagnosis and the causes of insanity. These were included in asylum medical reports throughout the 1880s and 1890s, and by the turn of the century, relatively sophisticated ways of visualising mental health statistics, such as those showing the rates of insanity across the country, appeared in the final sets of Lunacy Commission reports of the first years of the twentieth century. In-depth analysis of the statistics on diagnosis began to appear, with age, gender and recurrence of the disorder included in the reports between 1902 and 1909. This trend ends abruptly, without explanation. The 1911 report would be the last of the Commissioners in Lunacy that would breakdown data on the diagnosis of insanity into its different forms. Its replacement, the Board of Control, would not continue to routinely publish detailed information on the forms of insanity, with statistics on diagnosis only appearing occasionally under their stewardship. The reasons behind this are unclear, but they mark the end of over fifty years of development of nationally collated medical statistics on the psychological diagnosis of insanity.

This chapter has presented evidence to suggest that the sudden end occurred principally due to changes in attitudes to insanity and mental health statistics on psychological diagnosis apparent from statistical studies on insanity occurring at the time this shift occurred, and in light of changes to lunacy administration linked to the 1913 Mental Deficiency Act and the handing over of powers to the Board of Control. The influence of eugenics, then, on mental health statistics was largely responsible for ending the collation, analysis and publication of medical data on the forms of insanity.

CHAPTER 7

Amending a Melee of Contradictions: The 1934 Revisions to the Table of the Forms of Mental Disorder

On 8th July 1931, and in the face of growing despair about the prospects of psychiatric research, Dr Richard Leeper, then serving as the president of the Royal Medico-Psychological Association (RMPA), gave an address that asked whether clinical science had failed in its quest to understand and treat mental disease.[1] At the time of Leeper's address, the state of the art was divided, with new developments in psychoanalysis and psychology vying for position with the remaining dogmas of asylum psychiatry. Leeper, an evangelical representative of the latter, pointedly titled his speech 'Progress in Psychiatry' despite his vision of psychiatric classification being conservative, providing an impassioned defence of hereditarian theories of mental disease that had informed asylum medical treatment of the late nineteenth century. He complained that a lack of scientific progress in recent years was down to distractions from studies on constitution from the latest fads in psychological medicine that had avoided the inconvenient truth that 'nine out of ten forms of mental

[1] Richard Robert Leeper, 'Some Reflections on the Progress of Psychiatry: The Presidential Address at the Ninetieth Annual Meeting of the Royal Medico-Psychological Association Held in Dublin' in the *JMS*, vol. 77, no. 319, October 1931, pp. 683–691.

K. M. Jones, *Psychological Classification and Diagnosis in Asylum Statistics, 1800–1948*, Mental Health in Historical Perspective,
https://doi.org/10.1007/978-3-031-46154-5_7

disease are due to the ever-varying vagaries of hereditary defect'.[2] Psychoanalysis was the principal target of Leeper's attack, which he claimed had achieved nothing and was simply an ornamental luxury for the wealthy classes. Freud and his followers had provided little insight into the causes or treatment of mental disorders, and fewer still that could be used within large psychiatric institutions. Seduced by its glamour, psychiatrists who had dabbled with psychoanalysis had drawn attention away from a material account of the causes of madness that could explain predisposition through bodily constitution. Psychoanalysis was not the only target of Leeper's address, with focal sepsis theory, the view then in vogue that insanity was caused by bodily infections, also coming under criticism. The recent trend of focal infection theory had also wasted time, albeit in a different and more macabre manner, as research into it often entailed the painful removal of body parts suspected to be the focal point of an infection. In his attack on both movements, Leeper provided his vision of the future of mental science: one that was unwaveringly committed to research that would unearth the heritability of mental health disorders.

Leeper's favoured brand of psychiatry was deeply entrenched in degenerationist principles that went back to the middle of the nineteenth century. They had attracted a sizeable following by the end of the Victorian period and had dominated research during the early decades of the twentieth. The fundamentals of both psychoanalysis and focal sepsis were misguided, and instead of wasting time listening to patients to find the source of a trauma, or looking for the focus of an infection, Leeper believed that segregation and sterilisation were the most humane treatments. He described in dramatic tones the dangers posed by the mentally ill, which he regarded as products of hereditary defect, since 'neurotics breed neurotics, and unstable people breed insane people'.[3] As psychiatrists were distracting themselves with fripperies and novelties, the risks and costs to society were getting worse, as marriages between the mentally ill produced offspring who in turn clogged up asylums. Leeper thought that these 'terrible and disastrous unions' should be prevented at all costs, especially because the 'persecuted paranoiac [was] much more dangerous

[2] Ibid., p. 683.

[3] Ibid., p. 684.

to the public than a man with a smallpox rash'.[4] To further emphasise the risks posed by the insane, Leeper invoked the murderer of the English actor William Terriss, Richard Archer Prince. Terriss had enjoyed fame in the 1880s and had made the acquaintance of George Bernard Shaw and Thomas William Robertson before being stabbed to death in 1897 by fellow actor Prince.[5] Prince was found guilty but not responsible for his actions on the grounds of insanity, and as Leeper was speaking, would have been whiling away the rest of his days in Broadmoor mental hospital.[6] The danger posed by 'constitutionally psychotic' people like Prince could only be combatted by what Leeper regarded to be the one true form of 'scientific psychiatry', one that understood the causes and classification of mental disorder through heredity.[7]

The same year Leeper delivered his address, a committee established in 1929 was busy working on revisions to the Table of the Forms of Mental Disorder in an attempt to solve once and for all the problem of classification that had long blighted the association. By the end of the 1920s, the Table of the Forms came to be viewed by psychiatrists and hospital administration as a relic of a bygone era and drastically in need of a revision. The 1907 Revisions were largely considered inadequate, with the decision of the revisions committee not to include a set of definitions of disorders coming to be regarded as its main failure. Although the document was Kraepelinian in essence, it employed terminology that would be familiar to British asylum superintendents, making the Association's classification appear stale and out of date by the 1920s as psychoanalysis, Kraepelin's classification and focal infection had made their mark. The work of the revisions committee would be the final set of revisions to the Table of the Forms of Mental Disorder.

Speaking shortly before the committee published a draft of the revised classification, Leeper, as president of the association stated that he did not care much for the problem of classification or the work of the revisions committee for that matter, considering them a distraction from psychiatry's true purpose. He asked during his address whether the RMPA had 'a

[4] Ibid.

[5] Richard Foulkes, 'William Terriss [real name William Charles James Lewin] (1847–1897), Actor' in *Oxford Dictionary of National Biography*, OUP.

[6] Ibid.

[7] Daniel Pick, *Faces of Degeneration: A European Disorder c.1848–1918*, Cambridge University Press, 1993.

really satisfactory classification of insanity, or should not all mental abnormality be ascribed to one fact – hereditary mental aberration?'.[8] Leeper's call to understand all forms of mental disorder through the prism of heredity was a solution of sorts to the problem of classification, albeit rather a heavy-handed one. He cast doubt on the very notion of a disease entity in psychiatry as he stated that dementia praecox, manic depressive insanity, melancholia, neurosis, psychopathic constitutions and mental deficiency all stemmed from the same cause of 'insane inheritance'.[9]

Calls to Revise the Table of the Forms: 1919–1929

Throughout the 1920s, calls were made to revise the Table of the Forms. Broadly speaking, developments in the clinical and human sciences since the 1907 Revisions had led to pressure to revise the document. A revisions committee was appointed at the July 1929 annual general meeting of the Association, but calls to revise the classification were expressed immediately following the Great War. There were a number of reasons for this: recovery from the disruption to mental health services caused by the conflict, preparation for the 1926 Royal Commission on Mental Disorders and the subsequent 1930 Mental Treatment Act had pushed psychological classification and asylum statistics down the agenda.[10]

The immediate cause of the revisions was a presidential address made by J.R. Lord to the 1926 annual meeting of the Association.[11] As well as serving as president of the now Royal Medico-Psychological Association (RMPA) since it had been granted Royal Charter that same year, Lord was also serving as honorary secretary of the National Council for Mental Hygiene (NCMH), one of a set of mental health social services groups that had cropped up in the first decades of the twentieth century. Lord's presidential address was a wide-ranging reflection on the state of the clinical study of mental disorders in the United Kingdom, but he singled out the Table of the Forms for preventing the development of

[8] Ibid.

[9] Ibid.

[10] *The Eighth Annual Report of the Board of Control*, HMSO, 1922, p. 16.

[11] J.R. Lord, 'The Clinical Study of Mental Disorders: The Presidential Address at the 85th Meeting of the Royal Medico-Psychological Association' in *JMS*, vol. 72, no. (S)298, August 1926, pp. 1–79.

statistical knowledge on mental health.[12] He complained that the state of medical statistics had some impact on the goals of the NCMH, as he complained that the information that could assist public mental hygiene was hampered by a set of diagnostic terms that were 'confusing and meaningless'.[13] Despite efforts detailed in previous chapters, Lord worried that much of the important information recorded by psychiatrists in case notes and admissions registers 'would be hidden, perhaps for centuries, between heavy brass-mounted boards, and that would be the end of it'.[14] Effective communication of the information collected within asylum records had been partly stymied by a psychological classification that did not provide definitions for any of the disorders it listed.

To remedy the impasse, Lord called for a fundamental rethink of the purposes of classification. He contrasted his proposed approach with the descriptive endeavour that had characterised previous attempts to revise the classification, one he identified with an 'old order' committed to the descriptive symptomology that had characterised most attempts to classify insanity since the eighteenth century. He called for a break from it, and a fundamentally different approach, instead of simply replacing one set of descriptive categories with others, an error he accussed previous revisions committees of committing. Instead, he argued that the mental sciences needed to 'leave their static or descriptive stage of the observation and classification of phenomena' behind and develop a 'dynamic' method of classification that Lord proposed as being interactive in spirit.[15] It is difficult to know precisely what he had in mind since he offered little elaboration on what exactly he meant by 'dynamic', but it bears resemblance to an epistemic division the philosopher Gilbert Ryle was in the process of developing around the same time.[16] Ryle described the difference between knowing-that and knowing-how, or between propositional knowledge in the form of factual statements that describe the world, and practical knowledge, such as the ability to play an instrument or knowing how to ride a bicycle. Epistemic distinctions described by Ryle frequently

12 Ibid.

13 Ibid.

14 Ibid.

15 Ibid., p. 2.

16 Gilbert Ryle, 'Are There Propositions?' in *Proceedings of the Aristotelian Society*, vol. 30, 1929, pp. 91–126.

arose during debates over the Table of the Forms, with the oft-made charge being that descriptive concepts of psychological diagnosis failed to capture the tacit wisdom used to make a diagnosis, a form of knowing-how that had been accumulated over years of clinical experience. Lord also invoked a distinction between tacit and propositional knowledge in his judgment of the diagnostic concepts then in use, describing them as 'confusing and meaningless' precisely because they were divorced from the everyday practices of diagnosis developed during clinical experience. The sundering of knowledge garnered from experience led, according to Lord, to the fetishisation of concepts of diagnosis based on descriptive symptomology which populate modern classifications of psychological disorders. They had contributed to an unacceptable degree of ambiguity that prevented effective communication:

> On the broader issue, psychiatrists, not being able to understand each other, take their own lines, and hence the endless, confusing and seemingly contradictory psychological and clinical conceptions. The student, unable to make head or tail of this melee of contradictions, makes the best shift he can, and his psychology as a rule is peculiar and individual to himself.[17]

Descriptive classifications were, then, shaped by the biases of those devising them, and had led, conversely, to scientific communication over mental disorders breaking down. The source of the confusion was the way in which clinical classifications presented subjective judgements as universal categories. This created a situation where students, unable to understand the descriptions clearly, developed their own working knowledge during training and ostensibly employed abstract concepts in diagnosis and treatment, but for Lord the understanding and applications of them remained subjective. Sticking with symptomatic categories frequently led to communication breaking down, as subjective judgements parsed as universal categories became the implicit norm within the mental sciences. If classification continued to be caught on the descriptive level, thought Lord, then it would only serve to continue to produce incoherent classifications, which would in turn render statistics on psychological diagnosis useless. Lord cited George Robertson's 1926 Maudsley

[17] J.R. Lord, 'The Clinical Study of Mental Disorders: The Presidential Address at the 85th Meeting of the Royal Medico-Psychological Association' in *JMS*, vol. 72, no. (S)298, August 1926, pp. 1–79.

lecture 'The Prevention of Insanity – A Preliminary Survey of the Problem' to highlight his point.[18] Robertson pointed towards statistics in the Report of the Commissioners in Lunacy for New York State published by the American Psychiatric Association (APA) as being a model of well-executed statistics. The APA had implemented a standard table of forms for asylum statistics on diagnosis, and although it had not made a radical shift away from symptomology, it had at least included definitions of the disorders listed, reducing the extent to which subjective judgements were expressed in statistics. Lord concluded his own lecture by emphasising how the decision of the committee to not include similar definitions for the Table of the Forms had produced a melee of contradictions that had hindered the development of mental health epidemiology.[19]

Remnants of the old guard of asylum doctors still exerted influence after the Great War and threatened to stand in the way of the kind of radical revisions Lord had called for. At the same time, an emerging generation of psychiatrists, who took recent developments like psychoanalysis and focal infection seriously, was beginning to establish a new orthodoxy. Hereditarian theories of mental disorder that had characterised classification and diagnosis were still attractive to many, and those who reviled Freudian psychoanalysis held on to the idea that some form of physical cause for all types of mental disorder was yet to be discovered.

Candidates had arisen during the twenties to become this magic bullet. The malarial treatment developed by Julius Wagner-Jauregg of the syphilis spirochete that caused general paralysis of the insane inspired and sustained hopes throughout the interwar period for a miracle cure for all the forms of insanity. Developed in the wake of germ theory and the rise of bacterial medicine, focal infection had become popular during the 1920s as a candidate to become a magic bullet cure for most forms of insanity. Proponents of the theory held that the locus of an infection that caused illnesses like scarlet fever or typhoid might be quite far removed from the manifestation of the disease. Psychiatrists applied the principles of focal infection theory to insanity, and speculated that certain forms, including dementia praecox and manic-depressive insanity, could be directly linked to infections present in certain parts of the body.

[18] George M. Robertson. 'The Seventh Maudsley Lecture: The Prevention of Insanity—A Preliminary Survey of the Problem' in *JMS*, vol. 72, no. 299, 1926, pp. 454–491.

[19] Ibid., p. 10.

Opinion varied on the exact location of the infection that caused insanity, with principal candidates including gums, limbs and internal organs. One of the theory's most enthusiastic and evangelical popularisers, the American physician Henry Cotton, believed oral infection to be the seat of insanity. As Andrew Sculls describes, focal infection theory had motivated Cotton to forcefully remove the teeth of inmates in the asylum he ran, in painful procedures often carried out against the express will of his patients.[20] Before being disgraced at the hands of federal investigations prompted by concerned families, Cotton had been the talk of the town when he was invited to London to present his research at the Association's summer meeting.[21] His speech to the MPA in 1923 detailed the work he had carried out during his time as the director of the New Jersey State asylum at Trenton, at that time one of the largest institutions in the USA. Cotton's address heralded the public health potential of focal infection, and that it held the prospect of a quick and efficient treatment for cases that were considered beyond hope and written off as having a flawed hereditary constitution. Focal infection gained popularity throughout the 1920s, and by 1927, discussion at the Association's annual meeting centred on the prospects of focal sepsis.[22] Excitement about its potential spilled over into the public sphere, with a 1929 article in *The Manchester Guardian* citing one practitioner's belief that 'it was beyond doubt [that] focal sepsis was a cause of depression and suicide'.[23] At the meeting, the president of the Association, William Francis Menzies, stressed the importance of focal infection theory in establishing a 'relation [between] psychological medicine [and] general medicine, as expressed by

[20] Andrew Scull, *Madhouse: A Tragic Tale of Megalomania and Modern Medicine*, Yale University Press, 2005.

[21] Henry A. Cotton, 'The Relation of Chronic Sepsis to the So-Called Functional Mental Disorders' in *JMS*, vol. 69, 1923, pp. 434–465.

[22] 'The Royal Medico-Psychological Association: The Eighty-Sixth Annual Meeting, July 19th–22nd, 1927' in *JMS*, vol. 73, no. 303, pp. 691–728 (pp. 723–726).

[23] Patrick Watson-Williams, remarks recorded in 'The Royal Medico-Psychological Association: The Eighty-Ninth Annual Meeting of the Association: July 1st–4th' in *JMS*, vol. 76, no. 315, October 1930, pp. 860–894.

the link of bacteriology'.[24] The same year, the Edinburgh-based physician William Ford Robertson presented a paper on 'Chronic Bacterial Infections in Dementia Praecox' to the annual meeting of the MPA.[25] Those participating in the discussion following Robertson's paper called for more effort to be put into research which could establish strong links not only between dementia praecox and infection, but a 'multiplicity of mental symptoms', 'bacterial growth, and [...] the toxins [that] they produce'.[26] Robertson's research bore traces of unitary psychosis, for he theorised that mania, melancholia and other forms of insanity were different manifestations of one and the same disease entity, namely a bodily infection that corrupted the mind. Different forms of insanity were caused by the same infection but had different forms because of the constitution of the individual. This understanding of insanity gave rise to optimism that if insanity was caused by a single entity like a germ or an infection, then it could be possible to find one treatment for all its different forms.

By the time of Leeper's address in 1931, focal infection theory had begun its rapid fall from grace. Despite its promise as a magic bullet treatment with public health potentials to improve mental hygiene, it quickly faded from the scene and came to be associated with megalomania and quackery after the extent of Cotton's crimes was uncovered.[27] Cotton had removed the teeth of hundreds of patients, frequently without consent, in a desperate attempt to prove the connection between oral infection and insanity.[28] If it weren't for the misery and pain he had inflicted, Cotton might cut a sympathetic figure in his attempts to find a cure for insanity and to disprove the strong hereditarianism of those like Leeper who had doomed acute cases as untreatable. Indeed, professional interests had motivated Leeper's attack since he did not express concerns about the welfare of patients when he dismissed focal infection theory, but instead

[24] William Ford Robertson, 'Chronic Bacterial Infections in Dementia Praecox', lecture and responses recorded in Minutes from The Medico-Psychological Association of Great Britain and Ireland: Eightieth Annual General Meeting of the Association in *JMS*, vol. 67, no. 279, October 1921, pp. 511–556 (p. 543).

[25] Ibid., pp. 543–546.

[26] Ibid.

[27] Ibid.

[28] Andrew Scull, *Madhouse: A Tragic Tale of Megalomania and Modern Medicine*, Yale University Press, 2005.

questioned its scientific credentials to promote his own agenda. For all his criticism, Leeper acknowledged that treatments advanced in pursuit of the focal infection theory may possibly lead to a short-term improvement in the condition of the patient since they at least removed infected parts of the body, but they would never provide a cure for mental illness.

Psychoanalysis did not attract the same kind of popularity amongst British psychiatrists during the 1920s, as many considered it to be the reserve of the rich, and unlike focal infection theory, had little potential as a psychiatry for the masses. Yet, there were some who acknowledged that the methods of psychoanalysis could inform changes to psychiatric practice for the better. For instance, in a somewhat grudging acknowledgement of Freud's contribution to the field, the Scottish psychiatrist John Carswell conceded that psychoanalysis had at least forced physicians to pay more attention to the lived experiences of patients:

> It had always occurred to the speaker that Freud was particularly fortunate in the time at which his theories were presented [...] Probably some were getting a little tired of looking into test tubes and into microscopes to find an explanation for human conduct, even of insane human conduct [...] it could be said at any rate that Freud had projected a new idea into our methods. So that, instead of looking into the nerve structures and the influence of the fluids of the body on the nerve tissues, to find the explanation of morbid feelings and ideas they ought to look at conduct itself as an explanation. And so *Freud sent the minds of the psychiatrists back to the experiences of life*.[29]

Carswell was not alone in thinking that an over reliance on biological and scientific avenues of research had estranged psychiatrists from the experience of their patients. Research into physical causes had become a preoccupation that was distracting from the patient's psychological states and their lived experiences, and it was these experiences that had played a crucial role in the development of mental disorder. With a growing concern from some quarters that biological lines of enquiry were running dry, there was a sizeable section of the RMPA that became increasingly receptive to psychoanalysis. Those who it seriously believed that psychoanalytic methods could treat even extreme cases of neurosis, and they

[29] John Carswell, remarks recorded in 'Minutes from The Medico-Psychological Association of Great Britain and Ireland: Eightieth Annual General Meeting of the Association' in *JMS*, vol. 67, no. 279, October 1921, pp. 511–556.

appealed to developments made by figures such as C.S. Myers and his research into the treatment of war neurosis.[30]

Edward Glover articulated concerns about classification from a psychoanalytic perspective. As one of a generation of psychiatrists that emerged during the interwar years who sought to reconcile mainstream psychiatry with psychoanalysis, he proposed a new classification of mental disorders that was informed by psychoanalytic theory. He thought that a classification which incorporated psychoanalytic prniciples of causation could become the starting point for psychoanalysis to come into an 'increasingly close alliance with psychiatry'.[31] He asked his audience at the Royal Society whether medical professionals should be satisfied classifying symptoms based upon a 'purely clinical and descriptive terminology'.[32] Echoing Lord's concerns, Glover thought that descriptive classification could lead to confusions in diagnosis due to the changing nature of symptoms manifested in a patient, claiming that 'an apparently simple phobia may be a transient neurotic manifestation or the peak of a concealed paranoid construction'.[33] Glover questioned the way disease models of mental health disorders construed symptoms:

> To call the delusions of paranoia a symptom of disease, is as complete a reversal of the psychological truths as to call granulation-tissue an abrasion – granulation tissue is what we colloquially call the scab and is the first stage in the healing process of a wound.[34]

Glover deployed this metaphor to argue that by formulating disease categories from symptoms like delusions, Pinel and those that had followed in his footsteps were guilty of making a category error that confused

[30] The discussions contained in the minutes of the Annual General Meetings of the Association throughout the 1920s demonstrate this clearly, and although there were prominent members like John Carswell and William McDougall who had some time for Freud's ideas, for the main they were dismissed as being a luxury that could only be afforded by the rich.

[31] Glover in fact uses the term 'pure psychiatry' but he is using this in the sense of the biologically informed psychiatry that this chapter has described as 'mainstream': Edward Glover, 'A Psycho-Analytic Approach to the Classification of Mental Disorders' in *JMS*, vol. 78, no. 323, October 1932, pp. 819–842.

[32] Ibid.

[33] Ibid.

[34] Ibid.

the signs of a healing mind for the symptoms of a disease. Paranoia, then, was not the symptom of a disease but was the first sign of a mind healing from a trauma, and psychiatrists needed to assist with the healing process as opposed to preoccupying themselves with suppressing or managing the symptoms. By invoking psychoanalytic theories of causation, Glover was calling into question the dominance of symptom-based models and arguing for their potential to inform medical practice and public health measures. This was no easy task since for many in the mainstream of British psychiatry, psychoanalysis was too speculative and failed to live up to the scientific standards of modern medicine. Glover outlined the internal psychological drives and complexes that psychoanalytic theory claimed were behind the development of mental disorder. To better understand these drives and complexes, psychiatrists needed to end a fixation on symptoms alone, and analyse the thoughts, feelings and testimonies of the patient to search for clues of a concealed trauma.

Attempts by figures like Glover to combine psychoanalysis with mainstream psychiatry had some impact: as we will see later in the chapter, concepts of psychopathology compatible with psychoanalysis were included in the 1934 Revision, a classification that attempted to bring together diverging approaches to psychiatric diagnosis. This is because in the midst of these divisions, the RMPA saw itself as in the words of Lord, 'guardian and cultivator in these [British] Isles of psychological medicine'.[35] The Table of the Forms became the object of criticism to opposing factions, with the committee placed in charge of revising it tasked not only with merging differing theoretical commitments to classification, but also theories of disease and philosophies of mental disorder. New approaches were in contest with the hereditarian views that had gestated in the asylum, and which were given a new theoretical thrust by the eugenics movement. Robert Armstrong-Jones, who would become a vocal critic of the 1934 Revisions, celebrated Frederick Mott as being the foremost representative of biological and organic approaches to psychiatry that were informed by the work of Francis Galton and Karl Pearson.[36] Mott had established himself as a central figure in research attempting to connect heredity to neurasthenia and dementia praecox, and had been a

[35] Minutes from The Medico-Psychological Association of Great Britain and Ireland: Eightieth Annual General Meeting of the Association in *JMS*, vol. 67, no. 279, October 1921, pp. 511–556.

[36] Robert-Armstrong Jones, remarks recorded in ibid.

card-carrying member of the Eugenics Society from early on in its life.[37] By the interwar period, Armstrong-Jones was one of the Association's elders, having been involved in discussions surrounding classification that had taken place at the turn of the century.[38] He had praised Mott's quest to find the somatic seat of mental diseases by detecting congenital weaknesses in the endocrine system.[39] When presenting his vision of the genetics of mental disorder, Mott neatly outlined differing approaches to investigating dementia praecox:

> On the one hand there was the organic or the material school; and on the other the psychogenetic or mental school, [the] latter has been very much in evidence during and since the war. The latter school believed, among other things, that dementia praecox was entirely due to mental causes, and that epilepsy also had a similar origin. It was held by many that the abnormal mental states were due to subconscious complexes causing repression, and that this repression gave rise to conflicts involving a dissociated personality and so resulting in dementia praecox.[40]

He perhaps had in mind Jung's work on dementia praecox when criticising those looking for the psychological causes of it, with the Swiss psychoanalyst's ideas being very much the antithesis of his own hereditarian ideas.[41] Mott was interested in the inherited organic pathologies that gave rise to insanity, and he viewed dementia praecox as a sign of a congenital weakness.[42] He believed that research into the pathology of insanity undertaken since the Great War had placed a discovery of the

[37] Edgar Jones, 'An Atmosphere of Cure: Frederick Mott, Shell Shock and the Maudsley' in *History of Psychology*, vol. 25, 2014, pp. 412–421.

[38] See the discussions covered in the last chapter, and in particular Robert Armstrong-Jones' contributions.

[39] Minutes from The Medico-Psychological Association of Great Britain and Ireland: Eightieth Annual General Meeting of the Association in *JMS*, vol. 67, no. 279, October 1921, pp. 511–556.

[40] Frederick W. Mott, 'The Genetic Origin of Dementia Praecox' in *JMS*, vol. 68, no. 283, October 1922, pp. 333–347 (p. 333).

[41] Ibid.

[42] Ibid.

biological causes of dementia praecox within reach. Mott, like Armstrong-Jones, thought that identifying patterns of heredity within family lines was the first step in the discovery of dementia praecox's biological cause.[43]

Deliberations of the Revisions Committee: 1929–1934

In response to Lord's call for a new horizon for classification, a committee to revise the Table of the Forms was appointed in 1929. The clinical sub-committee in charge of the revisions comprised 'representatives from four London teaching hospitals, the School of Medicine for Women, the Post-graduate College, the Edinburgh and Welsh Universities, together with a commissioner of police'.[44] It included notable figures from the profession including Hubert Bond, David Henderson, Henry Yellowlees and Frederick Lucian Golla.[45] Four prison commissioners were also appointed, most notable being the forensic psychiatrist William Norwood East, the then Medical Inspector of Prisons. It was chaired by the Association's honorary secretary, G.W.T.H. Fleming, with Lord also participating in the development of the classification, but as Fleming noted in the final report published in 1934:

> Although he did not live to see the completion of this classification, his was the moving spirit in the last two years work.[46]

In contrast to the detailed minutes of the deliberations accompanying previous revisions to the Table of the Forms, there is comparatively little

[43] Ibid.

[44] Hugh Stott, 'The Royal Medico-Psychological Association's Classification of Mental Disorders' in *the Indian Medical Gazette*, vol. 70, no. 1, January 1935, pp. 33–36.

[45] The full composition of the committee was as follows: J. Brander, L.C.F. Chevens, K.K. Drury, W. Norwood East (Prison Commissioner), F.L. Golla, W. McCartan, Professor D.K. Henderson (Professor of Psychiatry, Edinburgh University), P.K. McCowan (Lecturer in Mental Diseases, Welsh National School of Medicine), D. McRae, W.F. Menzies, J.E. Nicole, W.D. Nicol (Lecturer on Psychiatry, London School of Medicine for Women), A.A.W. Petrie (Lecturer on Mental Diseases, Charing Cross Hospital and West London Post-Graduate College), M. Hamblin Smith, W.V.H.B. Stoddart, W.S.J. Shaw, B.H. Shaw, A. Walk, H. Yellowlees (Lecturer on Psychological Medicine, St. Thomas's Hospital).

[46] Ibid.

record of those conducted during this final set of revisions. It is not possible to say for certain why the revisions were not presented for debate at annual general meetings as with previous revisions. The members of the committee were certainly aware of the previous sets of debates, with Lord himself having participated in the debates that accompanied the 1907 Revisions, and the committee having penned a report summarising past disputes over the Table.[47] Similarly, it is difficult to say for certain the factors that influenced key decisions of the committee, but important clues on their theoretical allegiances are apparent from the lengthy review it conducted of literature surrounding psychiatric classification.[48] In it, the committee outlined the views of many of the figures we have already encountered in the pages of this volume: Pinel, Esquirol, Griesinger, Skae, Bénédict Morel, Daniel Hack Tuke, Thomas Laycock and John Charles Bucknill are all considered central characters in the story of classification. The report deemed Griesinger to be the founder of modern clinical classification, and lauded Skae's work for finding the physical seat of mental disorder, judging it to be of fundamental importance to asylum psychiatry. The influence of Pinel's symptom-based classification however was downplayed, despite it having dominated psychiatric classification during the second half of the nineteenth century. The committee judged Pinel's *nosographie* as being part of the 'early history of psychiatry' and therefore of little relevance to modern medical science, except perhaps as historical trivia.[49] As we have seen in the first part of this work, this isn't exactly accurate because Pinel's concepts of psychopathology were akin to a standardised classification for much of the second half of the nineteenth century, and they provoked debate that took up much of the Association's energy from the 1860s onwards. Instead, the report

[47] It is perhaps the case that the length and intensity of these debates had influenced their decision to keep their deliberations mainly behind closed doors, but it is impossible to say for certain due to the lack of a record. G.W.T.H. Fleming, 'The Revision of the Classification of Mental Disorders: Report by the Clinical Psychiatry Sub-Committee of the Research and Clinical Committee—Part II' in *JMS*, vol. 78, no. 321, April 1932, pp. 387–339.

[48] Adrian Wilson has recognised the importance of literature reviews in understanding science's conception of its own intellectual heritage: see Adrian Wilson, 'Viewpoint: Science's Imagined Pasts' in *ISIS*, vol. 108, no. 4, December 2017, pp. 814–826.

[49] R. Lord and G.W.T.H. Fleming, 'The Revision of the Classification of Mental Disorders: Report by the Clinical Psychiatry Sub-Committee of the Research and Clinical Committee' in *JMS*, vol. 78, no. 320, January 1932, pp. 177–201 (pp. 177–178).

emphasised the importance of figures from the heyday of asylum psychiatry including Morel, Laycock, Bucknill, Hack Tuke and Clouston. James Cowles Prichard's work was not mentioned.

The committee undertook a review of classifications published by the national psychiatric associations of Belgium, the Netherlands and the USA.[50] This was to arrive at an understanding of the way these had synthesised recent ideas in standardised diagnostic systems used in mental health statistics. The conclusion they reached was that many non-British classifications, including that drawn up by the APA were 'too complicated' for use by the RMPA.[51] They followed the association's established tradition of using simplicity and concision as guiding principles over technical detail. The classification committee grouped the classifications they had reviewed into four categories:

1. The psychological basis—[this approach] claims that this would be the primary factor in classifying mental states and their departure from normality.
2. The symptomatological basis—the principal basis of the classification [currently] used by the Association.
3. The aetiological basis—due to the number of factors offered by different psychiatrists for the [cause of a] manifestation of a particular case, this kind of classification would be too cumbersome for construction, and difficult to use practically.
4. The pathological basis—deemed the ideal scientific standard, but the factors for such a classification were meagre and failed entirely to illuminate symptomatology. Those anatomical and physiological data upon which a pathology could be founded were not yet sufficiently worked out.[52]

The clinical psychiatry sub-committee devoted most of its time in 1931 to discussing the revision of the classification of mental disorders, and it

[50] Ibid.

[51] Ibid.

[52] Ibid., p. 180.

presented a provisional classification in July 1931 at the Annual General Meeting (see Fig. 7.1).[53]

At a meeting of the research and clinical committee on Monday 23 November 1931, it was reported that the Clinical Psychiatry Sub-Committee had decided to arrange a meeting between a sub-committee of the Royal College of Physicians appointed to deal with the classification of mental disorders, and a small sub-committee of the Clinical Psychiatry Sub-Committee.[54] At the next meeting on 23rd February 1932 the draft report of the committee was presented to the council of the association. The Final Revisions that were passed in February 1932 are displayed in Fig. 7.2.

The final version of the table was published two years later. The final version of the table had been drafted by the clinical psychiatry sub-committee of the RMPA, and the table had been expanded and modified in the published version (see Table 7.1).[55] The committee had merged the Table of the Forms and the Table of the Causes into one classification with two parts. Although Lord had passed away during the revisions, the committee honoured his recommendation that definitions of the terms included in the final version should accompany the tables. As Table 7.1 shows, the Table had more categories than previous iterations, and included seven main classes of mental disorder that were divided into two or three sub-classes, with some having sub-sub-classes, and alcoholic psychosis having four sub-classes, itself being a sub-class of exogenous forms of toxic forms of insanity. It also included what may be labelled a residual or junk category as an eighth class, that allowed medical superintendents to include disorders they did not feel should be diagnosed according to any of the main classes.

The first section of the first part of the classification included one class, named both oligophrenia and amentia, which had replaced congenital

[53] 'The Royal Medico-Psychological Association: The Ninetieth Annual General Meeting of the Association: July 8th–11th 1931' in *JMS*, vol. 77, no. 319, October 1931, pp. 862–901 (p. 879).

[54] G.W.T.H. Fleming, 'The Revision of the Classification of Mental Disorders: Report by the Clinical Psychiatry Sub-Committee of the Research and Clinical Committee—Part II' in *JMS*, vol. 78, no. 321, April 1932, pp. 387–39 (p. 389).

[55] G.W.T.H. Fleming, 'The Revision of the Classification of Mental Disorders: Report by the Clinical Psychiatry Sub-Committee of the Research and Clinical Committee—Part II' in *JMS*, vol. 78, no. 321, April 1932, pp. 387–391 (p. 389).

PROVISIONAL CLASSIFICATION, 1931.

Part I: Amentia.

Part II: (1) Neuroses or psychoneuroses.
- (a) Mental inertia.
- (b) Anxiety states.
- (c) Hysteria.
- (d) Compulsions, obsessions and phobias.
- (e) Hallucinations.

(2) Schizophrenic psychoses.
- (a) Dementia præcox.
  1. Simple.
  2. Hebephrenic.
  3. Catatonic.
  4. Paranoid.
- (b) Paraphrenia.

(3) Affective and emotional psychoses.
- (a) Cyclothymic.
  1. Alternating.
  2. Non-alternating.
- (b) Involutional.

(4) Confusional or hallucinatory psychoses.
- (a) Toxic exhaustion.
  1. Acute.
  2. Chronic.
- (b) Psychogenic.

(5) Psychopathic constitution (including paranoia) or constitutional psychopathy.

(6) Epileptic psychoses.

(7) Organic brain disease psychoses.
- (a) General paresis.
  1. Acute.
  2. Chronic.
- (b) Arteriopathic psychoses.
  1. Presenile.
  2. Senile.

(8) Exogenous toxic psychoses.
- (a) Alcoholic psychoses.
  1. Delirium tremens.
  2. Subacute and chronic hallucinosis.
  3. Paranoia or delusional.
- (b) Other drug psychoses.

(9) Mental disorders not within the definitions of 1–8.

Fig. 7.1 Provisional classification presented in July 1931[56]

56 Ibid.

Fig. 7.2 Final classification approved by the RMPA[57]

FINAL REVISION (FEBRUARY, 1932).

Part I: Amentia (oligophrenia).
- (*a*) Idiocy.
- (*b*) Imbecility.
- (*c*) Feeble-mindedness.
  - i. Moral.
  - ii. Intellectual.

Part II: 1. Neuroses and psychoneuroses.
- (*a*) Exhaustion neurosis.
- (*b*) Anxiety states.
- (*c*) Compulsions, obsessions and phobias.
- (*d*) Hysteria.

2. Schizophrenic psychoses.
   - (*a*) Dementia præcox.
     - i. Simple.
     - ii. Hebephrenic.
     - iii. Catatonic.
     - iv. Paranoid.
   - (*b*) Paraphrenia.
3. Psychopathic constitution (including paranoia).
4. Affective and emotional psychoses.
   - (*a*) Manic-depressive insanity (cyclothymia).
     - i. Alternating.
     - ii. Non-alternating.
   - (*b*) Involutional melancholia.
5. Toxic psychoses.
   - (*a*) Endogenous.
   - (*b*) Exogenous.
     - i. Alcoholic.
       - α. Delirium tremens.
       - β. Mania *a potu*.
       - γ. Chronic hallucinosis.
       - δ. Korsakov's polyneuritic psychosis.
     - ii. Other drug psychoses.
6. Epileptic psychoses.
7. Organic brain disease psychoses.
   - (*a*) Syphilitic psychoses.
     - i. General paresis.
     - ii. Other types.
   - (*b*) Arteriopathic psychoses.
     - i. Presenile.
     - ii. Senile.
   - (*c*) Other types.
8. Other types of mental disorder not mentioned in 1–7.

57 Ibid.

Table 7.1 Classification of Mental Disorders—Part I to be used in conjunction with Part II (The Aetiological Factors)

Classification of Mental Disorders – Part I to be used in conjunction with Part II

(The Aetiological Factors)[58]

A. Oligophrenia (amentia, mental deficiency).		
	(a) Idiocy (b) Imbecility (c) Feeble-mindedness (moron) (d) Moral Deficiency	
B. Neurosis and psychoneurosis	(a) Exhaustion States (including neurasthenia) (b) Anxiety states (c) Compulsions, obsessions and phobias (d) Hysteria (e) Mixed and other forms*	
C. Schizophrenic psychoses	(a) Dementia praecox	(i) Simple (ii) Hebephrenic (iii) Katatonic (iv) Paranoid
	(b) Paraphrenia (c) Other forms*	
D. Psychopathic constitution (including paranoia)		
E. Affective psychoses	(a) Manic depressive psychosis (cyclothymia)	(i) elation (ii) Depression (iii) Stupor
	(b) Involutional melancholia.	
F. Confusional states*		
G. Epileptic psychoses		
H. General paralysis		
I. Other Psychoses associated with organic brain disease*		
J. Dementia*		
K. Undetermined types*		

(continued)

Table 7.1 (continued)

Classification of Mental Disorders – Part II: The Aetiological Factors

1. Heredity	(a) Psychotic* (b) Epileptic (c) Neurotic* (d) Alcoholic (e) Various organic nervous diseases* (f) Endocrine disease* (g) Tuberculosis	
2. Deprivation of special sense	(a) Sight (b) Hearing	
3. Critical periods	(a) Puberty (b) Puberty (c) Climacteric (d) Senility	
4. Child-bearing	(a) Pregnancy (b) Puerperium (not septic) (c) Lactation	
5. Mental factors	(a) Previous attacks of mental disorder (b) Sudden stress*	
	(c) Maladjustments of:*	(i) Social life (ii) Sex life
6. Physiological disturbances	(a) Malnutrition (b) Privation (c) Exhaustion*	
7. Trauma	(a) Injuries* (b) Operations* (c) Sun- or heat-strike (d) Electric shock	
8. Toxic Factors		
A. Chemical	(a) Alcohol (b) Narcotic drugs* (c) Mineral poisons* (d) Other poisons*	
B. Infective	(a) Syphilis	(i) Congenital (ii) Acquired
	(b) Puerperal fever (c) Influenza (d) The specific fevers* (e) Tuberculosis (f) Focal sepsis* (g) Other infections*	

(continued)

Table 7.1 (continued)

C. Metabolic*		
9. Deficiency of diseases (pellagra, beri-beri, etc)*		
10. Diseases of the nervous system*		
11. Diseases of other systems	(a) Haemopoietic system (b) Cardiovascular system (c) Respiratory system (d) Gastro-intestinal system (e) Genito-urinary system (f) Endocrine system	
12. No factor ascertained		
13. No History obtained		

deficiency from the 1907 Revision. This category was intended by the committee to include 'all classes of mental defectives'.[58] The committee expressed concerns about using amentia because its literal meaning in Greek, absence of mind, they viewed as not being entirely helpful since very few patients encountered by psychiatrists suffered a total obliteration of the mind. The committee returned to Cullen and John Thurnam's work in using the term amentia, and moved away from the Pinelean phrasing of dementia to avoid confusion with dementia praecox, which had been included in the Table, although as Table 7.1 shows, the term dementia was reintroduced into the final version of the Table published in 1934.[59] The committee thought that contemporary use of amentia had taken off since Theodor Meynert had used it to describe cases associated with confusional insanity, which had been employed in the 1907 Revision and was used around the time of the Great War to describe troops with temporary and permanent states of severe incoherence.[60] It had been used in clinical literature in Britain to describe patients who had 'an insane contrariness' and 'a purposeless resistiveness, confusion,

[58] G.W.T.H. Fleming, 'Definitions and Explanatory Notes on the Classification of Mental Disorders' in *JMS*, no. 80, April 1934, pp. 409–410.

[59] G.W.T.H. Fleming, 'Definitions and Explanatory Notes on the Classification of Mental Disorders' in *JMS*, no. 80, April 1934, pp. 409–410.

[60] C. Perris, 'Leonhard and Cycloid Psychosis: Clinical Section' in *A History of Clinical Psychiatry: The Origin and History of Psychiatric Disorders*, edited by Berrios and Porter, Routledge, 1995, pp. 421–430 (p. 424).

absence of emotion, and a facial expression which is perhaps best termed embarrassment'.[61] Physical symptoms associated with confusional insanity included leucocytosis, or increased white blood cells associated with infection, and irregular blood vessel contraction. It was thought to be linked to toxins of bodily constitution in the endocrine system or complications with lactation.[62]

The committee expressed a preference for Eugen Bleuler's use of the term oligophrenia to replace confusional insanity.[63] Like amentia, they presented the genealogy of the term, claimed that oligophrenia's literal meaning of small mind was preferable to the amentia, but opted to include both in their draft of the classification.[64] Treading the same ground as revisions committees before them, they wrote that a sizeable proportion of the members of the RMPA would be more familiar with amentia. Whilst the committee recommended that dementia be completely removed from any revised classification because they thought the term was deceptive since they noted a literal translation of it being 'out of the mind', deeming oligophrenia's lack, deficiency or small mind being more appropriate for clinical usage, but it was reintroduced into the final published version of the classification.[65] In using oligophrenia and amentia, the committee chose not to employ the term 'mental deficiency' in the revisions, the term then in use in law. In doing so, the committee split from the legal and administrative term that had been in use since the passing of the 1913 Mental Deficiency Act. Their efforts were part of a broader movement to review the language used in mental health legislation that had come into place since the publishing of the Report of the Royal Commission on Mental Disorder in 1926, which had called for a break from terminology that had informed Victorian and pre-war jurisprudence on mental health.[66] Their recommendations had been enacted into law with the passing of the 1930 Mental Treatment

[61] L.D.H. Baugh, 'Some Observations on Confusional Insanity' in *BMJ*, vol. 2, no. 2337, October 14th, 1905, pp. 949–951 (p. 949).

[62] Ibid., p. 950.

[63] G.T.W.H. Fleming, 'The Revision of the Classification of Mental Disorders: Report by the Clinical Psychiatry Sub-Committee of the Research and Clinical Committee—Part II' in *JMS*, vol. 78, no. 321, April 1932, pp. 387–391 (p. 390).

[64] Ibid., pp. 389–390.

[65] Ibid.

[66] *The Report of the Royal Commission on Mental Disorder*, 1926, HMSO.

Act, an amendment to the 1890 Lunacy Act, which stated that 'asylum' be recast as 'psychiatric hospital', and 'lunatic' as 'person of unsound mind', 'patient' or 'person'.[67] The committee had attempted to follow these trends by removing mental deficiency from the first draft of the Table, and in their 1931 provisional report they described oligophrenia as a state of 'arrested or incomplete development of mind, whether arising from inherent causes or induced by disease or injury'.[68] Despite the aim of breaking from the language of deficiency, it would also be reintroduced into the final version as an alternative term for oligophrenia. Heredity was introduced as a class in the second section of the classification, and this included epilepsy and endocrine disorders as sub-categories (see Table 7.1). Although heredity was represented well in both the Table of the Forms and the Causes that came from these revisions, they can hardly be said to dominate or define them. This reflected wider concerns brewing over heredity and eugenics. Despite Leeper's sensationalist address for radical solutions to break the degenerative chain, as well as the lasting influence of Mott's work, many psychiatrists were not especially committed to degeneration or the eugenics cause; in 1933 the association had distanced itself from the Eugenics Society by voting to not support their plans to lobby the MacDonald government to introduce voluntary sterilisation for mental defectives.[69] Although the vote was tight, it shows the divisions in feeling over the appropriate links a medical society should have with the eugenics movement. Despite prominent psychiatrists being committed eugenicists, including D.K. Henderson, A.F Treadgold and Carlos Patton Blacker, sterilisation had been a sticky subject that proved a step too far for the majority of the association.

Neurosis and psychoneurosis, the second main class of the first part of the Table, included the sub-classes of exhaustion neurosis, anxiety states, compulsions, obsessions and phobias, and hysteria. Understandings of this set of disorders had changed since the Great War, with

[67] Kathleen Jones, *Asylums and After: A Revised History of the Mental Health Services from the Early Eighteenth Century to the 1990s*, Athlone, 1993, p. 135.

[68] G.T.W.H. Fleming, 'The Revision of the Classification of Mental Disorders: Report by the Clinical Psychiatry Sub-Committee of the Research and Clinical Committee—Part II' in *JMS*, vol. 78, no. 321, April 1932, pp. 387–391 (p. 390).

[69] Richard Robert Leeper, 'Some Reflections on the Progress of Psychiatry: The Presidential Address at the Ninetieth Annual Meeting of the Royal Medico-Psychological Association Held in Dublin' in the *JMS*, vol. 77, no. 319, October 1931, pp. 683–691.

them frequently being included under the loose rubric of 'shell shock' in the report of the Royal Commission on Shell Shock published in 1919.[70] The report defined shellshock as including hysteria, anxiety neurosis and various insanities induced by the 'environment' or reactions to trauma.[71] It also claimed that these different forms of insanity may be co-morbid which confounded the difficulty in differentiating the forms of insanity from one another. The revisions committee also did not differentiate between neurosis and psychoneurosis, with the terms being interchangeable in the classification. They split this class into four sub-classes: exhaustion neurosis, anxiety states, compulsions, obsessions and phobias, and hysteria. Exhaustion neurosis they defined as 'abnormal mental states characterised essentially by mental or motor fragility; anxiety states they described as being characterised by symptoms of 'generalised fear'; the third class included 'phobia where the anxiety is attached to some definite object or situation'; and the fourth class of hysteria was 'a faulty reaction to environment characterised by a variety of i. motor symptoms, ii. sensory symptoms, iii. mental symptoms'.[72] The committee observed that patients:

> are bound together by their dependence upon fundamental psychological laws, and that any one case may be found to exhibit the characteristics of two or more types of reaction. Thus a hysteric may show signs of anxiety neurosis and may also exhibit evidence of congenital mental defect, while his irresponsibility in any specific conduct may be due more to his degree of mental defect than to his hysteria.[73]

The revisions committee had decided not to use neurasthenia despite it being favoured by a great number of the RMPA's members because it had, like shell shock, been used too loosely during the war 'as a dumping

[70] War Office 'Summary of Evidence of Witnesses Regarding the Influence of War Stress and 'Shell Shock' in the Production of Insanity' in *Royal Commission into Shell Shock*, HMSO, 1919.

[71] Ibid., p. 6.

[72] Ibid.

[73] G.W.T.H. Fleming, 'Definitions and Explanatory Notes on the Classification of Mental Disorders' in *JMS*, vol. 80, no. 329, April 1934, pp. 409–410.

ground for all sorts and conditions of mental disorders'.[74] They also did not want to confuse neurasthenia with its Freudian usage, and instead considered the term exhaustion neurosis to be clearer and more distinct. The committee considered hysteria's clinical usage as an environmentally caused trauma to be clear enough and did not provide a justification for its use, despite it being closely associated with psychoanalysis by the 1930s.

The classification committee used schizophrenic psychosis as a main category stating that it had come to 'occupy a permanent place in our vocabulary'.[75] They noted that there was still some instability to its reference, stating that 'this syndrome includes cases which show remissions and even recoveries in addition to cases which show progressive deterioration'.[76] Schizophrenic psychosis was split into two sub-categories, using dementia praecox for the first, and paraphrenia for the second, which Kraepelin had used in his 1913 *Lehrbuch der Psychiatrie* to describe delusional disorders that did not affect the personality of a patient.[77] Dementia praecox was first introduced as a clinical concept in its modern form in 1893 when Kraepelin used it in the fourth edition of his textbook; paraphrenia had first been used by Kahlbaum to describe a form of insanity that would develop in adolescence and early adulthood.[78] By the 1930s, Kraepelin's distinction between paraphrenia and dementia praecox was commonly used, and the committee wrote that the former described patients whose 'emotional and volitional disorder is slight' with '[d]elusions and hallucinations generally grandiose and phantastic but

[74] G.T.W.H. Fleming, 'The Revision of the Classification of Mental Disorders: Report by the Clinical Psychiatry Sub-Committee of the Research and Clinical Committee—Part II' in *JMS*, vol. 78, no. 321, April 1932, pp. 387–391 (p. 390).

[75] Ibid.

[76] G.W.T.H. Fleming, 'Definitions and Explanatory Notes on the Classification of Mental Disorders' in *JMS*, vol. 80, no. 329, April 1934, pp. 409–410.

[77] Lorenzo Pelizza and F. Bonazzi, 'What's Happened to Paraphrenia? A Case-Report and Review of the Literature' in *Acta Biomed*, vol. 81, no. 2, 2010, pp. 130–140.

[78] Ewald Hecker, cited in Kenneth Kendler and E. Engstrom, 'Kahlbaum, Hecker, and Kraepelin and the Transition from Psychiatry Symptom Complexes to Empirical Disease Forms' in *American Journal of Psychiatry*, vol. 174, no. 2, February 1st, 2017, pp. 102–109; see also P. Hoff, 'Kraepelin' in *A History of Clinical Psychiatry: The Origin and History of Psychiatric Disorders*, edited by Berrios and Porter, Routledge, 1995, pp. 261–279; J. Hoenig, 'Schizophrenia' in *A History of Clinical Psychiatry: The Origin and History of Psychiatric Disorders*, edited by Berrios and Porter, Routledge, 1995, pp. 336–348.

with little effect on ordinary conduct'.[79] The committee had followed Bleuler's terminology in using schizophrenia as the main category name, but they retained dementia praecox as a sub-class so that it could be differentiated from the milder paraphrenia and split into the 'time-honoured' Kraepelinian sub-categories of (i) simple, (ii) hebephrenic, (iii) catatonic and (iv) paranoid.[80] It provided the following definitions of each of these terms:

i. Simple—Cases characterised by defects of interest, gradual development of an apathetic state often with peculiar behaviour, but without expression of delusions or hallucinations.
ii. Hebephrenic—Cases showing prominently a tendency to silly-laughter, grimaces, mannerisms, together with grotesque ideas and erratic behaviour.
iii. Katatonic—Cases in which there is a prominence of negativistic-reaction or peculiarity of conduct, with phases of stupor or excitement, sometimes characterised by impulsive or stereotyped behaviour, and usually hallucinations.
iv. Paranoid—Cases characterised by unsystematised delusions, usually of persecution or grandeur. Hallucinations in various fields and a tendency to early dementia.

After the Great War, dementia praecox had become widely used as a disease concept in the United Kingdom, and it was used in debates surrounding the aetiology of mental disorder amongst troops returning from the conflict. In 1919, the War Office set up a committee to scrutinise mental breakdown amongst troops: mindful of a burgeoning pension bill, the commission asked prominent British psychiatrists including Frederick Mott and his Maudsley colleague Edward Mapother whether it was the war that was solely responsible for the development of psychoses in troops. Mapother testified that:

> His impression of the service patients seen by him since the war was that most of them would have been insane had there been no war.

[79] G.W.T.H. Fleming, 'Definitions and Explanatory Notes on the Classification of Mental Disorders' in *JMS*, vol. 80, no. 329, April 1934, pp. 409–410.

[80] Ibid.

> They suffered from insanity of the ordinary type; mostly from dementia praecox.[81]

Stanford Reade supported Mapother's view by testifying that:

> Of the service patients [by 1919 who were now] in asylums, he thought the majority are suffering from dementia praecox. He thought the majority would have broken down under any slight strain.[82]

This was by no means a uniform view, however, with G. Roussy having stated before the committee that there may have been a certain number of cases of manic-depressive insanity and dementia praecox only occurring in response to the combat environment. Roussy countered Mapother and Reade in claiming that instances of dementia praecox and manic depression were in fact rare, but he agreed with their view that the war had not been the sole cause of a spike in breakdowns. When asked by the commission whether it was a constitutional weakness aggravated rather than produced by the war, he answered:

> I think the war created nothing in the way of the psychoses. It simply aggravated or revealed these manifestations in people who were predisposed to them.[83]

Dementia praecox was invoked within deliberations like these concerning the awarding of war pensions to veterans, and it became the popular term to describe patients who tended not to recover from their condition. Manic depression and dementia praecox were associated with constitution and proved to be powerful shorthand, deployed to refer to those destined for insanity, and those for whom the war had played a role in the development of mental disorder.[84] Neurasthenia, in contrast, was viewed as being a temporary condition caused by physical fatigue and shock to the body, as Dr W. Johnson testified:

[81] War Office 'Summary of Evidence of Witnesses Regarding the Influence of War Stress and 'Shell Shock' in the Production of Insanity' in *Royal Commission into Shell Shock*, HMSO, 1919, p. 146.

[82] Dr Stanford Read in ibid.

[83] Ibid., p. 145.

[84] Ibid.

> He thought the psychoses were revealed rather than produced by the war. He did not get many cases who, having been diagnosed with neurasthenia, later developed mental symptoms.
> The 15 service patients [still] at present in his hospital [in 1920] were all cases of dementia praecox. None of these cases was sent in as neurasthenic.[85]

To receive a diagnosis of dementia praecox as a veteran from the Great War meant facing a bleak future, and its use in the War Report was influential during the interwar period. It came to be wrapped in meaning from degeneration theory, which was popular amongst those with eugenic and social Darwinist leanings before the Great War. As a result, patients could find themselves left without a veteran's pension, with the authorities deeming that the psychosis suffered was not caused by the war and was therefore not the responsibility of the state. As absurd as it sounds, the government held individuals responsible for their physical and mental constitution: if someone received a diagnosis of dementia praecox, they were viewed as being the kind of danger that Leeper would come to refer to in his presidential address nearly a decade after the shell shock committee sat.

Likewise with the concept of 'psychopathic constitution', which had been introduced to the Table to distinguish certain forms of 'paranoiac conditions which do not end in intellectual impairment [...] from the schizophrenic psychoses'.[86] This class included 'a large group of pathological personalities, such as may be found amongst criminals, tramps, sex perverts, drug addicts, mattoids, agitators, etc. [...] The prison psychoses should be included in this group'.[87] Briefly put, three different strands of thought are realised in the concept: Pinel's work on *manie sans délire*, built upon by Prichard to formulate *moral insanity*, described as a disorder of emotion that saw no cognitive impairment;[88] Morel's work on degeneration and the increasing popularity of eugenics and hereditarian

[85] Ibid., p. 147.

[86] G.W.T.H. Fleming, 'Definitions and Explanatory Notes on the Classification of Mental Disorders', *JMS*, no. 80, April 1934, pp. 409–410.

[87] Ibid.

[88] Greg Eghigian, 'A Drifting Concept for an Unruly Menace: A History of Psychopathy in Germany' in *ISIS*, vol. 106, no. 2, 2015, pp. 283–309 (p. 285).

views of insanity's causation as being down to inherited constitution;[89] and finally, the German origins of the term itself, with J.L.A Koch first using psychopathy in his 1889 textbook *Leitfaden der Psychiatry* to describe a state that existed between the normal and pathological, and could be functional or biological, claiming that 'psychopathic inferiority did not corrupt personality [but] produced an isolated mental weakness of the faculties of intellect, emotions, or willpower'.[90] Emil Kraepelin and Karl Birnbaum would, during the earlier decades of the twentieth century, employ Koch's term to describe a category of patient whose mental illness led to disturbances in personality and in emotions, yet did not seem to have an impact upon cognitive abilities such as problem solving and speech abilities and rarely led to hallucinations. Furthermore, both Kraepelin and Birnbaum were influenced by Lombroso, and as a result sought to link the disorder to early ideas from criminology about the psychological make-up of criminal types.[91] In his 1909 paper on degeneration, Kraepelin associated psychopathy with increased instances of depression, anxiety and neurosis, conceptualising it as a hereditary disorder.[92] He used the term degenerative psychosis (*Entartungsirresein*), which he grouped together with a set of disorders that could lead to:

> The weakening drive for self-preservation [which] is shockingly evident in the continuous decline in the birth-rate, [and] has already begun to take the French people down the path towards extinction, and no less so in the prevalence and tolerance of all sorts of unnatural sexual aberrations.[93]

'Psychopathy' was widely used during the interwar period, with interest growing since the First World War. Mott argued that the largest sub-group of shell-shocked patients were those servicemen who had 'an inborn timorous or neurotic disposition' or an 'acquired neuropathic or

[89] Henry Werlinder, 'Psychopathy: A History of Concepts', *Acta Universitatis Upsaliensis*, no. 6, Stockholm, Almqvist & Wiksell, 1978, 8vo, pp. 218–25).

[90] Greg Eghigian, 'A Drifting Concept for an Unruly Menace: A History of Psychopathy in Germany', *ISIS*, vol. 106, no. 2, 2015, pp. 283–309 (p. 286).

[91] Ibid., p. 287.

[92] Emil Kraepelin, 'On the Question of Degeneration' in *History of Psychiatry*, vol. 18, no. 3, 2007, pp. 399–404.

[93] Ibid., p. 401.

psychopathic taint'.[94] Mott believed that conscription had led to people being admitted to the services who possessed an inherent vulnerability to mental strain. It had been used as an administrative category in military records, with the term 'borderline psychopathic states' being used as a diagnostic category in statistics collected by the War Office.[95] The historian Ben Shepherd points out in anticipation of a Second World War with aerial bombardment of large cities that psychiatric preparations under the lead of Francis Prideaux were being carried out which included provisions for citizens with borderline psychopathic states.[96] Psychotic and psychopathic were widely used in the United Kingdom from the interwar period onwards, with 'psychopathic' eventually becoming a medico-legal category under the terms of the 1959 Mental Health Act.

The clinical psychiatry sub-committee did not provide definitions for toxic psychosis and its sub-categories. It was split into two parts: endogenous and exogenous. Despite its waning influence, focal infection was given a place in the classification through the inclusion of endogenous to describe the toxins from within the body that were responsible for a mental disorder. Investigations into the link between the endocrine system and psychoses were still thought to be a potentially fruitful line of research, and disorders thought to be caused by an endocrine disorder would also be classed as endogenous. Exogenous included sub-categories of alcoholism and Korsakoff's psychosis, a distinct delusional disorder characterised by false memories that were believed to be linked to alcohol consumption. Korsakoff's psychosis would be removed in the final version of the classification published in 1934, and moved to Table of the Causes. The final version of the classification, with codes for the purposes of filling in statistical returns, was published in the *British Medical Journal* in 1934, with some adjustments to take into consideration the table of causes, that had been drafted between spring 1932 and spring 1934.[97]

[94] Edgar Jones, 'An Atmosphere of Cure: Frederick Mott, Shell Shock and the Maudsley' in *History of Psychology*, vol. 25, 2014, pp. 412–421 (p. 415).

[95] Ben Shepherd, ''Pitiless Psychology': The Role of Prevention in British Military Psychiatry in the Second World War' in *History of Psychiatry*, vol. 10, October 1999, pp. 491–524.

[96] Ibid.

[97] G.W.T.H. Fleming, 'Classification of Mental Disorders' in *BMJ*, vol. 1, no. 3834, June 2nd, 1934, p. 991.

Reactions to the 1934 Revisions

Did the revisions and the definitions included in the revision committee's report do anything to reinvigorate asylum statistics, clinical classification and psychological diagnosis? An address given by Henry Yellowlees in 1934, shortly after the publication of the latest set of revisions, indicates not. A prominent and influential member of the Association's clinical psychiatry sub-committee, he said shortly after the publication of the classification that:

> It is simply the case that unfortunately research in psychiatry bears, on the whole, far less relation to clinical work with and for patients than in any other branch of medicine [...] the research aspect and the clinical aspect of present-day psychiatry are so far apart from each other that any amount of so-called research can be and is carried out far away from any mental hospital. Further, a very large number of the more junior research workers in our speciality, even though working in a mental hospital, have not, in spite of their undoubted talents, the slightest practical acquaintance with what most of us call clinical psychiatry.[98]

The address received a mixed reaction, with some agreeing with the spirit of Yellowlees's concerns but disagreeing on specific details, and others taking exception to a proposal he had put forward at the same meeting that had a distinct whiff of eugenics about it: to separate those with severe mental illness from borderland cases. Yellowlees's proposal, to create a kind of hospice for chronic patients, showed that hope was beginning to be abandoned for patients who were doomed to their natural fate. The following year, news that Yellowlees had resigned from his position on the clinical psychiatry sub-committee for research was announced at the summer 1935 general meeting, and the Association seemed to be thrown back into the therapeutic nihilism that had characterised the years before the Great War.[99] Yellowlees was not alone in his despair. That same year an address by that year's president, Reginald Worth, chief superintendent

[98] Henry Yellowlees, 'Modern Psychiatry and Mental Hospitals', address recorded in 'The Royal Medico-Psychological Association' in *JMS*, vol. 80, no. 331, 1934, pp. 757–780.

[99] 'The Royal Medico-Psychological Association: Ninety Fourth Annual Meeting, July 3rd–5th, 1935' in *JMS*, vol. 81, no. 335, pp. 970–991 (p. 981).

of Springfield Mental Hospital, also criticised the research coming from the Association, but in much stronger terms:

> At the risk of bringing the whole of the elegant fabric of this learned society about my ears, I am going to make a bold statement. I maintain, whilst heartily deploring therapeutic nihilism, that we have advanced but little in the diagnosis and treatment of mental disorder: in fact, I am inclined to the view that some cases that have fallen within my purview have recovered in spite of, not because of, the treatment. We are plodding along, some of us desperately in earnest, experimenting with this and that in an empirical fashion, now a new drug and now a new electrical gadget, and so forth, and I express the view, again with all due humility, that I am after all this long time just as bewildered when confronted with a psychosis as I was at the outset of my career.[100]

The freshly revised classification did nothing to cure these concerns. On 30 June 1936, the Research and Clinical Committee of the RMPA put forward a request to the Council of the Association to approach the Board of Control to adopt the classification of mental disorders.[101] It was reported at the 1938 meeting that the Board of Control was not entirely happy with the classification, and had expressed concern about its potential use in asylum statistics because it was too complicated.[102] The classification sub-committee pledged to make amendments in the hope of satisfying the requirements of the board, and sent through an amended classification for their certification. By 1940, the committee had not heard anything other than a formal acknowledgement of receipt from the Board of Control, and due to the emergency conditions imposed by warfare, the committee decided not to pursue the matter any further.[103]

[100] Reginald Worth, 'Four Decades of Psychiatry: The Presidential Address at the Ninety-Fourth Annual Meeting of the Royal Medico-Psychological Association', held in the Middlesex Guildhall, Westminster, July 3, 1935. *In JMS*, vol. 81, no. 335, pp. 755–765 (p. 757).

[101] Royal Medico-Psychological Association, Minutes of the Meeting of the Research and Clinical Committee, June 30th, 1936, in RCPSYCH/L10—Records of the Research and Clinical Section, 1927–1970, held by The Royal College of Psychiatrists, London.

[102] Royal Medico-Psychological Association, Minutes of the Meeting of the Research and Clinical Committee, 10th July 1938 in RCPSYCH/L10—Records of the Research and Clinical Section, 1927–1970, held by The Royal College of Psychiatrists, London.

[103] Dr Strom-Olsen, remarks recorded in Royal Medico-Psychological Association, Minutes of the Meeting of the Research and Clinical Committee, July 17th, 1941, in

The classification was too Freudian for the old guard of British psychiatry, and not Freudian enough for modernisers. Robert Armstrong-Jones, by then in his late seventies and one of the last of the old generation of RMPA members involved in drafting the 1907 Revision, criticised the latest set of revisions for its psychoanalytic influences and for being unsettlingly 'continental' in flavour.[104] Armstrong-Jones took issue with the inclusion of Bleuler's term schizophrenia, which although beginning to replace the Kraepelinian dementia praecox was still objectionable, at least for him.[105] He also took exception to the use of Latin and Greek terminology, complaining that the use of oligophrenia and amentia unnecessarily complicated the classification:

> apart from the uneasiness, and even fear, which many medical men entertain about introducing the Greek Gods and other's into their patients, whether they be Oedipus, Electra, Narcissus or any other, I fail to see the necessity for complicating an English terminology with the use of classical names when the English equivalents can express the full meaning very well.[106]

Behind these gripes with terminology, Armstrong-Jones was airing similar concerns to those of the Board of Control, who also judged the revisions committee's classification to be unnecessarily complicated and unwieldy. Armstrong-Jones thought that the new classification placed an unreasonable requirement to fill in statistical returns using what he termed 'hieroglyphs', and appealed for another revision that simplified the tables.[107] A reply signed by the secretary of the clinical committee was published two weeks later that curtly stated in response that the classification had been

RCPSYCH/L10—Records of the Research and Clinical Section, 1927–1970, held by The Royal College of Psychiatrists, London.

[104] Robert Armstrong-Jones, 'Correspondence: Classification of Mental Disorders' in *BMJ*, June 16th, 1934, pp. 1091–1092 (p. 1091).

[105] The historical instability of *schizophrenia* is an area that needs further research, but Richard Noll's work questions the conceived linear relationship between it and dementia praecox. See: Richard Noll, American Madness: The Rise and Fall of Dementia Praecox, Routledge, 2011.

[106] Ibid.

[107] The Nomenclature of Diseases. Drawn Up by a Joint Committee Appointed by the Royal College of Physicians of London. Sixth Edition, Etc. London, 1931.

approved by the Association one year earlier and that no further work would be conducted to revise the tables.[108]

In contrast, the authors of one of the most influential and longest running textbooks of British psychiatry considered the 1934 Revisions to be crude and retrograde, with the diagnostic concepts it included unbecoming of a classification that had aimed to offer new avenues for psychological diagnosis. I.R.C. Gillespie and D.K. Henderson's damning verdict of what they termed 'the British classification' was that:

> This scheme can hardly be held to reflect modern psychiatric teaching as fully as might have been achieved. Confusional insanity is not a clinical entity on an equal footing with the other categories of part I; it is nearly always, if not always, a symptom of some of the other mental disorders. We have never seen a case which could not be more profitably designated as something else. In actual practice there have been grouped under this heading such diverse diseases as alcoholic, toxic and exhaustion states, senile confusion and dementia praecox. A given case will therefore sometime fall not only into a category of Part II, but into two categories of Part I. A similar criticism applied to the allocation of dementia to a separate category on an equal footing with, for example, schizophrenia, and the affective psychoses, of either of which type of dementia is a terminal state.[109]

As if this was not damning enough, they had also recommended instead the mental health section of the sixth edition of the 'Royal College of Physicians' Nomenclature of Diseases' for use in mental health statistics, one that would eventually formulate the basis of the first clinical classification of mental health disorders issued by the World Health Organization shortly after the Second World War. It is perhaps less surprising that both had sat on the committee that had drawn up the College's classification of mental health conditions.

[108] G.W.T.H. Fleming, 'Correspondence: Classification of Mental Disorders' in *BMJ*, June 30th, 1934, p. 1187.

[109] It is apparent that Henderson and Gillespie were commenting on the earlier 1931 draft of the classification when they target 'confusional insanity', which was reformulated as 'confusional states' in the final classification. As mentioned above, confusional insanity was most notably used during the 1920s in the War Office commission into shellshock, but it was also used by a generation of RMPA members who had experience training and working in asylums: D.K. Henderson and R.D. Gillespie, *A Textbook of Psychiatry for Students and Practitioners*, 3rd edition, OUP, 1932, p. 13.

In their attack on the Table of the Forms, Gillespie and Henderson represented a new wave of psychiatrists who had trained in out-patient wings of general hospitals and would view themselves as internationalist in their approach, looking beyond the narrow parochialism of the British asylum. Indeed, both Henderson and Gillespie had spent time abroad, working with Emil Kraepelin in Germany and Adolf Meyer at the John Hopkins Hospital in Baltimore.[110] The alternative classification that they presented in their textbook bore the marks of these influences, with them being one of the central lines of communication to British Psychiatry for Meyer's psycho-biological approach to the theory and treatment of mental disorder, or the New Psychiatry as it was sometimes called. Henderson and Gillespie questioned the category of 'psychopathic constitution' claiming that it was outdated, and that there was little justification for tying paranoia to hereditary factors.[111] They favoured the American Psychiatric Association's schema, which they judged to be more faithful to the spirit of Kraepelin's work, albeit with modifications that were largely down to Meyer's influence. In their classification, they stressed that they were not describing different kinds of mental disorders or diseases, but were instead describing what they termed 'different types of reaction'.[112] Their rationale for talking about 'reaction types' was to incorporate into their own work on classification that incorporated environmental causes, and wrote how 'the individual as a psycho-biological individual [is] perpetually called upon to adapt to a social environment'.[113] Whilst appearing to break from past tradition in calling for attention to be paid to the psychological make-up of the individual, the pair still made concessions to heredity when they stated that 'in many instances the constitutional element is the important factor [and] that the environmental influences in a number of cases are of relatively minor importance'.[114] What marks their work as historically significant is that they acknowledged an internal psychological environment, and argued

[110] K. Loughlin, 'Henderson, Sir David Kennedy (1884–1965), Psychiatrist' in *Oxford Dictionary of National Biography*, September 23rd, 2004.

[111] K. Henderson and R.D. Gillespie, *A Textbook of Psychiatry for Students and Practitioners*, 3rd edition, OUP, 1932, p. 16.

[112] Ibid., p. 21.

[113] Ibid.

[114] Ibid.

that 'what is regarded as a constitutional type of mental disorder may often be the reaction of the mind to inner-stimuli to which it finds difficulty in maintaining a healthy adjustment'.[115] Psychopathic constitution is the most obvious of the psychopathologies open to their criticism since it was the most clearly linked of the psychological categories included in the first part of the classification to hereditarian causation. It was very likely that this was in fact the target of their criticism since Henderson was at this time conducting research on psychopathy which culminated in his textbook in 1939 which listed different types of the disorder that had given consideration to both developmental and constitutional factors in the development of psychopathy (Table 7.2).

The pair also expressed regret that the RMPA's classification isolated forms of exhaustion-based insanity from others, claiming in their textbook that exhaustion was a symptom 'which on further analysis will be found to express either an anxiety or a hysterical psychoneurosis or some other form of mental illness'.[116] For both, the classification committee had made a grave error in confusing symptoms with disease types, which was something that the pair sought to resolve by referring to reaction types instead of disease entities:

> The truth is that no attempt at classification is entirely satisfactory, and consequently that 'diagnosis', or the placing of the patient in the appropriate class, is on an unstable foundation. But, fortunately, it is not diagnosis that matters, but the understanding of the disorder, and of the patient who suffers from it—under what circumstances it arose, how it is related to the patient's normal condition, what the disorder means, what light is shed on his problems, and what can be done to help towards a favourable outcome. In Adolf Meyer's words, it is not the patients we are told to sort out, but the facts; and while in the following pages the case records will be arranged in groups for the sake of more or less systematic description, the disorders exhibited will be considered as the individual reactions of a specially endowed, and often constitutionally loaded, organism to the environment.
>
> Nevertheless, classification is useful and even necessary; first for the student; that he may more readily grasp and arrange his cases; and second, for the compilation of a uniform set of statistics by institutions and administrative authorities, in order to make comparison possible. It seems to me that it

[115] Ibid.

[116] Ibid.

Table 7.2 Classification of mental diseases as included in Henderson and Gillespie's *A Textbook of Psychiatry*

SECTION III

Mental Diseases.

- Mental deficiency (Amentia.)
  - Simple
  - Mongolian
  - Microcephalic.
  - Amaurotic
  - Sclerotic
  - Hydrocephalic
  - Inflammatory
  - Syphilitic
  - Paralytic
  - Epileptic
  - Cretinous
  - Due to sensory deprivation
- Idiocy
- Imbecility
- Feeble-mindedness
- Dulness and backwardness
- Moral deficiency
- Psychoses accompanying Organic diseases
  - Toxic
    - Endogenous (*e g.*, uræmia, eclampsia, &c)
    - Exogenous
      - Due to alcohol
        - Mania a potu
        - Chronic alcoholism
        - Delirium tremens
        - Alcoholic hallucinosis (acute and chronic)
        - Alcoholic dementia
        - Korsakow's polyneuritic psychosis
      - Due to Opium
      - Due to Lead
      - Due to other poisons
- Infection-exhaustion psychoses.
  - General
    - Prefebrile, febrile and post-febrile delirium
    - Exhaustion-psychoses
    - Puerperal psychoses
    - Psychoses associated with chronic organic disease.
  - Local brain-infections.
    - Syphilis
      - Cerebral syphilis
      - General paralysis
        - (Dementia paralytica)
    - Encephalitis (including Epidemic encephalitis)
    - Meningitis
    - Abscess.
- Psychoses with Primary Degenerative Brain-changes
  - Senile dementia
  - Presenile sclerosis.
  - Arteriosclerotic brain-disease.
  - Huntington's chorea
- Psychoses with Brain-trauma
  - Traumatic delirium
  - Traumatic constitution
    - (Explosive diathesis)
  - Traumatic mental enfeeblement
- Psychoses with Organic Brain-disease (*e g.*, Tumour, Multiple sclerosis, Thrombosis, Embolism, &c)
- Psychoses associated with Metabolic and Endocrine disorders
  - Pellagra
  - Myxœdema.
  - Other metabolic disorders

13

14 MENTAL DISEASES

Mental Diseases—*continued*

- Functional psychoses.
  - Manic-depressive
    - Mania
      - Hypomania.
      - Acute mania
      - Acute delirious mania
    - Depression
      - Simple retardation
      - Acute depression
      - Depressive stupor
      - Hypochondriacal depression
    - Stupor
      - Manic stupor
      - Depressive stupor
    - Mixed type (*e g.*, agitated depression)
    - Circular type
    - Alternating type.
    - Recurrent type
  - Cyclothymia
  - Involution melancholia
  - Hypochondriasis.
  - Paranoia
  - Paranoid state.
  - Hallucinatory paranoid state
  - Paraphrenia.
  - Schizophrenia.
    - (Dementia præcox)
    - Simple
    - Hebephrenic
    - Paranoid
    - Catatonic
    - Periodic.
- Epileptic psychoses
  - Epileptic dementia.
  - Epileptic confusion
  - Epileptic dream-state.
  - Epileptic automatism.
  - Epileptic hallucinatory paranoid state.
  - Epileptic depression.
  - Epileptic excitement.
- Psychopathic personality.
  - Temperamental instability.
  - Pathological lying.
    - (Pseudologia phantastica)
  - Pathological swindling
  - Kleptomania
  - Contentious (litigious) type
  - Sexual perversions
- Psychoneuroses
  - Neurasthenia †
  - Anxiety-neurosis
    - (Psychoneurotic anxiety-state)
  - Phobia
    - Agoraphobia
    - Claustrophobia.
  - Hysteria.
  - Obsessive-compulsive psycho-neurosis (Psychasthenia)

† This term is used in various senses and should therefore be avoided.

> would be a great help to British psychiatry if a uniform type of classification were adopted similar to that [of the APA]. The Royal College of Physicians (England) has lately recognised this and has tried to adopt, in its Nomenclature of Diseases, a classification similar to that which follows [in this textbook].[117]

The Table of the Forms would be criticised by two additional future doyens of British psychiatry in Bernard Hart and Eliot Slater. Both had served on the revisions committee for the Nomenclature of Diseases of the Royal College of Physicians, which as mentioned would formulate the basis of the first classification of mental diseases used by the World Health Organization. Slater would also write a textbook with the German émigré Wilhelm Mayer Gross and Michael Roth that again would, like Henderson and Gillespie, call for attention to be paid to the psychological terrain of a patient in the treatment of mental health disorders.[118] Mayer Gross was an influential figure in British psychiatry since his arrival in the British Isles in 1933, and he would come to be regarded as the founder of 'The British School of Psychiatry', a form of psychiatric inquiry that was informed by the phenomenology of Henri Bergson, Edmund Husserl, Max Scheler and Karl Jaspers.[119]

The classification did however receive one of the few positive reviews from an unexpected source. Hugh Stott, the Principal and Dean of King George's Medical College in Lucknow, India, wrote in the *Indian Medical Gazette* that the RMPA had 'presented the medical profession with a practical scheme of classification' that was 'helpful in its ease of application, so elastic in its provision for future extension and so stimulating towards the fuller investigation of the cause of each individual case of mental disorder that it appears worthy of the widest adoption'.[120] It is unclear whether the Table of the Forms was a curate's egg for Stott, but if his remarks are taken at face value, then they constitute perhaps the only

[117] Ibid., p. 16.

[118] William Meyer-Gross, Eliot Slater and Martin Roth, *Clinical Psychiatry*, Cassell, 1954.

[119] Rhodri Hayward, 'Germany and the Making of 'English' Psychiatry: The Maudsley Hospital 1908–1939' in *International Relations in Psychiatry: Britain, Germany and the United States to World War II*, edited by Volker Roelcke, Paul J. Weindling and Louise Westwood, University of Rochester Press, 2013, pp. 67–90.

[120] Hugh Stott, 'The Royal Medico-Psychological Association's Classification of Mental Disorders' in *the Indian Medical Gazette*, vol. 70, no. 1, January 1935, pp. 33–36.

review that took the classification seriously. Despite Stott's overtures, he had one minor criticism, albeit a constructive one; he suggested revision of category D of the classification from 'Psychopathic Constitution and Paranoia' with the sub-categories of pathologic constitution and paranoia, to 'Systematised Delusional Psychosis' with paranoia retained as a sub-category, and paraphrenia added replacing pathologic constitution. Stott also considered paraphrenia a 'half-way link' between delusional psychosis and the forms of dementia praecox included in the RMPA's classification in Part I, category C. He wrote that '[i]f paraphrenia is placed in the above relationship with paranoia, the paranoid type of dementia praecox in which delusion occurs becomes the connecting link with group C'.[121] Stott's criticisms, as well-intentioned as they appear, were some of the only positive noises made towards the RMPA's 1934 Revision.

Conclusion

This chapter has outlined how competing schools of thought during the interwar period shaped the last version of the Table of the Forms, published in 1934. Figures such as the RMPA president Richard Leeper had little time for approaches to psychiatry that diverged from hereditarian theories of causation, and although his dogmatic views are by no means representative of all members of the Association, they do indicate the stark differences within British psychiatry during the interwar period. For every psychiatrist who understood mental disorder primarily as a product of congenital weaknesses, the solution to which was prevention, containment and isolation from the rest of society, there were as many who sought to establish newer approaches to diagnosis and classification that could reform or replace the institution. In an attempt to pave over theoretical and professional differences, the classifications committee produced a document that sought to bring together different approaches to diagnosis in one classification. The final version of the classification was a curious mélange of the fashions of the time, with its inclusion of focal infection, hereditarian concepts of diagnosis and Koch's psychopathy, along with the usual Kraepelinian and Freudian suspects and remnants of nineteenth-century symptomology.

Although admirable in its ambition, the attempts to incorporate different approaches and satisfy conflicting attitudes severely weakened

[121] Ibid., p. 35.

the coherence of the system produced. Unfortunately, as we see with the examples of Leeper, Glover and Cotton, these approaches were in many ways incompatible and mutually exclusive: for Leeper, any form of classification was pointless given that all mental disorders are caused by constitution, whereas Glover's attempts to reconcile psychiatry and psychology through psychoanalysis would have been dismissed by Cotton as pointless because mental disorders were caused by infections of the body. As noble as the intentions were to create a universal classification to bring these schools together, they also made the last revision to the Table unpopular, with the version published in 1934 attracting near universal scorn. It failed to convince prominent members of the British psychiatric profession and the Board of Control that it would serve as a useful document for diagnostic purposes, and it would never become implemented in practice. As we will see in the next chapter, this would be the last set of revisions that would be made to the Table of the Forms, and during planning for the new nationalised health system that took place from 1942 onwards, it was decided to use the Nomenclature of Diseases of the Royal College of Physicians for the purposes of diagnosis in mental health statistics, which would formulate the basis for the concepts of mental health included in the *International Classification of Diseases* upon its introduction in 1948.

The circumstances surrounding the last revision to the Table of the Forms, as well as the diagnostic categories it contained, represent not only structural changes to medicine, but also cultural attitudes to mental disorder. Prevailing orthodoxies that had informed asylum psychiatry were challenged, but as we have seen, these still informed much of the work on classification that had been carried out during the interwar years. At the same time as there were those like Leeper, whose views bore the stamp of Victorian asylum and eugenics, there were those who were working in modern research institutes and out-patient clinics who sought to establish ways to treat psychiatric patients without admittance and a lengthy stay within an institution. The last set of revisions came at the crossroads of the remaining vestiges of the diagnostic categories commonly used in the Victorian asylum with the rising popularity of Kraepelinian classifications and Freudian notions of the psychological significance of trauma as a cause of neurosis and psychosis. The concepts included in the 1934 Revisions were the last flourish of professionals like Leeper and Armstrong-Jones who had practised for much of their career in the asylum.

CHAPTER 8

The 'Mesozoic' Table of the Forms: Admissions Reform 1942–1948

By November 1944, the balance of power in the Second World War had tipped towards the allies, and peace, although not certain, was becoming an ever-closer prospect. The huge reforms to health and social care that had been proposed in Beveridge's 1942 report were by this point in full motion, with special commissions appointed by the war cabinet to look at ways to realise a universal social and health service for the post-war world.[1] These projects and fact-finding exercises were commissioned by the government during the final phases of the war to assess the current state of health services to help realise this grand vision, and they were often led by prominent medical professionals, including psychiatrists.[2] As cities and infrastructure were beginning to be rebuilt, the profession turned its attention to the role psychiatry would play in a better society. At the summer meeting of the association, Lt Col. Andrew Petrie, serving as president, gave an address that provided a quite extraordinary vision of the role that psychiatry would play in the post-war world.[3] Not only

[1] Frank Honigsbaum, *Health, Happiness, and Security: The Creation of the National Health Service*, Routledge, 1989.

[2] Kathleen Jones, *Asylums and After: A Revised History of the Mental Health Services: From the Early 18th Century to the 1990s*, Athlone Press, 1993, p. 143.

[3] Charles Webster, *The Health Services Since the War vol. 1*, London, HMSO, 1988–1996, pp. 11–12.

K. M. Jones, *Psychological Classification and Diagnosis in Asylum Statistics, 1800–1948*, Mental Health in Historical Perspective,
https://doi.org/10.1007/978-3-031-46154-5_8

would a new and better society emerge after the war, but also a new and better psychiatric profession, one that would go beyond the clinic and would be wound into the fabric of social life.[4] Petrie's plan was grounded in his conviction that psychiatry should no longer preoccupy itself with heredity and degeneration, but instead pay an increased attention to how environmental factors caused mental health conditions.[5] If psychiatry were to shift its focus, then a radical social psychiatry would follow, one that saw mental health services incorporated into education, industry, the Church, advertising, the arts and politics. Petrie used changes in his own attitudes during his time in the military to stress the point, with the observations on the trauma of pilots and sailors that he treated prompting a re-evaluation of the role of hereditary constitution as a deciding factor in the causes of mental illnesses. If the profession as a whole could learn similar lessons from the war, then it could seize opportunities it had not taken advantage of during the inertia of the interwar period. To realise these ambitions, Petrie proposed plans that included every major political party appointing a psychiatric advisor to enable a better understanding of the desires of the general population:

> A psychological bureau attached to each of the great political parties is an obvious suggestion, and such parties would be more likely to guide their followers widely if influenced by sound psychological principles. With a given party in power such a bureaux [*sic*] would become advisors to the Cabinet, a position occupied by the soothsayers of the ancient world.[6]

Petrie went on: 'although ancient soothsayers were superstitious, they had some psychological understanding of the masses, and their advice allowed politicians to be more effective leaders'.[7] The occult magic of soothsayers, with their mystical ability to tune into the frequency of the public and understand their desires, could now be practised by the modern psychiatrist.

[4] A.A.W. Petrie, 'Psychiatric Developments: The Presidential Address Delivered at the One Hundred and Third Annual Meeting of the Association on Wednesday November 29th 1944' in *JMS*, vol. 91, no. 384, July 1945.

[5] Ibid.

[6] Ibid., p. 269.

[7] Ibid.

Although Petrie's grand vision did not quite work out as planned, reforms were in the process of being made to psychiatric services that would expand their purview beyond the established boundaries of former asylums.[8] The introduction of the health service saw a number of developments that brought psychiatry closer to general medicine, at least within the British context, with mental hospitals—no longer referred to as asylums—being brought into a unified health care system.[9] Changes to mental health statistics would coincide with the amalgamation of mental hospitals into the nationalised health system, with health records from psychiatric institutions being combined with those of mental health wards in general hospitals to produce new frameworks that would define mental health statistics during the years immediately after the war and beyond. The changes described in this chapter would mark the end of the functional life of the Table of the Forms, since mental health statistics would no longer be published in asylum annual reports and instead would be published in statistical health reports issued by the Registrar-General's office. The Board of Control was replaced by the Ministry of Health as overseeing body of former asylums under the new National Health Service, and similarly mental health statistics became aligned to general health statistics. The Table itself came to be deemed a relic of the asylum era, a document that was nothing more than a part of the fossil record of mental health diagnosis and public health statistics.

As a result of the redesign of admissions procedures and medical data collection that were conducted in anticipation of a new health service, the enactment of the National Health Service Act in July 1948 would signal the end of the operational life of the Table of the Forms. The Mental Health section of the World Health Organization's *International Classification of Diseases* (*ICD*) would be chosen as the standard set of psychological diagnoses used in mental health statistics derived from new admissions procedures. The data on admissions would be returned to the General Record Office, the same agency that processed them prior to the

[8] Kevin Matthew Jones, 'A National Social Care Service beyond COVID-19: Lessons from the History of Mental Health Social Work and the Origins of the NHS' in History and Policy, 14 June 2021, Available Online:https://www.historyandpolicy.org/policy-papers/papers/a-national-social-care-service-beyond-covid-19-lessonsfrom-the-history-of-mental-health-social-work-and-the-origins-of-the-nhs

[9] Charles Webster, 'Psychiatry and the Early National Health Service: The Role of the Mental Health Standing Advisory Committee' in *150 Years of British Psychiatry*, edited by Berrios and Freeman, Gaskell, 1991, pp. 103–106.

establishment of the Lunacy Commission under the terms of the 1845 Lunacy Acts.

This chapter will present the conclusion to the story of the Table of the Forms. It will outline changes that led to the end of its operational existence, which were linked to the broader institutional alignment of psychiatry to general medicine due to mental health services being brought within the remit of the National Health Service (NHS). Reflecting the optimism of Britain's role in international affairs towards the end of the war and immediately after, the redesigns to NHS admissions data collection were viewed to be a part of a vision of global psychiatry, and a key development in the realisation of a transnational psychiatric epidemiology. The adoption of the *ICD* for new NHS procedures for recording patient data on psychological diagnosis therefore signalled wider changes to the collection and publication of medical statistics that would define the post-war period.

From 1942, plans were being made to reform the processes used to collect the data of psychiatric patients as a part of a set of measures to develop mental health statistics beyond the asylum and lunacy administration. Data on mental health were not to be kept distinct from the rest of medicine, as had been the case since the passing of the 1845 Lunacy Acts, which had made the collection and publication of asylum statistics a responsibility of the Commissioners in Lunacy.[10] Mental health policy was no longer predominantly focused on the asylum, but had become viewed by policymakers as a part of daily life, and accordingly, mental health statistics must be reformed to, as the sociologist Nikolas Rose phrases it, 'chart the neurotic topography of the population'.[11] In a report on mental health records conducted as a part of these measures to reform mental health data collection, the psychiatrist and eugenicist Carlos Patton Blacker deemed the Table of the Forms to be 'Mesozoic'.[12] To improve the data collection procedures on psychological diagnosis,

[10] For a full account of the initial steps to integrate psychiatry and general medicine, see Kathleen Jones, 'First Steps in Integration' in *Mental Health and Social Policy, 1845–1959*, Routledge, 1960, pp. 135–147.

[11] Nikolas Rose, *Inventing Ourselves: Psychology, Power and Personhood*, Cambridge University Press, 1996, p. 134.

[12] Carlos Patton Blacker, 'Mental Health Records: What We Can Learn from Them?', 27th February 1947, in Papers by Carlos Paton Blacker on Mental Health Records, Carlos Paton Blacker Collected Papers, held by The Wellcome Collection.

Blacker thought it necessary to replace the Table of the Forms with a classification of diseases that included mental health disorders within a general nosology of all human medical conditions: this would be the simplest way of resolving the difficulties that had plagued asylum statistics since their introduction in 1845, and bring medical records pertaining to mental health together with those of general health.

Mental health statistics, records, classification and diagnosis would come under the scrutiny of the research conducted by Blacker and the biologist Lionel Penrose. Their research was one project amongst many that was commissioned to explore ways to bring general and psychiatric medical services under a unified health service, services that had long been divided administratively and institutionally.[13] These moves were prompted by recent trends towards treating psychiatric patients in general hospitals, with some suggesting that better recovery rates were seen in patients admitted to general hospitals than to specialised psychiatric institutions.[14] Patients who suffered the kinds of transitory anxiety and neurotic states that had been seen throughout the war, and those demonstrating early signs of psychosis, could have 'avoided prolongation of illness, subsequent certification, and economic loss' with early admission and treatment, but this would remain difficult to achieve given the association the public had of lengthy stays in asylums, and the many other stigmas associated with psychiatric treatment.[15]

Vivian Quirk and Jean-Paul Gaudillière note that the period immediately following the Second World War had also started an era of global biomedicine, characterised by attempts by national and international medical societies to forge stronger links between the laboratory and the clinic.[16] Adopting the *ICD* for medical records was part of a wider vision to realise a transnational project in global psychiatric epidemiology that was modelled on previous attempts to trace illnesses and disease on a global scale. It would be the classification of mental health conditions of

[13] Kathleen Jones, 'First Steps in Integration' in *Mental Health and Social Policy, 1845–1959*, Routledge, 1960, pp. 135–147.

[14] D.E. Sands, 'Treatment of Psychiatric Patients in General Hospitals: A Social Experiment' in *BMJ*, May 22nd, 1943, p. 628.

[15] Ibid.

[16] Vivian Quirk and Jean-Paul Gaudillière, 'The Era of Biomedicine: Science, Medicine, and Public Health in Britain and France After the Second World War' in *Medical History*, vol. 52, pp. 441–452.

the Royal College of Physicians that formulated the basis of the mental health section of the *ICD*, not the classification of the RMPA. This is because of the near-universal scorn poured on the final version of the Table, and as outlined in the last chapter, it had come to be regarded with derision by a younger generation of psychiatrists.

The *ICD* itself was based on previous international classifications of the causes of death that were published first by the Office International d'Hygiène Publique upon its formation in 1907, and subsequently by the League of Nations' Health Organisation during the interwar period. Although these documents included neurological disorders and a select few concepts of mental disorder, they primarily functioned to standardise the recording of causes of death, and not those made in medical diagnosis. The change in 1948 to it being a classification of recognised diseases allowed the inclusion of concepts of mental disorder, bringing psychological diagnosis into a standard general medical nosology which aimed to reflect a global medical consensus.

In his analysis of psychiatric journals from 1950 onwards, John Burnham claims that the 'extreme national isolation of psychiatric communities' of the pre-war period 'gave way to a substantial transnationalisation' of psychiatric discourse.[17] Focusing on the *Journal of Mental Science* during this period, Burnham claims that the journal functioned as an important communication channel between the ideas in Europe and the Americas, and was also tied to Britain's former colonies of Australia, New Zealand and Canada. Burnham's view that there was extreme isolation prior to the war is to some extent questioned by the work of Rhodri Hayward, Paul J. Weindling and Mark Jackson, who in their work identify the permeable boundaries between European, British and American psychiatry during the interwar years.[18] As we have seen, the development of psychiatric epidemiology was to some extent a transnational project,

[17] John C. Burnham, 'Transnational History of Medicine After 1950: Framing and Interrogation from Psychiatric Journals' in *Medical History*, vol. 55, no. 1, 2011, pp. 3–26.

[18] See Rhodri Hayward, 'Germany and the Making of 'English' Psychiatry: The Maudsley Hospital 1908–1939'; Mark Jackson, 'Permeating National Boundaries: European and American Influences on the emergence of Medico-Pedagogy in Late Victorian and Edwardian Britain'; Paul J. Weindling, 'Alien Psychiatrists: the British Assimilation of Psychiatric Refugees, 1930–1950' in *International Relations in Psychiatry: Britain, Germany and the United States to World War II*, edited by Volker Roelcke, Paul J. Weindling and Louise Westwood, University of Rochester Press, 2013, pp. 67–90.

albeit confined largely to European medical circles during the period of this study. As we have seen throughout this work, there were important differences between, and distinctive features of, the mental sciences in France, Germany, Italy, the United Kingdom and the USA, with each developing tables of psychological diagnosis for use in official statistics. At the same time, the concepts used were often exchanged between national and linguistic boundaries, with cross-pollination being facilitated at least as far back as the first decades of the nineteenth century through the translation of textbooks. As medical journals developed in the mental sciences during the second half of the nineteenth century, reviews of textbooks served as a means to circulate ideas on psychological diagnosis. The development of the Association from its establishment in 1841 saw the further proliferation of cross-border exchanges on medical diagnosis, with psychiatrists from outside the United Kingdom being frequently invited to present at meetings, and the participation of Association members in international conferences and statistical organisations. The post-war period saw the resumption of international co-operation after the interregnum caused by European fascism's disruption of measures to create a transnational project that could develop a global medical epidemiology. Measures before 1945 had been limited to causes of death and diseases, but the first classification of the WHO had introduced a section on mental disorders with the view to developing ways to collect and publish vital statistics pertaining to mental health. This was to build on earlier work conducted by the International Statistical Institute and the Health Organisation of the League of Nations, both of whom had made attempts to develop ways to collect and collate medical statistics from countries with national statistical bureaux, although there was still no clear vision on how this would be achieved with psychological diagnosis. Individuals including Blacker believed that the United Kingdom, with its well-established and centralised bureaucracy, could and indeed should work to develop a models for the collection of medical statistics that could be applied further afield.

Psychiatrists from the United Kingdom and the other Allied powers played a prominent role in the formulation of an international psychiatry that would come to define the post-war era. They sought to bring about greater standardisation of practice, treatment and classification. After the Second World War, Britain enjoyed a period of international influence, with notable scientists and public administrators appointed to leading roles within global organisations. Julian Huxley was perhaps the most prominent of these figures, being appointed head of UNESCO in 1946, with John Boyd-Orr serving as the first Director-General of the United Nations Food and Agriculture Division, and the British-trained Canadian psychiatrist Brock Chisholm acting as the first head of the WHO.[19] With its establishment in 1948 replacing the health bodies of the League of Nations, the WHO ushered in what Iris Borowy calls a 'third phase' of international health co-operation; the first phase being the rise of international societies during the nineteenth century, and the second being marked by the work of the League of Nations Health Organisation after the Great War.[20] This third period was marked by heightened interest in mental health care which, until this point, had been neglected on an international level since the League of Nations did not have a well-established policy towards mental health, and instead philanthropic organisations such as the Rockefeller were largely responsible for the development and funding of global mental hygiene initiatives.[21] This began to change after the war, with psychiatry attracting interest from transnational medicine due to its links to wider political and social concerns. The rise of fascism was understood by some as being a form of mass psychosis, with psychologists and psychiatrists in the Allied countries coming to view themselves as playing some role in preventing extremist political forces coming into power again.[22] The Sheffield-based German émigré Erwin Stengel and the Tavistock-affiliated head of psychiatry for the British Army, T.P. Rees, were pivotal figures in these movements, with Stengel viewing a shared international terminology of mental disorders as indispensable for a global psychiatry that would lead to universal human betterment.[23]

[19] Allen Irving. *Brock Chisholm: Doctor to the World*, Fitzhenry & Whiteside, 1998.

[20] See Iris Borowy, *Coming to Terms with World Health: The League of Nations Health Organisation 1921–1946*, Peter Lang, 2009.

[21] The Rockefeller foundations, for instance, had helped to fund the first training course for psychiatric social workers in the United Kingdom and possibly in Europe; Noel Timms, *Psychiatric Social Work in Great Britain, 1939–1962*, Humanities Press, 1964.

[22] F.A. Jenner, 'Erwin Stengel: A Personal Memoir' in *150 Years of British Psychiatry: 1841–1991*, edited by German Berrios and Freeman, Gaskell, 1991.

[23] Attempts to psychologise fascism and understand it as a mental disorder began with Wilhelm Reich's work, *The Mass Psychology of Fascism*, which was published in 1933, although it would not be translated into English until 1946. In this work, Reich offered the theory that fascism was a product of a repressed sexual urge, and this was the key to understanding why it had come to triumph in Germany and not in other nations.

The establishment of the NHS provided an opportunity for the improvement of the quality of admissions diagnosis data, which in turn could improve mental health statistics and could contribute to transnational projects. The hope was to emulate and improve upon the successes of book-keeping methods in the United States and Germany, and use the power of a centralised bureaucracy to provide new avenues for medical records.[24] As we have seen in previous chapters, the tricky question of what forms of insanity should be used in statistical tables was the catalyst for debate over classification, psychological diagnosis and medical statistics, and after one hundred years of such debate, the question had still not made much headway. Speaking at the first annual general meeting convened by the Royal Medico-Psychological Association (RMPA) after the Second World War, Penrose commented on this lack of progress, and provided his own suggestions on how to improve the collection of medical statistics.[25] Penrose focused upon what he called the social impact of mental illness: the burden placed upon families caring for relatives, associates within the workplace and the wider community.[26] Penrose called for improvement in the collection of mental health statistics because it was only through these that the social impact of mental health disorders could be understood. He thought that the figures could be garnered from, firstly, cases treated in both mental hospitals and psychiatric wards, and secondly from the general population, who were treated at home and in out-patient clinics. According to Penrose, in-patients were, or at least ought to be for the most part, 'psychotic' and 'mentally deficient patients', with neurotic patients tending to be treated in out-patient

Although Reich's view is highly questionable, this, and the large number of psychiatrists who emigrated from the Nazi regime, triggered attempts by the human sciences to understand the psychology of fascism. Another highly problematic study, *The Authoritarian Personality*, which has become infamous for its association with the Frankfurt School philosopher Theodor Adorno, was also influential during the 1940s and 1950s, and the work that these studies prompted had some influence on global health policies. See Wilhelm Reich, *The Mass Psychology of Fascism: Translated from the German Manuscript*, translated by Mary Boyd Higgins, Orgone Institute Press, 1946; Theodor Adorno et al., *The Authoritarian Personality*, Harper and Row, 1950.

24 Volker Hess, 'A Paper Machine of Clinical Research in the Early Twentieth Century' in *Isis*, vol. 109, no. 3, 2018, pp. 473–493.

25 L.S., Penrose, 'Social Aspects of Psychiatry: The Importance of Statistics' in *JMS*, vol. 9, no. 389, October 1946, pp. 713–718.

26 Ibid.

wards and in the home.[27] He emphasised that at present, the mental health statistics garnered from the medical records of patients diagnosed by medical authorities were the best guide available to public health authorities on the impact of psychological illness upon society.

He noted that British psychiatry's preoccupation with heredity had proved to be an obstacle to a nuanced approach to understanding mental health amongst the general population. He singled out Frederick Mott as one of the most recent and evangelical adherents, and that research corrupted by eugenics had hindered scientific progress.[28] Penrose argued that psychiatrists like Mott had misinterpreted their data by placing an unwarranted emphasis on heredity as a cause of mental disorder. In doing so, they had overlooked social and environmental circumstances as causing factors. As we have seen from this work, no attempts were made by those involved in the discussions to develop a Table of social or environmental causes, or integrate either into diagnostic concepts. Penrose thought psychiatry and mental health statistics as a whole had overlooked important causing factors that were social in nature, such as parents with undiagnosed mental health problems causing developmental problems in their children.[29] Psychiatric social work could remedy the situation, and provide solutions including breaking the cycle of intergenerational mental health problems by supporting parents suffering from a mental health condition they themselves may never recognise they have. Penrose proposed that such a system would need data collection procedures that would go beyond capturing data at the point of admittance to a hospital, with the notes drawn up by psychiatric social workers and other professionals involved in the development of mental health social care requiring new procedures that would amalgamate these data points. The work involved would have powerful returns, with increased infrastructure and better data in diagnosis providing more visibility of social and mental health problems. Penrose hoped that in turn this would raise awareness of mental health disorders and could lead to an increase in those seeking treatment, which, thereby would increase the data captured on diagnosis amongst the population.

[27] Ibid.

[28] Ibid.

[29] Ibid.

Penrose acknowledged that such a service was a long way off. Until the day came when psychiatric social services could be employed to collect data on mental disorders amongst the public, inferences based upon the data gathered from hospital admissions would have to suffice. Although acknowledging that these numbers had their limitations, Penrose claimed that even very basic data could be used to provide imperfect but useful inferences that could provide insights into the mental disorders suffered by the population.[30] He thought it possible to make predictions based upon basic data such as the age of a patient's first admission and their gender, and that these would have a good degree of reliability: a case certified below the age of twenty was, according to Penrose, most likely a 'defective'. As the age increased over twenty, it would become likely that they were a 'schizophrenic' if they were a male, however this would be up to thirty-five in females. Affective psychosis would see its peak at forty-five for women and fifty-five for men. Anyone diagnosed for the first time after sixty-five would most often be suffering with 'senile or organic' disorder.[31]

Blacker similarly thought mental health statistics needed an overhaul. He had collaborated with Penrose in research undertaken to reform mental health records from 1942, which was implemented into admissions procedures for psychiatric patients into general and psychiatric hospitals from 1948. In remarks to the Psychological Group of the British Medical Association, Blacker gave his view of the admissions system that had been in place since the establishment of the Board of Control in 1913, which used the Schedule of Aetiological Factors and the MPA's Table of the Forms. He criticised the inclusion of masturbation in the 'Schedule of Aetiological Factors' as a cause of mental disorder and thought that it demonstrated the ignorance of psychiatric knowledge from before the time when the causes of General Paralysis of the Insane were known. He poured equal scorn on the Table of the Forms of Mental Disorder with the damning judgement that it was a relic from 'the Mesozoic age of psychiatry', expressing distaste at its continued use in reports issued by the Board of Control.[32] In his report on the state of mental health records, explored in this chapter, he expanded upon this geological metaphor in his judgement of the history of psychiatric records, and

30 Ibid.

31 Ibid.

32 Carlos Patton Blacker, 'Mental Health Records: What We Can Learn from Them?', 27th February 1947, in Papers by Carlos Paton Blacker on Mental Health Records, Carlos Paton Blacker Collected Papers, held by The Wellcome Collection.

meticulously broke down the development of the Table into different periods, with the period before the 1890 Lunacy Act described as the Paleozoic era, the Mesozoic era running from the passing of the 1890 act until the passing of the 1930 Mental Treatment Act, and the Caenozoic era running from 1930. Blacker labelled the Table 'Mesozoic' because he took exception to it not including schizophrenia as a diagnostic category. This suggests he was reviewing the 1907 Revision and not the 1934 Revisions, the latter of which, as the last chapter showed, had in fact included it as a main category. Further clues that Blacker was in fact reviewing the 1907 Revision are apparent in remarks in the same report that criticise the main headings of delusional, volitional and moral insanity as inappropriate for their time, but none of which are in the 1934 Revision.

Although he deployed a natural and somewhat determinist metaphor to describe the development of mental health records, he also apportioned blame for their glacial progress. The chaotic handling of mental health records by lunacy bureaucracy and the failure to publish useable statistics on mental health diagnosis were both down to perfunctory administration that did not seem to understand how to complete the task:

> Clerical staff have little in common with the Light Brigade, but there is one feature in common: 'Theirs was not to reason why'. They compiled knowing that compilations could never be published. In-coordination of forms and returns. *Without ridicule* [underlined in pencil].[33]

Blacker had a point. When I myself went through the mental health records during the research for this volume, I was surprised that detailed breakdowns of admissions by diagnosis were only sporadically published in annual reports from 1845. Blacker considered this not just a problem for mental health statistics, but one that had stymied the development of psychiatric knowledge:

> the fact that the information, laboriously collected and assiduously compiled, was never published, may have been responsible for the continuation into the caenozoic [*sic*] era of psychiatry of habits characteristic of its Mesozoic age.[34]

[33] Carlos Patton Blacker, 'Mental Health Records: What We Can Learn from Them?', 27th February 1947, in Papers by Carlos Paton Blacker on Mental Health Records, Carlos Paton Blacker Collected Papers, held by The Wellcome Collection.

[34] Ibid.

Blacker blamed these problems on an administrative culture that failed to adopt technologies allowing efficient data collation. Manual processing of statistical returns had continued despite the introduction of new counting technologies such as tabulating machines. Systems using punched cards, resembling those proposed by Charles Babbage in 1848 and developed by the United States Census Bureau during the 1890s, were used to compile the 1911, 1921 and 1931 British censuses.[35] Blacker blamed 'tradition, custom and inertia' within lunacy administration for the lack of adoption of similar technologies to assist in the compilation of asylum medical statistics. He speculated that members of the Board of Control may have not raised these issues in parliament because of some odd sense of loyalty to fellow commissioners on the board. Blacker did commend the 1914 Board of Control Reports for providing some of the most comprehensive statistics on diagnosis, with complex breakdowns of information on diagnosis amongst other things, and he puts the end of the short-lived successes down to the economic pressures imposed by the Great War. Despite the success of the 1914 report, he somewhat sardonically remarks that established procedures and an unwillingness to change them had prevented further progress. The unwillingness led to a lack of interest in adopting new technologies, with the paper technologies of pen and paper not having given way to electrical methods, remarking that 'old pen and ink methods [were] like using hand plough when a high-powered tractor was standing by'—the tractor was new Hollerith technology which could speed up information processing.[36] He also warned of the danger of the new system becoming fixed, judging the Board of Control for treating both the Table of the Forms and the Causes of Insanity as having become regarded as 'immutable and sacrosanct' by asylum administration, who made few changes to the categories used in statistical collection in between revisions to the document. To remedy this, he suggested a mechanism be built into statistical returns whereby changes could be made by administrative bodies on an annual basis in the light of new developments in psychological and demographic research. He signed off his address with

[35] John P. Mandeville, 'Improvements in Methods of Census and Survey Analysis' in *Journal of the Royal Statistical Society*, vol. 109, no. 2, 1946, pp. 111–129.

[36] Carlos Patton Blacker, 'Mental Health Records: What We Can Learn from Them?', 27th February 1947, in Papers by Carlos Paton Blacker on Mental Health Records, Carlos Paton Blacker Collected Papers, held by The Wellcome Collection.

the hope that 'the way was now clear for the mental health statistics [in the UK] becoming the best in the world'.[37]

Penrose also expressed frustration with procedures and classifications of mental health statistics. In a paper published in 1944, he complained that 'though they may be of constant sources of irritation or of fascination to the psychiatrist according to his type of mind, [classifications] are useless for the research worker'.[38] He called for improvements, stating that 'we cannot distinguish between schizophrenia and affective psychosis with any certainty'.[39] Penrose believed that a comprehensive collection of statistics, for analysis by specialists who would not necessarily be psychiatrists, would enable the data to be understood, and allow for patterns such as those based upon the age of a patient, and their diagnosis. Inferences such as these can in turn assist inquiries into aetiology, which ultimately would allow understandings of the causes of the forms of mental disorder to be improved by establishing clearer differences between the categories used in statistical returns.

As we have seen throughout the course of this volume, debates surrounding the concepts of psychopathology that were used by the Lunacy Commission or Board of Control and the Association had taken place since the very birth of the beginnings of mass psychiatric treatment in the British Isles in the mid-nineteenth century. These concepts were tied to statistical enquiry, with the concepts that were employed affecting the quality of the data returned. Blacker and Penrose saw the potential this system offered for new and modernised epidemiological data to be produced by entries to the hospitals, but hoped that with broader application, it may provide insights into mental illnesses affecting those who would never be admitted to a hospital. This project relied upon an improvement in the quality of data that was produced by mental hospitals: by gaining better understandings of the acute disorders that were treated there, and by linking this data to genetics and aetiology, the prevalence of disorders amongst certain sectors of the population could be predicted and early treatment could prevent the onset of an acute disorder.

[37] Ibid.

[38] L.S., Penrose, 'Social Aspects of Psychiatry: The Importance of Statistics' in *JMS*, vol. 9, no. 389, October 1946, pp. 713–718.

[39] Carlos Patton Blacker, 'Mental Health Records: What We Can Learn from Them?', 27th February 1947, in Papers by Carlos Paton Blacker on Mental Health Records, Carlos Paton Blacker Collected Papers, held by The Wellcome Collection.

In the plans that were made to record admissions to psychiatric hospitals and psychiatric wards, Blacker and his Eugenics Society colleague Lionel Penrose sought to realise these goals. They argued for the importance of a well-designed admissions system that would record the diagnosis that had been given to a patient.[40] Although mental health statistics had been the centre of a great deal of labour undertaken by the Association since 1845, they were still considered crude and underdeveloped, and the classification that had been at the centre of debate for decades had been condemned as useless. Blacker's plans to revolutionise the way in which data was collected from mental health patients had been in development from 1942.[41,42] Blacker had to make the best out of what was available however, since the inclusion of mental health services was an 'afterthought'[43] within the initial planning for the NHS: this had resulted in mental health services being spread across a tripartite system that had sought to nationalise services, yet at the same time compromise with GPs and dentists by allowing them to continue private practice. For the most part, the mental health services, then, had to make the best out of the existing infrastructure of statistical collection from the ageing Victorian asylum buildings.

[40] Carlos Patton Blacker, 'Redhill Hospital—Notes on Visit Paid by Dr Harris and Dr Blacker on Monday, 16th December 1946 in Papers by Carlos Paton Blacker on Mental Health Records, Carlos Paton Blacker Collected Papers, held by The Wellcome Collection; Daniel Kevles provides a great deal of biographical information in his chapter on Penrose: 'Lionel Penrose and the Colchester Survey' in *In the Name of Eugenics: Genetics and the Uses of Human Heredity*, University of California Press, 1986, pp. 148–163.

[41] Chris Renwick makes the argument that it is somewhat of a misnomer to talk about the *establishment* of the NHS and the welfare state, but rather social work agencies and health services that had been developed during the nineteenth and early twentieth centuries were standardised and brought together in post-war planning. There is a convincing case for this to be applied to psychiatric social work, by looking at the formation of the National Association for Mental Health (NAMH) (later Mind the Mental Health Charity) from organisations that were founded in the Edwardian period, including the Central Association for Mental Welfare, the National Council for Mental Hygiene, and the Child Guidance Council. They were initially brought together on the eve of the Second World War in the form of the Emergency Mental Health Services to assist Emergency Medical Services and billeting operations but would be renamed the NAMH in 1946. See: Chris Renwick, *Bread for All*, Macmillan, 2017.

[42] Francis Pilkington, 'Review: W.H.O. and Mental Health 1949–1961. W.H.O. Geneva 1962' in *JMS*, vol. 109, no. 458, January 1963, p. 154.

[43] Charles Webster, *The Health Services Since the War*, vol. 1, HMSO, 1996, p. 55.

Mental hospitals were included in the new NHS and were given the same legal and administrative status as general hospitals. They were to come under the authority of the Ministry of Health, and were no longer overseen by the Board of Control.[44] Social services were covered by what the historian Kathleen Jones judged to be a 'vague' requirement placed upon local authorities within section 28 of the NHS Act.[45] In reality, no clear obligations were placed upon local authorities to provide mental health social care services, and although there existed areas, predominantly big cities, in which psychiatric social services had developed during the late 1940s, it still remained for most part the case that these services did not have the kind of state resources made available to the clinical care of those with mental disorders; medical superintendents of mental hospitals, as well as psychiatrists who served in out-patient units, were employed by hospital boards, whereas psychiatric social workers and other primary care professionals would usually work for a voluntary organisation such as the National Council for Mental Health, whose services were contracted by local authorities.

Having been low on the agenda for those leading health reforms, the inclusion of clinical services relating to mental health care within the NHS was perhaps only achieved so quickly due to it being a convenient and a rather straightforward matter: since clinical care for mental disorders was delivered primarily through mental hospitals or out-patient units in general hospitals. Since all general hospitals were set to be nationalised, it was not hard to include clinical psychiatric services within the measures of the 1946 National Health Service Act. Clinical mental health services, along with ophthalmic services and dentistry, however, soon led to spiralling costs for the fledging health service. Even with this spending, Aneurin Bevan acknowledged the overcrowding of beds in mental hospitals,[46] and had warned cabinet colleagues about the possibility of a scandal

[44] M. Crowther, 'From Workhouse to NHS Hospital in Britain 1929–1948' in *The Poor Law and After*, edited by Hillam and Bone, Liverpool: Liverpool Medical History Society, 1999, pp. 38–49.

[45] Kathleen Jones, *Asylums and After: A Revised History of the Mental Health Services: From the Early 18th Century to the 1990s*, Athlone Press, 1993, p. 144.

[46] Ibid., p. 160.

arising due to the poor conditions in mental hospitals: mental healthcare services were, as Klein remarks, 'the slum of the NHS'.[47]

Attention was drawn to Bevan's slums only after the dust had settled from the negotiations that had taken place between the Ministry of Health and professional bodies like the British Medical Association and RMPA during the formation of the NHS act.[48] The poor state of mental hospitals and the fragmented nature of social services led to calls for the kind of wholesale reforms in psychiatry that had been made to general medical services immediately after the war. Mental health services had been pushed to the back of the queue when it came to funding and available resources, and despite the enthusiasm from members of the medical profession to bring about reform, political will dwindled as soon as the costs of the NHS began to spiral out of control. This would lead to legal reform of mental services coming only after almost a decade since the establishment of the NHS, in the form of the 1959 Mental Health Act.

Whilst these developments were ongoing, Penrose and Blacker, still prominent members of the British Eugenics Society, were working on their research to link psychiatric disorders to genetics and population numbers. Meanwhile, a medical committee appointed by the United Kingdom's General Registry Office (GRO) had taken over the collection of general medical statistics during and after the Second World War from the Board of Control.[49] The GRO had also taken over the duties of collecting data on admissions to mental hospitals and in-patient units. This was in line with statistics collected for general hospitals and other sorts of clinics, and what had started as a wartime measure was made official under the NHS act. The act did not make provisions for mental hospitals aside from bringing them directly under the control of the Ministry of Health: they were not subject to the same kinds of inspections that general hospitals were by the local health authorities, and instead, the Board of Control was retained for these purposes until the passing of the 1959 Mental Health Act.

[47] Rudolf Klein, *The New Politics of the NHS: From Creation to Reinvention*, 3rd edition, Longman, 1995, p. 59.

[48] This was a lengthy process which took place between the initial white paper published in 1944 and the NHS amendment act made in 1949. For a full treatment, see Charles Webster, *The Health Services Since the War*, vol. 1, HMSO, 1996.

[49] Carlos Patton Blacker, 'Redhill Hospital—Notes on Visit Paid by Dr Harris and Dr Blacker on Monday, 16th December 1946 in Papers by Carlos Paton Blacker on Mental Health Records, Carlos Paton Blacker Collected Papers, held by The Wellcome Collection.

Mental hospitals had a similar but distinct policy to asylums on collecting data relating to admissions. Work had begun on amalgamating and redesigning this during the war, with Blacker as head, and this was due to him serving within the Ministry of Health during the conflict. The team led by Blacker conducted field trips to existing mental hospitals to review their admissions policies, making observations on how to improve the efficiency of the collection of data.[50] Meticulous planning to derive a system that would record patient data accurately was undertaken. They drew up proposals to produce index cards to record the data coming back from institutions. Two versions of the card were designed: yellow for those diagnosed as mentally deficient and pink for those diagnosed with a mental illness, with both having a small box in which the *ICD*'s code for the diagnosis of the patient would be entered. In doing so, they made the distinction between congenital disorders and mental illness that informed the revisions to the Table of the Forms going all the way back to the first set of revisions covered in this volume from the 1860s onwards. Despite developing plans for recording patient data through index cards that could be processed with the latest mechanical computing technology, and elaborate measures for storing, rotating and ordering them, the conceptual distinction between congenital and acquired disorders that informed the system was hardly new (Fig. 8.1).

The questions that Blacker posed to the data were also hardly novel, though four crucial questions have cropped up throughout this study in one form or another:

1. Is the mental health of the country improving, remaining stationary or deteriorating?
2. What good are the mental health services doing?
3. How do the mental health services vary throughout the country?
4. Are specific forms of mental illness or defect becoming commoner or rarer?[51]

[50] Carlos Patton Blacker, 'Redhill Hospital—Notes on Visit Paid by Dr Harris and Dr Blacker on Monday, 16th December 1946 in Papers by Carlos Paton Blacker on Mental Health Records, Carlos Paton Blacker Collected Papers, held by The Wellcome Collection.

[51] Carlos Patton Blacker, 'Redhill Hospital—Notes on Visit Paid by Dr Harris and Dr Blacker on Monday, 16th December 1946 in Papers by Carlos Paton Blacker on Mental Health Records, Carlos Paton Blacker Collected Papers, held by The Wellcome Collection.

Psychosis (300)

300 Schizophrenic disorders (dementia praecox)
300.0 Simple type
300.1 Hebephrenic type
300.2 Catatonic type
300.3 Paranoid type
300.4 Acute schizophrenic reaction
300.5 Latent schizophrenia
300.6 Schizo-affective psychosis
300.7 Other and unspecified
301 Manic-depressive reaction
301.0 Manic and circular
301.1 Depressive
301.2 Other
302 Involutional melancholia
303 Paranoia and paranoid states
304 Senile psychosis
305 Presenile psychosis
306 Psychosis with cerebral arteriosclerosis
307 Alcoholic psychosis
308 Psychosis of other demonstrable aetiology
308.0 Resulting from brain tumour
308.1 Resulting from epilepsy and other convulsive disorders
308.2 Other
309 Other and unspecified psychoses
(310-318) Psychoneurotic disorders
310 Anxiety reaction w/out mention of somatic symptoms
311 Hysterical reaction without mention of anxiety reaction
312 Phobic reaction
313 Obsessive-compulsive reaction
314 Neurotic-depressive reaction
315 Psychoneurosis with somatic symptoms (somatisation reaction) affecting circulatory system
315.0 Neurocirculatory asthenia
315.1 Other heart manifestations specified as of psychogenic origin
315.2 Other circulatory manifestations of psychogenic origin
316 Psychoneurosis with somatic symptoms (somatisation reaction) affecting digestive system
316.0 Mucous colitis specified as of psychogenic origin
316.1 Irritability of colon specified as of psychogenic origin
316.2 Gastric neuroses
316.3 Other digestive manifestations specified as of psychogenic origin
317 Psychoneurosis with somatic symptoms (somatisation reaction) affecting other systems
317.0 Psychogenic reactions affecting respiratory system
317.1 Psychogenic reactions affecting genito|urinary system
317.2 Pruritus of psychogenic origin
317.3 Other cutaneous neuroses
317.4 Psychogenic reactions affecting musculoskeletal system
317.5 Psychogenic reactions affecting other systems
318 Psychoneurotic disorders, other, mixed and unspecified types
318.0 Hypochondriacal reaction
318.1 Depersonalisation
318.2 Occupational neurosis
318.3 Asthenic reaction
318.4 Mixed
318.5 Of other and unspecified types
(320-326) Disorders of character, behaviour, and intelligence
320 Pathological personality
320.0 Schizoid personality
320.1 Paranoid personality
320.2 Cyclothymic personality
320.3 Inadequate personality
320.4 Antisocial personality
320.5 Asocial personality
320.6 Sexual deviation
320.7 Other and unspecified
321 Immature personality
321.0 Emotional instability
321.1 Passive dependency
321.2 Aggressiveness
321.3 Enuresis characterising immature personality
321.4 Other symptomatic habits except speech impediments
321.5 Other and unspecified
322 Alcoholism
322.0 Acute
322.1 Chronic
322.2 Unspecified
323 Other drug addiction
324 Primary childhood behaviour disorders 325 Mental deficiency
325.0 Idiocy
325.1 Imbecility
325.2 Moron
325.3 Borderline intelligence
325.4 Mongolism
325.5 Other and unspecified types
326 Other and unspecified character, behaviour and intelligence disorders
326.0 Specific learning defects
326.1 Stammering and stuttering of non-organic origin
326.2 Other speech impediments of non-organic origin
326.3 Acute situational maladjustment
326.4 Other and unspecified.

Fig. 8.1 Mental Health Section, *ICD*[52]

[52] Manual of the International Statistical Classification of Diseases, Injuries and Causes of Death: 6th Rev. of the International Lists of Diseases and Causes of Death. Adopted 1948 [by the International Conference for the Sixth Decennial Revision of the International Lists of Diseases and Causes of Death]. Geneva, 1948.

As we have seen in Chapter 4, the associated questions of the state of mental health amongst the general public and the benefit of mental health services were posed by lunacy administration and psychiatrists during the nineteenth century, with no conclusive answer ever being reached. To help answer the first question, Blacker thought that mental health statistics needed to be collected which were of at least the same quality as existing epidemiological data that gave public health authorities clues on the physical health of the nation, namely: numbers relating to 'deficiency diseases such as rickets, infant mortality, and the weight of children'.[53] Possible 'finger-pointers' or clues based on data points that could be arrived at by existing public records included divorce rates, numbers of suicides and 'juvenile delinquency'.[54] The second question was one that had potential political capital—with the subsuming of mental health services into the NHS and it being funded by public finances, Blacker believed that there was a responsibility to demonstrate how public money was being spent and whether it was making a difference, not only in the treatment of acute psychological disorders, but also increasing contentment amongst the population and the maintenance of a good level of mental health.[55] When it came to his third question about how mental health services varied across the United Kingdom, Blacker followed in a long tradition of those viewing statistics as crucial for comparison and eventual improvement to standardise the levels of treatment across rural and urban areas.

To answer his fourth question, concerning the different forms of mental disorder, Blacker resorted to a comparison between mental health and known facts relating to somatic disorders:

> The answer is available of many physical conditions. Typhoid is now a rarity. Plague, typhus and leprosy are now practically non-existent. Industrial diseases diminish as conditions of work improve [...] Tuberculosis and rheumatic disease fluctuate in incidence.[56]

[53] Ibid.

[54] Ibid.

[55] Ibid.

[56] Ibid.

Mental diseases associated with clearly discernible health conditions such as GPI, lead encephalopathies, pellagra, cretinism, myxoedema and alcoholic psychoses were less prevalent than they had been, making it harder to identify mental diseases. Again, Blacker hoped that a new system of mental health data collection would provide the means to improve the statistics and open up new questions. In 1946, when planning of this new system was at an advanced stage, publication of the *ICD* was on the horizon, and Blacker's committee decided that it was to be used for the purposes of admissions diagnosis in their new system.[57] This was after the Board of Control has been consulted by Lionel Penrose to discuss possible classifications that could be used.[58] There is no evidence to suggest that the Board considered the 1934 Revisions to the Table of the Forms as an option, although Penrose did consider the use of a classification used by the Medical Research Council instead of the *ICD*.[59] The classification had the qualities of simplicity and concision that were long valued by lunacy administration, but he acknowledged that it must be expanded upon to be useful within a new data collection framework (Fig. 8.2).

One of the benefits of using the *ICD* was that each disorder had a numerical code, and having that as the standard meant that little work would be needed to submit data from British hospitals to contribute to transnational mental health statistics. The numerical system of classification also meant that hole punch reading technology could be used to speed up the collation of the information gathered, and use processes the GRO had developed in counting census data. The cards were introduced for service on 1 January 1949, and the booklet dispatched accompanying the cards instructed users to fill them in with the diagnostic codes contained in the *ICD*, emphasising that this would make it possible to correlate the returns with those from other parts of the country, and countries from across the world.[60] The manual dismissed the MPA's Table of the Forms as being out of date, and that the data returned from the Board of Control based upon this classification were 'too meagre to

57 Ibid.

58 Ibid.

59 Lionel Penrose, Correspondence to R. Tomsett, the Board of Control, in Mr Corbett's proposals for revising the Index Cards. Diagnostic Lists, Carlos Paton Blacker, Collected Papers.

60 General Register Office, 'Mental Health Statistics' in RG 41/46, held by The National Archives.

satisfy present day requirements'.[61] It stated that although the knowledge on admissions to mental hospitals collected by the Board of Control was satisfactory, one of the goals of the new system was to improve the dataset to include those who were in out-patient wings, and the progress of long-stay patients. An early draft of the manual provided with the new patient index cards stated that the exact number of long-stay patients in mental homes was not known, but this was removed from the final version for fear that the Ministry of Health being ignorant of these figures would face controversy. When it came to diagnosis, the manual instructed that the physical condition be given as the first diagnosis, with any accompanying mental condition being labelled as a secondary one (Table 8.1).

Improving this data would, it was hoped by Blacker, fulfil the goal articulated by Penrose to improve understandings of mental disorder through statistical analysis. As we can see from the cards above, detailed

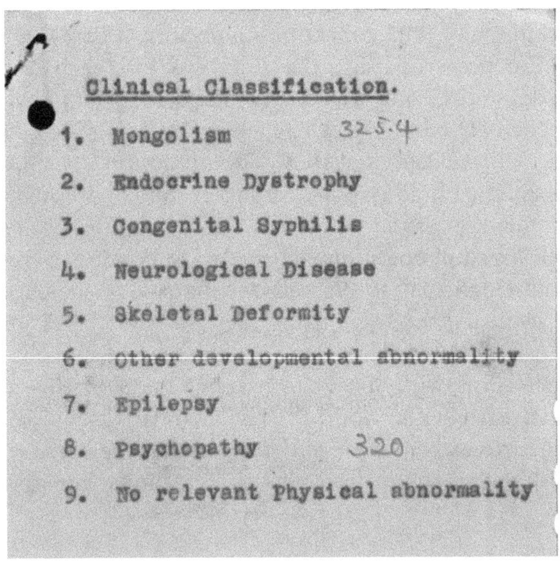

Clinical Classification.

1. Mongolism 325.4
2. Endocrine Dystrophy
3. Congenital Syphilis
4. Neurological Disease
5. Skeletal Deformity
6. Other developmental abnormality
7. Epilepsy
8. Psychopathy 320
9. No relevant Physical abnormality

Fig. 8.2 Draft classification of the Medical Research Council proposed by Penrose[62]

[61] Ibid.

[62] Ibid.

Table 8.1 Mental illness and Mental Deficiency Index cards

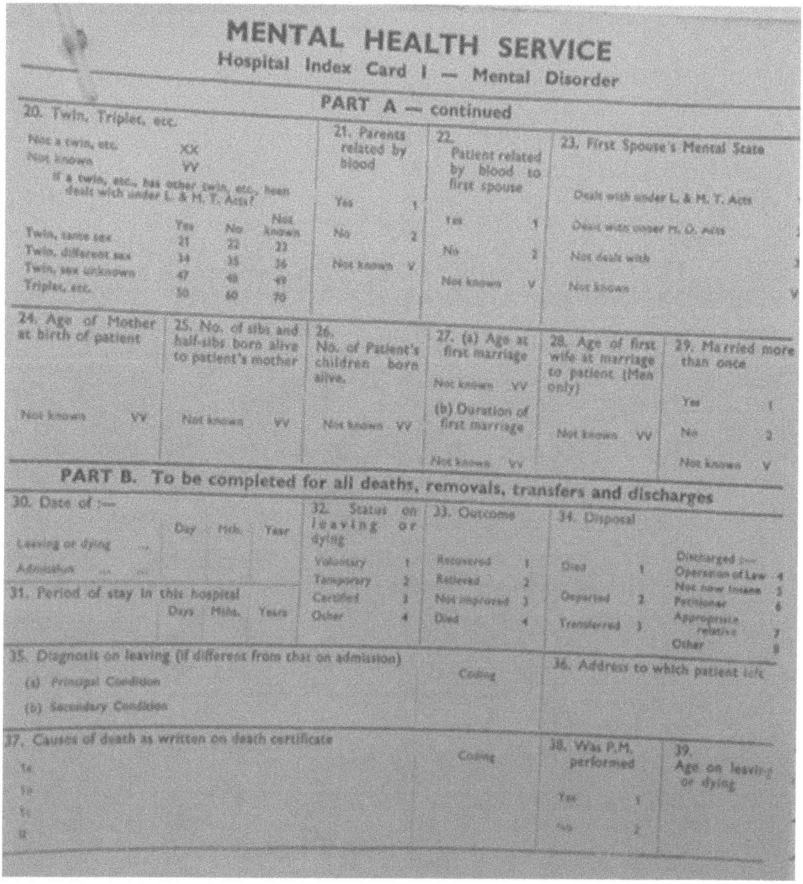

MENTAL HEALTH SERVICE
Hospital Index Card I — Mental Disorder

PART A — continued

20. Twin, Triplet, etc.
Not a twin, etc. XX
Not known VV
If a twin, etc., has other twin, etc., been dealt with under L. & M. T. Acts?

	Yes	No	Not known
Twin, same sex	21	22	23
Twin, different sex	34	35	36
Twin, sex unknown	47	48	49
Triplet, etc.	50	60	70

21. Parents related by blood
Yes 1
No 2
Not known V

22. Patient related by blood to first spouse
Yes 1
No 2
Not known V

23. First Spouse's Mental State
Dealt with under L. & M. T. Acts
Dealt with under M. D. Acts
Not dealt with
Not known V

24. Age of Mother at birth of patient
Not known VV

25. No. of sibs and half-sibs born alive to patient's mother
Not known VV

26. No. of Patient's children born alive.
Not known VV

27. (a) Age at first marriage
Not known VV
(b) Duration of first marriage
Not known VV

28. Age of first wife at marriage to patient (Men only)
Not known VV

29. Married more than once
Yes 1
No 2
Not known V

PART B. To be completed for all deaths, removals, transfers and discharges

30. Date of :—
Day Mth. Year
Leaving or dying ...
Admission ... ...

31. Period of stay in this hospital
Days Mths. Years

32. Status on leaving or dying
Voluntary 1
Temporary 2
Certified 3
Other 4

33. Outcome
Recovered 1
Relieved 2
Not improved 3
Died 4

34. Disposal
Died 1
Departed 2
Transferred 3
Discharged :—
Operation of Law 4
Not now insane 5
Petitioner 6
Appropriate relative 7
Other 8

35. Diagnosis on leaving (if different from that on admission)
(a) Principal Condition
(b) Secondary Condition
Coding

36. Address to which patient left

37. Causes of death as written on death certificate
Ia
Ib
Ic
II
Coding

38. Was P.M. performed
Yes 1
No 2

39. Age on leaving or dying

(continued)

Table 8.1 (continued)

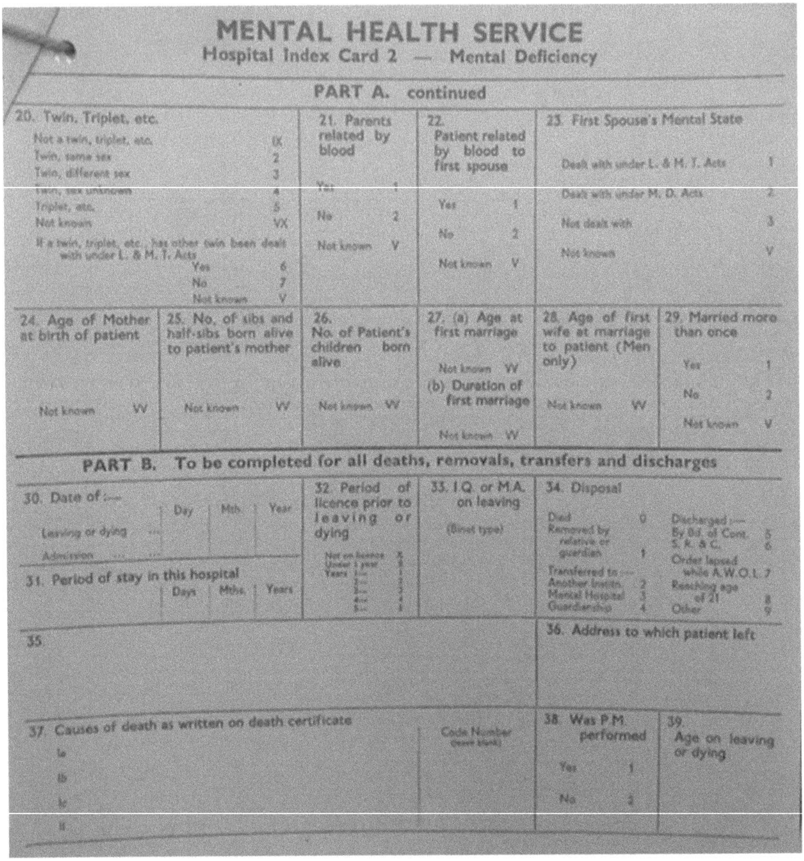

MENTAL HEALTH SERVICE
Hospital Index Card 2 — Mental Deficiency

PART A. continued

20. Twin, Triplet, etc.
Not a twin, triplet, etc. X
Twin, same sex 2
Twin, different sex 3
Twin, sex unknown 4
Triplet, etc. 5
Not known VX
If a twin, triplet, etc., has other twin been dealt with under L. & M. T. Acts
Yes 6
No 7
Not known V

21. Parents related by blood
Yes 1
No 2
Not known V

22. Patient related by blood to first spouse
Yes 1
No 2
Not known V

23. First Spouse's Mental State
Dealt with under L. & M. T. Acts 1
Dealt with under M. D. Acts 2
Not dealt with 3
Not known V

24. Age of Mother at birth of patient
Not known W

25. No. of sibs and half-sibs born alive to patient's mother
Not known W

26. No. of Patient's children born alive
Not known W

27. (a) Age at first marriage
Not known W
(b) Duration of first marriage
Not known W

28. Age of first wife at marriage to patient (Men only)
Not known W

29. Married more than once
Yes 1
No 2
Not known V

PART B. To be completed for all deaths, removals, transfers and discharges

30. Date of:—
Day | Mth. | Year
Leaving or dying
Admission

31. Period of stay in this hospital
Days | Mths. | Years

32. Period of licence prior to leaving or dying
Not on licence X
Under 1 year 0
Years 1— 1
2— 2
3— 3
4— 4
5— 5

33. I.Q. or M.A. on leaving
(Binet type)

34. Disposal
Died 0
Removed by relative or guardian 1
Transferred to:—
Another Instn. 2
Mental Hospital 3
Guardianship 4
Discharged:—
By Bd. of Cont. 5
S. K. & C. 6
Order lapsed while A.W.O.L. 7
Reaching age of 21 8
Other 9

35.

36. Address to which patient left

37. Causes of death as written on death certificate
Ia
Ib
Ic
II
Code Number (leave blank)

38. Was P.M. performed
Yes 1
No 2

39. Age on leaving or dying

social information concerning a patient's family background and marital status was included.

The first set of statistics on psychological diagnosis to be produced by these revised processes appeared in the *Registrar-General's Statistical Review of England and Wales for the Year 1949: Supplement on*

General Morbidity, Cancer and Mental Health.[63] Published in 1953, the document provided a detailed breakdown of diagnosis according to the categories of the *ICD* but noted caution on the validity of the application of the diagnostic terms. The statistics presented in this document provided the most comprehensive breakdown of mental health statistics by psychological diagnosis. They were the product of the century of chequered development of asylum medical statistics outlined in this volume. Although the 'asylum' had come to an end as a legal entity under the terms of the 1930 Mental Treatment Act, the publication of mental health statistics in the report signals the beginning of mental health epidemiology in the British context. Given Britain's links both to international agencies and the use of the *ICD*, the reforms undertaken by Blacker and Penrose would be noticed by those developing transnational mental health statistics. The introduction of the cards was judged to be a success, at least by those involved in the project. A letter from 25 September 1953, dispatched from Penrose's office at the Galton institute, congratulated the GRO on the statistics they had gathered on mental health diagnosis and consanguinity, stating that the numbers would provide useful information for further research.[64] For so-called mental defectives, Blacker and the eminent statistician Percy Stocks took the decision to record the I.Q. of the patient.[65] IQ was key because aside from being used to diagnose mental deficiency, it was used in education policy to detect mental and moral deficiency in children, and detect whether they should be sent to the increasing numbers of special schools, a measure to reduce juvenile delinquency. Classification would be done through the concepts of psychopathology that were used in the *ICD*.

[63] Registrar-General's Statistical Review of England and Wales for the Year 1949: Supplement on General Morbidity, Cancer and Mental Health, London, Her Majesty's Stationary Office, 1953.

[64] Correspondence, L.S. Penrose to Ruth M. Loy, 25th September 1953 in MH RG 41/46 held by the National Archives, Kew Gardens.

[65] Mental Health Statistics, Minutes of Meeting, Wednesday February 18th, 1948, in MH RG 41/46, held by National Archives, Kew Gardens.

Conclusion

International health and medical epidemiology following the war would contribute to bringing psychiatry, the ideas it used, the treatments it employed and the spaces in which mental health care was carried out closer to general medicine. Ambitions to reform mental health statistics were partly down to the eugenic aims of those involved, but also the template a country with a centralised bureaucracy and a nationalised health system could provide. By 1942, plans were being made for a new welfare state of which a nationalised health service was central in ensuring the health of the state's inhabitants from cradle to grave. They viewed the lack of such a system as being part of the reason why there had been a lack of progress in psychiatric knowledge in British mental science. They viewed the opportunity provided by the new health service as a chance to redesign the admissions system to improve mental health data collection procedures, and the standard classification recommended in these reforms was the *ICD* because Blacker considered the Table of the Forms an outdated relic of the asylum era.

The abandonment of the Table of the Forms signals wider institutional and conceptual changes in psychiatry that would lead it closer to general medicine. The restructuring of the health services, the appointment of psychiatrists to prominent government roles, and the adoption of a general, international medical nosology would spell the end of the RMPA developing the standardised concepts of mental disorder to classify admissions. The categories of the *ICD* would be used to record the disorder suffered by a patient upon admission to the nationalised mental hospitals of the NHS, or into the psychiatric wards of general hospitals. The end of the Table of the Forms then reflected wider changes to psychiatric diagnosis and practice in the United Kingdom.

The collection of psychiatric statistics would return to the GRO after the Second World War. This ended a century of division between the general medical statistics collected by the GRO and admissions data collected by Poor Law authorities, firstly the Lunacy Commission and, from 1914, the Board of Control. At the same time, this would end the era of the Table of the Forms, leading to its abandonment in favour of a general medical nosology that had a mental health section in the form of the *ICD*. This document would be published by the WHO in 1948; its adoption by the planning exercises outlined in this chapter formally ended the hundred-year history of the Table of the Forms that was published by the Medico-Psychological Association (MPA). Members of the MPA would not congregate or appoint committees to draw up new standard psychiatric classifications with such breadth and coverage as the Table of the Forms, with the era of a general and global medical nosology replacing the era of what may be called an asylum classification.

The events charted in this chapter signal the moves psychiatry made towards general medicine that occurred on a conceptual level and an institutional level. The conceptual shift is marked by the move from a specialised psychiatric nosology in the form of the RMPA's Table of the Forms and towards a new international and general nosology in the form of the *ICD* that would include a section on mental disorders. This is in one way a return of mental disorder to general nosology as seen in the work of William Cullen from the second chapter of this volume—like the *ICD*, Cullen aimed to give a comprehensive list of all known human ailments that included a section on the versanies, or nervous disorders. On the institutional level, the post-war reforms re-unified the collection of psychiatric statistics with those relating to general medicine, since these duties were taken away from the specialised organisation of psychiatric administration, the Board of Control, and they were returned to the GRO. The changes would define the classification that was used in mental health statistics during the immediate post-war period and would set the foundations for the paradigm of international classification used in statistical enquiry that still exists today.

CHAPTER 9

Conclusion

This study has offered the thesis that the development of asylum medical statistics, an oft-overlooked aspect of the history of psychiatry, is far from being an adjunct to the clinic, but helped to motivate the development of the fundamental categories used for diagnosis. The history charted in this book shows that classification is not simply a tale of scientific development, but incorporates professional politics as well as a series of considerations on the relationship between public health bodies and expert medical circles. Through an examination of the fundamental categories used to gather the data of madness and their placement in relation to larger systems of health data collection, this study has explored the links between the history of psychiatric classification and public health administration, governmentality and population studies. The Table of the Forms was then not merely a list of mental disorders but constitutes the way a European society with complicated public data collection frameworks and an expansive bureaucracy divided madness for statistical understanding.

The debates that were conducted over the Table of the Forms were part of a wider picture of the development of psychiatric knowledge that was enabled in part through the development of mental health statistics. By the 1860s, the psychological diagnostic concepts of melancholia and mania that were included in the set of terms recommended in the 1845 Lunacy Commission report came to be viewed as dated and

K. M. Jones, *Psychological Classification and Diagnosis in Asylum Statistics, 1800–1948*, Mental Health in Historical Perspective, https://doi.org/10.1007/978-3-031-46154-5_9

out of touch with a medical science that demanded scientific explanations for psychological illnesses which were rooted in the mechanisms of the body. This is part of the project of the human sciences that emerged from the nineteenth century onwards to study the mind and to explain it in scientific terms.[1] Many of the individuals engaged in discussions over classification and statistics sought to understand the unpredictable nature of insanity through the development of statistical data that displayed trends on causation and prognosis. However, many were also asylum medical superintendents who were trained in the causal, mechanistic and physical explanations for illnesses. The clashes were often between those who held on to the idea that mental health conditions could and should be explained through deterministic causal mechanisms, and those who remained agnostic but thought that imposing scientifically unproven causal relations could undermine statistical methods that were still in a nascent phase. Physicians like Skae attempted to apply these kinds of bodily explanations to insanity in their classifications, whereas others like Crichton-Browne thought that the diagnostic concepts were over-determined by a theory of mind–body causation—this was especially pertinent by the 1870s as alienists had largely failed to prove an indubitable and incorrigible link between the two. Skae's classification of aetiology faced resistance because the categories it included did not match the experience of many medical superintendents, and the tacit knowledge they had accumulated through medical practice. The first-hand contact with the freewill of patients defied the neat causal explanations of a system builder like Skae. Although many wanted a scientific classification in theory, asylum psychiatrists were somewhat hostile when presented with one, or at least the elaborate version presented by Skae. Instead, and again as Crichton-Browne argued, Pinel's symptomology was useful for statistics because it did not profess to present an exhaustive natural compendium of all the insanities.

Drives to count and classify mental disorder were linked to the development of psychiatric knowledge, and the attempts to understand chance and risk. The risks changed during the hundred year history of the Table of the Forms, and these were tied to the social and economic context, the state of the clinic and wider cultural anxieties. Victorian pessimism and

[1] Roger Smith, 'The History of Psychological Categories' in *Studies in History and Philosophy of Biological and Biomedical Sciences*, vol. 36, 2004, pp. 55–95.

degeneration theory linked declining standards of health in new industrial centres to the gradual collapse of a human civilisation that many had thought had past its peak in post-Enlightenment Europe of the later nineteenth century. These anxieties were frequently in response to sociopolitical events that many viewed as harbingers of the end of empire, such as British defeat in the Boer War, or fears of the inner-city criminal classes depicted in novels such as *Oliver Twist*. Accompanying these fears of social problems was an optimism about the powers of rational thought and scientific endeavour to understand and solve them, and improve society. Breakthroughs in biology and understandings of the human emerging from Darwinian biology, Mendelian genetics and the modern synthesis increasingly came to be seen as providing the tools for society to help itself: in many ways we still live with the implications of this faith in finding neat scientific answers to complex social problems. Alienism had sought to define itself in relation to these risks as asylums were beginning to be seen as iatrogenic and causing more problems than they solved. Interest in prognosis and diagnosis was partly driven by asylum superintendents themselves acknowledging the likely harm, shame and destitution resulting from a stay in an asylum, and that avoiding an unnecessary stay was in the interests of all. This placed them in the awkward position of acknowledging the failure of the asylum system by calling for diagnostic tools that would lead to only those absolutely in need of help being admitted to an asylum. Similarly with the 1882 Revision including not only the term 'incurables', but having a whole section devoted to incurable disorders, which was a tacit acknowledgement of the pessimism surrounding the abilities of medical psychology to assist sets of patients who were being admitted to asylums. The eugenic movement's interest in asylum statistics coincided with this therapeutic despair, as researchers from the Galton Institute applied methods of statistical analysis to asylum populations to extrapolate broader findings about mental health at the beginning of the twentieth century. In addition, the direct involvement of prominent figures in mathematical statistics including Karl Pearson and Francis Galton in revisions undertaken by the MPA to their statistical tables further shaped the history of mental health statistics during this period.

Far from the aim to find the ideal classification being an abstract endeavour that was solely contained in the pages of medical textbooks and scientific journals, this volume has shown that concepts of psychopathology were hotly contested in meetings and discussions, and this was in part due to their application in asylum medical statistics. In analysing the attitudes towards insanity that informed these debates on classification, this book has presented considerations on the function of classification from a historical perspective. Cultural assumptions about the individual and their role in society shaped the classifications that were published by subsequent revisions committees, who, in their pursuit of the most appropriate classification, were responding to changing social and economic conditions. Saying this, far from being a homogeneous body who were defined by these external factors, Victorian, Edwardian and interwar psychiatrists were a fairly diverse *thought collective* whose assumptions, ideas and convictions on how mental disorder should be classified were often heated and divisive—the first set of debates were drawn along various lines, and took place over nearly twenty years. The debates ended with a short-lived truce in 1882 primarily because the main antagonists had died or had retired. The debates, along with the subsequent set of discussions that commenced in 1902, touched on grander questions about what it meant to classify a mental disorder, whether such an enterprise would improve practice, and how to most effectively standardise diagnosis. The discussions that surrounded the Table of the Forms reveal insights that are difficult to gather from the analysis of historical textbooks and journals alone, and by exploring the discussions from meetings of the Association, this volume has outlined the discursive cultures that existed within British psychiatry during this hundred-year period. The discussions demonstrate how knowledge was communicated amongst mental scientists during the early years of psychiatry, with concepts of psychopathology functioning to allow communication to occur between members of the MPA. This allowed communication beyond the limits of asylum practice, to public health administration, psychiatric social work and primary health care.

The Table of the Forms constituted the shared terminology that was used to communicate between lunacy administration and the clinic. Although a melange of German, French, Latin and Greek derived terms were employed within the research papers that populated the pages of the MPA's *Journal of Mental Science*, the terms used in official documents, diagnosis and statistics were for the most part based on symptomology. Many viewed the aetiological concepts offered by Skae as being flawed, and it was hoped by many members of the MPA that data on diagnosis returned from asylums across the British Isles would establish causal links between the forms of insanity and the causes that were recorded in asylum admittance books. This demonstrates that aetiology during this period constituted the historical *a priori* that determined what statements were admissible within the discussions.[2] The grounding assumption to the deliberations that accompanied the Table of the Forms was that insanity could be given a causal explanation, even if the precise mechanisms were beyond the current grasp of understanding. The notion that there could be another form of explanation for insanity other than that of the physical and mechanistic was not admissible to the debates surrounding classification. Despite there being some individuals who were receptive to statistics and indeed used admissions data in their research, studies were usually based on the assumption that statistics would eventually reveal causal explanations, be they in the form of the natural history of the disease of Skae, or pathological explanations as in the classification offered by Batty Tuke. In short, the discovery of such bodily causes was seen by many as an eventuality and remained undoubted, even when the promise of anatomy was fading and attention turned towards using statistical research to understand prognosis. This steadfast believe in causal relationships between physical and mental illnesses thereby formed the historically constituted *a priori* conditions upon which rested the debates on classification and diagnosis undertake by alienists for much of the nineteenth century, and the first part of the twentieth.

Although this study has focused on a document principally used by medical specialists and administrators, the differences between so-called lay understandings and those of professionals were not as dramatic as is often assumed. Many of the diagnostic concepts of the Table of the Forms in its first editions would have been recognisable to a non-specialist, with melancholia and mania finding expression in everyday language, literature and the press. As the psychiatric profession matured, later iterations of the Table would include technical terminology that would be unfamiliar to non-specialists and even those within the profession; indeed, we have frequently seen concerns expressed by revisions committees over new terminology being alien to certain members of the medical profession. The terms included in the 1934 Revision, for example, would have been the most unfamiliar to a non-specialist, with the classification reflecting a well-established medical discipline that had developed

[2] Michel Foucault, *The Order of Things: An Archaeology of the Human Sciences*, Routledge, 2002.

its own technical vocabulary. Whether the sophistication of the terminology indicates a more advanced understanding of mental disorder is a matter for debate, but it is telling that many of the diagnostic categories of the 1934 Revision are no longer in use, with the theory informing concepts like 'psychotic heredity' and focal sepsis having been largely discredited since. It is also the case that the 1934 Revision caused as much if not more division than previous iterations of the document, which may indicate a degree of stasis in the development of diagnostic categories, with professional divisions proving to be an insurmountable challenge to standardising concepts of psychological diagnosis.

Viewing the impasses that characterised the Table of the Forms as simply a professional turfwar between rival factions would be a hasty reading however, and turning to work from historical epistemology is key to understanding why.[3] Broadly speaking, historical epistemology seeks to bring together the concerns of social history and history of knowledge to study the contingent practices that generate scientific understanding and simultaneously shape objects of study. By turning to historical epistemology, this study has aimed to combine the history of lunacy administration, largely a reserve of the social history of medicine, with that of psychiatric classification, conventionally the reserve of the history of scientific knowledge. In so doing, I have tried to prove that the history of psychological terms, including their standardisation, cannot be told meaningfully when divorced from their use in bureaucratic processes and asylum medical statistics. In turn, by outlining the processes and discussions that shaped data on psychological diagnosis from the years covered by the study, I have attempted to place scientific discussions from the early history of mental health statistics within their social context. Social values arose during these scientific discussions, and although the Table of the Forms purported to list disease entities and develop scientific knowledge, it also listed categories of mental health service users, who were frequently defined by their condition in the clinical literature, with service users often being referred to as melancholics, dements, maniacs, schizophrenics,

[3] Alain Desrosières, *The Politics of Large Numbers: A History of Statistical Reasoning*, Harvard University Press, 1998; George Canguilhem, *The Normal and the Pathological*, translated by Carolyn R. Fawcett, MIT Press, 1991; Ian Hacking, *The Taming of Chance*, Palgrave, 1990; Michel Foucault, *The Order of Things: An Archaeology of the Human Sciences*, translated by Alan Sheridan, Routledge, 2002; Lorraine Daston, *The Empire of Chance: How Probability Changed Science and Everyday Life*, Cambridge University Press, 1989.

psychotics and so on. Terms like these are awkward reading now, but they were how service users were objectified by a medical science that largely excluded the voices of patients as unworthy from scientific deliberations over psychological diagnosis.

Attempts to understand the historical conditions that gave rise to scientific knowledge, broadly conceived, are linked to the ways they structured communicative practices amongst what Ludwik Fleck called 'thought collectives', or a community of scientists mutually exchanging ideas and maintaining intellectual interaction.[4] The agreed assumptions of these thought collectives ultimately helped to formulate the shared horizon of beliefs and theories which would be used to comprehend experiences, structure communication between scientists and formulate scientific facts. Fleck claimed that specific problems within research communities are written into fact through communication practices such as the writing of pedagogical texts. The drafting of a medical classification as an aid to teaching and training has a long history, at least going back to William Cullen, and perhaps even to antiquity.[5] The classification offered by David Skae, that became a candidate to be the standard classification and which features prominently during the first half of the book, was designed initially to assist in medical training. Dissatisfied with the vagueness of the nosographies offered by French alienists, Skae developed a classification that attempted to use physical conditions as a foundation. This approach, developed in his teaching, was furthered by his students, who held that replacing the standard classification with Skae's would improve the precision of asylum medical statistics on psychological diagnosis. Skae's classification, then, transcended its initial design as a training document to become a classification that communicated knowledge of the physical causes of insanity. The reluctance of some to adopt the work was not out of a suspicion of the effectiveness of a science of the mind, or what may now be termed the medical model of mental health, but out of concerns that it would not live up to the ideal of a scientific classification.

Psychiatric classification was a medium of communication, one characterised by ordering mental disorders and diagnostic categories in tables

[4] Ludwik Fleck, *Genesis and Development of a Scientific Fact*, translated by Fred Bradley, Robert K. Merton and Thaddeaus J. Trenn, University of Chicago Press, 2008.

[5] Michael Barfoot, 'Philosophy and Method in Cullen's Medical Teaching,' in *William Cullen and the Eighteenth-Century Medical World*, edited by A. Doig, J.P.S. Ferguson, I.A. Milne and R. Passmore, Edinburgh: Edinburgh University Press, 1993.

and figures. The Table of the Forms can be understood as what Gianna Pomata calls 'epistemic genres', or 'kinds of texts that develop in tandem with scientific practices'.[6] These function in many ways like literary genres, but instead of having aesthetic characteristics that create meaning, epistemic genres have formal characteristics that are defined largely by convention, and thereby establish a set of expectations amongst an audience. Classifications of insanity functioned as epistemic genres in that they adopted certain conventions to produce and transmit scientific knowledge, and for a great portion of the nineteenth century, the project of psychiatric classification resembled a kind of Tower of Babel as alienists far and wide formulated their own classifications based upon their own observations and experiences. Many of these tinkered with existing terminology drawn along symptomatic lines, but as in the examples developed by Batty Tuke and Charles Mercier considered in this study, there were radical departures that sought to eschew existing symptomatic terminology. The epistemic genre of the classification relied on the expectation that a grounding principle, explicit or implicit, organised the disorders it listed, be it according to aetiology, pathology or symptomology. As with the Table of the Forms, a classification would attract criticism when it did not conform to a coherent grounding principle, or when the categories and sub-categories it employed were incoherently structured. Furthermore, classifications were expected to provide a valid diagnosis that could be replicated, making a diagnosis objective and relying as little on the individual judgement of an alienist as possible. Although arguably having roots in works of antiquity, the modern exercise of classifying nature was relatively novel and fresh at the beginning of the nineteenth century.[7] As the century wore on however, the genre became tired due to the sheer number of psychological classifications offered by individual authors. Each had an organising principle, such as aetiology or pathology, but the prevailing expectation underlying the genre in clinical discussions was that a classification ought to describe natural things, although how a classification represented them differed. Some sought to represent natural histories, others causal relations or unknown natural properties of diseases that could be detected by the outlook of a patient. The accusations of

[6] Gianna Pomata, 'The Medical Case Narrative: Distant Reading of an Epistemic Genre' in *Literature and Medicine*, vol. 32, no. 1, Spring 2014.

[7] Stefan Müller-Wille, 'Names and Numbers: "Data" in Classical Natural History, 1758–1859' in *Osiris*, vol. 32, no. 1, 2017, pp. 109–128.

Cartesianism directed towards works influenced by Pinel were a result of expectations that had arisen surrounding the epistemic genre of the classification. As the genre became exhausted, classification increasingly became a matter of committees reconciling existing work rather than individual authors offering new ways of representing natural divisions between different mental health disorders. The reason why Kraepelin's work stood out despite the plethora of classifications issued by the 1880s and 1890s was because it marked a departure from the tired genre of psychological classifications being based on symptomatic descriptions. The popularity of his work was partly down to the use of statistical data to map trends in outlook that chimed with the growing popularity of the sciences of chance during the last quarter of the nineteenth century.

The ideas expressed in the debates over the Table of the Forms have shaped the history of public data on mental health and have established lasting views on the purposes of mental health statistics that were drawn from administrative procedures and records. This study has sought to contribute to the expanding literature that looks at the role of administrative procedures in shaping scientific knowledge by bringing together psychiatric classification and diagnosis through a *longue durée* history that examines the role that the document played in the quantitative representation of mental health. The function of tables showing statistics on psychological diagnosis varied over time, but broadly speaking, they were linked to the most useful ways that public health authorities thought mental disorders should be represented for the purpose of statistical data. As Bowker and Star demonstrate in their critical work on the *ICD*, the medical training of those involved in revising classifications of disease can lead to documents that emphasise biomedical causes, and overlook the decisive social determinants of health conditions such as accessibility to sanitation and running water.[8] In the case of the Table of the Forms, the assumption that the proper representation of the physical aetiology of insanity was the task of a scientific classification was informed by the medical training of those who participated in these debates. Although social causes of mental health disorders were of some interest to alienists and lunacy administration, with occupation, environment and the family background included in asylum medical statistics, there were no attempts

[8] Geoffrey Bowker and Susan Leigh Star, *Sorting Things Out: Classification and Its Consequences*, Cambridge, MA: MIT Press, 1999.

to implement social considerations into concepts of psychological diagnosis. An emphasis on biomedical considerations was also seen in an early form through the criticisms directed towards Pinel's work, which was considered Cartesian by some because it remained unacceptably ambivalent on the physical causes of mental health conditions.

Accordingly, the ideas expressed in the debates over classification outlined in this volume have shaped the history of public health data and have established lasting views on the purposes of collecting statistics on mental health. As we have seen, authorities have typically used mental health statistics to understand the cost of mental health on society. 'Cost' can be understood in a number of ways, but when it came to the responsibilities of individual institutions and lunacy administration as a whole, it was frequently invoked to understand the resources needed to maintain patients in asylums. Statistics were used to conduct assessments of any potential increase in the numbers of insane to decide whether existing facilities were sustainable, or whether there was any requirement to expand or decommission services.[9] As we have seen, the turn of the century saw a move towards diagnostic concepts that sought to provide indications of the prognosis of a condition, and these would be reflected in mental health statistics after the 1907 Revision. Public health reports published afterwards included mental health statistics that were broken down according to psychological categories that provided some indication of the outlook of a patient. The increased sophistication of analysis appearing in Lunacy Commission reports up until 1914 would, with these categories, provide not only an indication of the future outlook of the patient, but also some indication of the future cost of asylum populations. These same reports presented forecasts on the future rates of insanity, with statistical studies from the same period attempting to assess the costs of mental health on society beyond the asylum walls. As we saw in Chapters 6, 7 and 8, statistical studies on insanity were framed as part of wider projects to assess the impact of insanity on society. Those suffering from mental health conditions were inhumanely dubbed a public health risk by eugenicists, be they psychiatrists like Frederick Mott, or population researchers like Karl Pearson. The insane were accused of having a detrimental impact on the public and on national interests. Although degeneration and psychiatry had been linked at least

[9] A. Scull, *Decarceration: Community Treatment and the Deviant: A Radical View*, Polity, 1984.

since Bénédict Morel's work in the mid-nineteenth century, the involvement of eugenicists with the development of statistical studies drew upon the data contained in asylum records. The medical statistics published by the Lunacy Commission could provide the data required to further eugenic campaigns to push through reforms that would encourage the bright to procreate and prevent the insane from having families. As we saw in Chapter 6, the work of Karl Pearson and David Heron had framed insanity as a cost on the psychic abilities of the nation and they sought to develop ways that utilised bureaucracy to minimise it. Conversely, due to the influence of eugenics, asylum statistics decreased in definition and ceased to be broken down according to psychological diagnosis as priorities shifted towards identifying the 'diathesis' or mark of insanity when assessing the cost of mental health to society. Anxieties over the cost of insanity continued on into the interwar period, with fears of the psychopathic constitution informing the decision of the 1934 Revisions committee to include it and a lengthy section on hereditary insanity in the Table of the Forms.

What are sometimes referred to as the sciences of chance have left an indelible but often underappreciated mark on scientific, social and cultural conceptions of psychological diagnosis. Work presented by a number of the characters encountered in this study have attempted to understand the unobservable mechanisms of the human mind through statistical data developed in asylum records.[10] This is often when anatomical or pathological studies, the typical reserves of medical research, have been exhausted. We have seen throughout this study how the act of diagnosis draws the mind and the body under abstract categories that can track patterns of behaviour when clear-cut physical explanations are lacking. We have seen how these categories are formulated from the initial observation of symptoms, and how they gain traction through social activities like the completion of public records and the publication of asylum statistics. We have also seen how changes to legislation associated with the 1845 lunacy laws led to diagnosis becoming a legal obligation for admissions to asylums, and this not only formalised diagnosis in asylum records, but essentially laid the ground for psychiatric epidemiology in the form of asylum medical statistics. As diagnostic concepts were circulated through usage in records, reports and debates on classification, they

[10] Ian Hacking, *The Taming of Chance*, CUP, 1993.

gathered meaning and had a looping effect as they filled up the pages of case notes, public health reports and medical journals. The Table of the Forms therefore shows how categories used in the clinic are linked to legislation and public health administration. Captured within the history of the Table of the Forms is a detailed story of the intertwined development of psychiatric knowledge, public health administration and mental health statistics that emerged from the middle of the nineteenth century. The sciences of chance used asylum statistics as the main set of data, be it the national statistics published by the Commissioners in Lunacy, or studies such as Robert Armstrong-Jones's work on those admitted to his Claybury asylum, assessed in Chapter 5. By presenting the history of the Table of the Forms, this study has attempted to show the under-appreciated impact of attempts to understand mental disorder through the abstractions used in statistical research and analysis. The standardised concepts were a vital part of the practice of science communication in the clinic, and this had a vital impact on the development of psychiatry as a medical discipline. Far from the requirement to keep records from being a 'deadening bureaucracy' that stifled care, the requirement to keep detailed information on a patient played a central role in the development of clinical knowledge.[11]

The classifications used in admissions diagnosis were a product of the social activity carried out by scientific communities. Asylum superintendents throughout the United Kingdom and Ireland were legally required to use the terms included in the Table of the Forms when diagnosing admissions. Assumptions that went beyond individual psychiatrists, structured debates that helped to formulate the concepts used in the Table of the Forms. During the second half of the nineteenth century, many who participated in discussions over classification held the grounding assumption that mental disorders were natural entities with a physical basis that existed independently of human knowledge, society and culture. Finding out the physical causes of the different forms of insanity would enable the nascent psychiatric community to formulate a classification that would resemble the kinds used by the other branches of general medicine. This is perhaps unsurprising given the medical background of those engaged in the debates, which helped to shape prophesies frequently aired during discussions about the future of psychological diagnostic categories. Some

[11] Kathleen Jones, *Asylums and After: A Revised History of the Mental Health Services*, the Athlone Press, 1993. (p. 91).

members of the MPA were certain that accurate predictions about the course of an illness based upon the detection of physical symptoms would be the ideal way to conduct psychiatric diagnosis, and that a firm understanding of the natural processes causing the different forms of insanity was just around the corner. The bone of contention was frequently over how far away this future was—as in the debates covered in Chapter 4 some camps believed that the future was decades away, others thought the future had already arrived, whereas the most sceptical quarters believed it to be perhaps a century away. What was common to these camps was the belief that concepts that described symptoms, such as melancholia and mania, would come to be less relied upon as the natural mechanisms of the body that gave rise to the different forms of insanity became better understood. Aspirations to provide a scientific classification of mental disorder would close the gap between the mind and the body, an epistemological dualism that many viewed to be a product of a lack of research would evaporate as the natural kinds of insanity came to be better understood.

The Table of the Forms was shaped by cultures of science during the nineteenth century that reached some degree of consensus on the forms of insanity that should be used in standard diagnostic procedures linked to asylum statistics. This book has explored how social and cultural factors helped to fuel discoveries that changed psychiatric knowledge and has demonstrated this through its treatment of the MPA's Table of the Forms. Historical accounts of classification have tended to emphasise the role of scientific discovery and clinical breakthrough in the development of concepts of psychopathology. The first that arose in the middle decades of the twentieth century gave priority to the discoveries made by medical science in charting the advancement of psychological knowledge, and these overlooked the role of communication amongst medical communities in forging the fundamental concepts of psychopathology that informed these investigations.[12] The emphasis on the role of discoveries recorded in textbooks in the advancement of classification and practice is partly explained by the clinical background of many early historians of psychiatry, with them presenting valuable resources that provide an in-depth analysis of the development of psychiatric ideas, and are still

[12] Richard Hunter and Ida McAlpine, *Three Hundred Years of Psychiatry 1535–1860: A History Presented in Selected English Texts*, LLC, 2013; Gregory Zilboorg, *A History of Medical Psychology*, W.W. Norton and Company, 1967.

useful to some extent to historians writing today. At the same time, the limitations of restricting investigation to the developments of clinical knowledge recorded in the great textbooks of Pinel, Esquirol, Hack Tuke, Kahlbaum and Kraepelin are perhaps obvious to many but are still worth restating: they can become 'Whiggish', with the assumption underlying these works being that less advanced concepts of insanity and mental illness were simply replaced with more advanced ones as knowledge was published in textbooks, and the classifications offered by these figures developed in their complexity. The priority given by these historians of this persuasion to scientific and clinical discoveries has narrowed history to the charting of some important but limited considerations from the history of clinical knowledge.

The knowledge that shaped psychiatric classification was propelled by social factors surrounding the practice of medicine, and as this volume has indicated, they were embedded within legal and public health frameworks that provided classifications of mental health. The diagnosis of insanity performed a social function in a variety of contexts, be it to admit an individual to an asylum or a hospital, or to make one eligible for psychiatric social services, or to be granted certain legal or duty-bound exemptions. The provisions made for those receiving a diagnosis of one of the forms of insanity were outlined in law: for instance, it was necessary to be given the status of a pauper lunatic until the passing of the 1930 Mental Treatment Act to receive state supported mental health treatment, and for the most part, 'treatment' would mean admittance and confinement within an asylum. Since the passing of the 1845 Lunacy Act, it was necessary for asylum superintendents to record a psychological diagnosis in an asylum's records. It was because of this legal requirement that the bureaucracy surrounding asylum regulation acted as a catalyst for discussions on psychiatric classification that frequently led to scientific aspirations being aired. Despite these hopes for the science of the mind, discussions would continue to be underpinned by cultural assumptions on what constituted the healthy and what defined the sick.

The literature on how the social and cultural factors have shaped our understandings of mental health is well-established, but these can become harder to trace when mental health statistics are the object of enquiry. In outlining the processes that shaped mental health data published between the nineteenth and twentieth centuries, this study has established how cultural attitudes shaped the categories used to break down the information on psychological diagnosis included in public health reports. As

Elaine Showalter argued in *The Female Malady*, madness was a social construct predominantly identified with women during the Victorian period, with diagnoses serving gendered political purposes and formulating a gendered views of subjectivity.[13] In her challenge to Showalter's thesis, Joan Busfield employs asylum admissions statistics in her claim that Showalter overemphasised the identification of madness with women and that she was mistaken in her claim that madness was a female malady.[14] Busfield's analysis indicates that there was no significant difference, statistically speaking, in the rates of diagnosis amongst admissions to asylums amongst men and women. Busfield showed how women had slightly higher ratios of admissions than men in 1879 and 1889, but lower in 1869 and 1895.[15] Busfield expands on this by presenting the statistics for individual asylums including the York Retreat, concluding again that there was no significant difference in the genders of asylum populations. However, as this study's interrogation of the discussions surrounding the psychological categories has shown, there was a preoccupation with the female body in the development of classifications used in asylum statistics on psychological diagnosis: as we saw in early versions of Skae's classification presented in Chapter 3, five classifications of madness were based on diagnostic categories that were rooted in Victorian notions of gender, with four being considered to exclusively relate to women—mania of pregnancy, mania of lactation, Ovario-Mania or Utero-Mania, Puerperal Mania—and one relating exclusively to men—Satyriasis. Skae's classification was used in admissions to the Edinburgh Royal Asylum, and at one point was a serious candidate to be the standard set of psychological diagnostic terms used in asylums across the British Isles. The looping effects the categories employed in asylum public records are hard to measure precisely, but given the widespread coverage of asylum statistics, and the debates over them included in popular publications, it is possible that they have contributed to the cultural attitudes described by historians of madness like Showalter.

I hope that this historical case study will provide an opportunity for reflection for those interested in the ongoing debates between social

[13] Elaine Showalter, *The Female Malady: Women, Madness and English Culture, 1830–1980*, Virago, 1987.

[14] Joan Busfield, 'The Female Malady? Men, Women and Madness in Nineteenth Century Britain' in *Medical Sociology*, vol. 28, no. 1, February 1994, pp. 259–277.

[15] Ibid., p. 264.

constructivists and biological naturalists on the nature of mental disorder. At risk of sounding circular, the Table of the Forms attempted to describe the forms of insanity, that is to say, the essence or core of a disorder that it was thought could be identified through different manifestations of symptoms. As we have seen, there have been tensions between those who viewed the Table of the Forms as a tool for diagnosis and those who wanted the implementation of a classification that carved the nature of mental disorder at the joints—that is to say, hope that a classification could provide an accurate representation of the essence of mental disorder. These debates were caught within a set of metaphysical assumptions that bear some resemblance to those behind current debates but have important context-bound differences. The most striking example is that in Skae's notion of a natural history of a mental disorder, which bears some resemblance to the notion of natural kinds of biological dysfunction that underpin more recent conceptions of mental disorder, but the important divergence being that he still used the language of forms. Like many of the hereditarian eugenicists who came later, he thought that insanity was one disease that had different manifestations depending upon the state of the body and the person's constitution. It is very difficult to say exactly when the tide turned against unitary insanity towards an understanding of the kinds of mental disorder, but the deliberations outlined in Chapter 5 suggest that this occurred sometime around the 1907 Revisions, despite the language of forms being preserved in the title of the table. Before these revisions, the tensions between those who thought insanity to be one illness that had different forms depending on the bodily constitution of the patient and the stage of the illness, and those who thought them to be different diseases with differing physiological causes, would characterise debates that surrounded the document until the turn of the century. Some understand insanity itself to be a heuristic that had institutional meaning; an influential example being Charles Mercier, who believed 'insanity' to have a predominantly social and cultural meaning that meant an illness which admitted one to an asylum and cautioned against it being used in reference to all mental disorders suffered by human beings.

I would like to end this study by turning for a moment to the United States of America, and a study conducted by the social psychologist Shirley A. Star shortly after the Table of the Forms had been replaced by the *ICD* in psychological diagnosis and mental health statistics. She delivered her findings on social and cultural perceptions of mental health at the 1955 Annual General Meeting of the American National Institute of Mental Health.[16] Through 3,500 interviews with members of the public, Star concluded that 'there is an old, socially-sanctioned, well-established set of views which supports the identification of mental illness only with violent, extreme psychosis', and that for many of those interviewed, 'mental illness emerges more or less as the ultimate catastrophe that can befall a human being'.[17] Star emphasised that this was not due to 'human capriciousness, mass stupidity, or any such dismissing epithet'.[18] To the contrary, she stressed that those interviewed as a part of her study provided in-depth and nuanced responses to her questions, and that many echoed the concerns of mental health professionals, including psychiatrists, social workers and psychologists. Star described to her audience how some interviewees had discussed the nature of rationality, others had veered-off on tangents on how to detect conventional and abnormal behaviour, the nature of mind–body dualism, relationships between physical and mental illnesses, or the differences between culturally sanctioned and clinical notions of self-control and propriety. She emphasised the significance of cultural perceptions of mental health and illness to her audience of clinicians, claiming that they shaped medical practices and psychiatric social services since those interviewed participated in elections and other aspects of civil society that influenced the formulation of mental health policy. Social attitudes also shaped psychiatric treatment in more subtle ways: according to Star, they helped to determine how and when an individual may seek treatment for themselves or for a family member.

This monograph has explored the old, socially-sanctioned and well-established views that emerged through an interrogation of the history of mental health statistics and psychological diagnosis. The attitudes Star described were shaped by many people only coming into first-hand contact with psychological diagnosis when they, a friend or a relative were at the point of being admitted to an asylum. How far attitudes have shifted since the age of the Table of the Forms and Star's study is difficult to say for certain, but the catastrophic impact of mental illness for many is still an economic burden that many fear. Developed in the

[16] Shirley A. Star, 'The Public's Ideas About Mental Illness' in *Report of the Annual Meeting of the National Association for Mental Health*, Indianapolis, IN, November 1955.

[17] Ibid., p. 5.

[18] Ibid.

years immediately before and after the COVID-19 pandemic, I hope this study can provide new opportunities for reflection on the worth of mental health statistics currently used to understand the prevalence of mental health conditions, and, perhaps more importantly, what is not captured by the definitions currently used. Despite the tired-old parity of esteem trope often deployed by politicians near election time, the lack of tangible progress on alleviating the economic costs of mental disorder by governments in the United Kingdom makes the associations between mental health, ruin and catastrophe persist into the twenty-first century.

Bibliography

Primary Sources

Archives Consulted

Archives and Manuscripts, Wellcome Library, London.
Archives of the Royal Society of Medicine, London.
Archives of the Royal College of Psychiatrists.
Parliamentary Archives, Hansard.
Manuscripts and Archives, The British Library.
Mass Observation Archives.
The National Archives at Kew Gardens.
Wakefield Collections, West Yorkshire Archives.
Special Collections, University of Leeds.

Reports and Minutes

'Annual Meeting of the Association of Medical Officers of Asylum and Hospitals for the Insane'. *JMS*, vol. 10, no. 51, October 1864, pp. 448–469.

'Association of Medical Officers for the Asylums and Hospitals for the Insane: Official Report of Proceedings at the Annual Meeting held at the Freemasons' Tavern, Thursday, July 5th, 1860'. *JMS*, vol. 7, no. 35, pp. 23–49.

'British Medical Association Annual Meeting'. *JMS*, vol. 26, no. 115, October 1880, pp. 460–471.

'Dr James Murray Lindsay'. *JMS*, vol. 58, no. 240, January 1912, p. 197.

K. M. Jones, *Psychological Classification and Diagnosis in Asylum Statistics, 1800–1948*, Mental Health in Historical Perspective,
https://doi.org/10.1007/978-3-031-46154-5

General Register Office, 'Mental Health Statistics'. MH 99/34, held by The National Archives.
'Medico-Psychological Association of Great Britain and Ireland'. *JMS*, October 1906, pp. 809–838.
'Medico-Psychological Association of Great Britain and Ireland'. *JMS*, vol. 52, no. 219, October 1906, pp. 809–838.
'Medico-Psychological Association of Great Britain and Ireland: Annual Meeting July 21st 1904'. *JMS*, vol. 50, no. 211, October 1904, pp. 784–805.
'Medico-Psychological Association of Great Britain and Ireland: Annual Meeting of the Association, July 20th, 1905'. *JMS*, vol. 51, no. 215, October 1905, pp. 773–789.
'Medico-Psychological Association: Quarterly Meeting January 1882'. *JMS*, vol. 28, no. 121, April 1882, pp. 136–146.
'Medico-Psychological Statistics: the Desirability of Definition and Correlation, with a View to Collective Study' to the Annual General Meeting of the Association in 1902 (check this)
'Mental Health Statistics, Minutes of Meeting, Wednesday February 18th, 1948'. MH 99/34, held by National Archives, Kew Gardens.
'Minutes from The Medico-Psychological Association of Great Britain and Ireland: Eightieth Annual General Meeting of the Association'. *JMS*, vol. 67, no. 279, October 1921 pp. 511–556.
'Minutes from The Medico-Psychological Association of Great Britain and Ireland: Ninetieth Annual General Meeting of the Association'. *JMS*, vol. 77, no. 319, pp. 862–901.
'Minutes from The Medico-Psychological Association of Great Britain and Ireland: Ninety-First Annual General Meeting of the Association'. *JMS*, vol. 78, no. 323, pp. 973–999.
Minutes from The Medico-Psychological Association of Great Britain and Ireland: Ninety-Second Annual General Meeting of the Association. *JMS*, vol. 79, no. 327, October 1933, pp. 800–817.
'Minutes of the Annual Meeting of The Medico-Psychological Association of Great Britain and Ireland, July 1902'. *JMS*, vol. 48, no. 203, October 1902, pp. 795–805.
'Minutes of the Meeting of the Research and Clinical Committee', July 17th, 1941 in RCPSYCH/L10 - Records of the Research and Clinical Section, 1927–1970, held by The Royal College of Psychiatrists, London.
'Occasional Notes: The Annual Meeting of the Medico-Psychological Association'. *The Journal of Mental Science*, vol. 49, no. 207, October 1903, pp. 703–705.
'Occasional Notes: The Annual Meeting'. *JMS*, vol. 50, no. 11, October 1904, pp. 750–751.

'Part IV: Notes and News: Medico-Psychological Association of Great Britain and Ireland: Annual Meeting 1903'. *JMS*, vol. 49, no. 207, October 1903 pp. 749–774.

'Proceedings of the Twenty-sixth Annual General Meeting of the Medico-Psychological Association, held at the Royal College of Physicians of London (by permission of the President and Fellows), on Thursday, August 3rd, 1871, under the Presidency of Henry Maudsley'. *JMS*, vol. 17, no. 79, October 1871, pp. 438–468.

'Report of a Meeting of Members of the Medico-Psychological Association, held at Glasgow, April 27th, 1870'. *JMS*, July, 1870, vol. 16, no. 74.

'Report of a Meeting of Members of the Medico-Psychological Association, held at Glasgow, April 27th, 1870'. *JMS*, July, 1870, vol. 16, no. 74, p. 304.

'Report of the Thirty-fifth Annual Meeting of the Medico-Psychological Association'. *JMS*, October 1880, pp. 444–460.

'Report of the Thirty-Seventh Annual General Meeting of the Medico-Psychological Association'. *JMS*, vol. 28, no. 123, October 1882, pp. 437–462.

'Reports of Societies: Royal Medical and Chirurgical Society, Tuesday, May 14, 1861'. *Medical Times & Gazette*, May 25th, 1861, pp. 562–565,

'Review: *Psychiatrie: ein Lehrbuch für Studirende und Aerzte* (Psychiatry: A Manual for Students and Physicians). Von Dr Emil Kraepelin'. *JMS*, vol. 45, no. 190, July 1899, pp. 581–583.

'Reviews: The Lunacy Blue Books'. *JMS*, vol. 25, no. 112, January 1880, pp. 557–574.

'Royal Medico-Psychological Association, Minutes of the Meeting of the Research and Clinical Committee, June 30th, 1936'. RCPSYCH/L10 - Records of the Research and Clinical Section, 1927–1970, held by The Royal College of Psychiatrists, London.

'Royal Medico-Psychological Association, Minutes of the Meeting of the Research and Clinical Committee, 01st September 1938 in RCPSYCH/L10 - Records of the Research and Clinical Section, 1927–1970, held by The Royal College of Psychiatrists, London.

'Statistical Intermission'. *JMS*, vol. 6, no. 56, January 1916, pp. 182–183.

'The Home Care of the Insane Poor in England'. *JMS*, vol. 49, no. 207, pp. 708–711.

'The Late C.A. Mercier'. *JMS*, vol. 67, no. 276, January 1921, p. 146.

'The Medico-Psychological Association of Great Britain and Ireland: Quarterly Meeting November 15th 1906'. *JMS*, vol. 53, no. 220, January 1907, pp. 214–217.

'The Medico-Psychological Association of Great Britain and Ireland: Eighty-Second Annual General Meeting of the Association'. *JMS*, vol. 69, no. 287, October 1925, pp. 528–580.

'The Medico-Psychological Association: Proceedings at the Annual Meeting of the Association, held at the Rooms of the Royal Society, Edinburgh, on Tuesday, July 31st, 1866'. *JMS*, vol. 12, no. 59, October 1866, pp. 415–437.
'The Medico-Psychological Association: The Eighty Fourth Annual General Meeting of the Association, July 7th–10th'. *JMS*, vol. 7, no. 295, October 1925, pp. 797–855.
'The Royal Medico-Psychological Association: The Eighty-Ninth Annual Meeting of the Association: July 1st–4th'. *JMS*, vol. 76, no. 315, October 1930, pp. 860–894.
'The Royal Medico-Psychological Association: The Eighty-Sixth Annual Meeting, July 19th–22nd, 1927. *JMS*, vol. 73, no. 303, pp. 691–728, (pp. 723–726).
'The Statistical Tables'. *JMS*, vol. 28, no. 124, January 1883, p. 653.
War Office 'Summary of Evidence of Witnesses Regarding the Influence of War Stress and 'Shell Shock' in the Production of Insanity'. *Royal Commission into Shell Shock*, HMSO, 1919.
The Medico-Psychological Association Proceedings at the Annual Meeting of the Association, held at the Royal College of Psychiatrists.
'The Report of the Commissioners in Lunacy'. *The Times* [London, England], August 16, 1888, no. 32466, p. 7.
Armstrong-Jones, Robert. 'Correspondence: Classification of Mental Disorders'. *BMJ*, June 16th, 1934, pp. 1091–1092, p. 1091.
Blacker, Carlos Patton. 'Mental Health Records: What We Can Learn from Them?', 27th February 1947, in Papers by Carlos Paton Blacker on Mental Health Records, Carlos Paton Blacker Collected Papers, held by The Wellcome Collection.
Blacker, Carlos Patton. 'Redhill Hospital–Notes on Visit Paid by Dr Harris and Dr Blacker on Monday', 16th December 1946 in Papers by Carlos Paton Blacker on Mental Health Records, Carlos Paton Blacker Collected Papers, held by The Wellcome Collection.
Bond, Hubert, and Yellowlees, David. 'Report of the Statistical Committee, Appointed at the Annual Meeting Held at Liverpool in 1902, Presented to the Annual Meeting of the Association, July 21st, 1904'. *JMS*, vol. 51, no. 215, October 1905, pp. 799–826.
Campbell, J.A. 'Proposed Statistical Tables'. *JMS*, vol. 28, no. 122, July 1882, pp. 318–319.
Campbell, J.A. and Todd, J. 'Uniformity in Public Asylum Reports'. *JMS*, vol. 19, no. 85, April 1873, pp. 67–78 (p. 69).
Cooper, Anthony Ashley, Earl of Shaftesbury, et al. *The Report of the Metropolitan Commissioners of Lunacy*, Bradbury and Evans Printers, 1844
Farr, William. 'Report upon the Mortality of Lunatics'. *Journal of the Statistical Society of London*, vol. 4, no. 1, April 1941, pp. 17–33.

Fleming, G.W.T.H. 'Classification of Mental Disorders'. *BMJ*, June 2nd, 1934, p. 991.

Fleming, G.W.T.H. 'Correspondence: Classification of Mental Disorders'. *BMJ*, June 30th, 1934, p. 1187.

Fleming, G.W.T.H. 'Definitions and Explanatory Notes on the Classification of Mental Disorders'. *JMS*, no. 80, April 1934, pp. 409–410.

Fleming, G.W.T.H. 'The Revision of the Classification of Mental Disorders: Report by the Clinical Psychiatry Sub-Committee of the Research and Clinical Committee–Part II'. *JMS*, vol. 78, no. 321, April 1932, pp. 387–391.

Hack Tuke, Daniel. 'Lunacy Statistics: To the Editor of the Times'. *JMS*, vol. 34, no. 147, October 1888; *The Times* [London, England], August 30, 1888, no. 32478, p. 6.

Hack Tuke, Daniel, et al., 'Report of Committee on the Statistical Tables of the Medical-Psychological Association'. *JMS*, October 1882, pp. 463–464.

Mercier, Charles. 'Correspondence: Proposed Sterilisation of Certain Degenerates'. *BMJ*, April 2nd, 1904, p. 808

Yellowlees, David. 'Definitions of Terms Used in the Report and the Statistical Tables'. *JMS*, vol. 51, no. 215, October 1905, pp. 834–856.

Yellowlees, David. 'Report of the Statistical Committee, Appointed at the Annual Meeting Held at Liverpool in 1902, Presented to the Annual Meeting of the Association, July 21st, 1904'. *JMS*, vol. 51, no. 215, October 1905, pp. 799–826.

Academic Papers, Textbooks, Treatise, Nosologies, Published Correspondence

'The Classification of Causes of Death'. *BMJ*, April 20th, 1940, p. 661.

Allen, Matthew. Essay on the Classification of the Insane John Taylor, 1837.

Andreasen, N.C. 'Linking Mind and Brain in the Study of Mental Illnesses: A Project for a Scientific Psychopathology'. *Science*, vol. 275, no. 5306, pp. 1586–1593.

Andriezen, William Lloyd. 'On the Bases and Possibilities of a Scientific Psychology and Classification in Mental Disease'. *JMS*, vol. 45, no. 189, April 1899, pp. 257–290.

Armstrong-Jones, Robert. 'Correspondence: Classification of Mental Disorders'. *BMJ*, June 16th, 1934, pp. 1091–1092, p. 1091.

Armstrong-Jones, Robert. 'Prognosis in Mental Diseases'. *BMJ*, December 16th, 1905, pp. 1578–1582.

Arnold, Thomas. Observations on the Nature, Kinds, Causes, and Prevention of Insanity, Lunacy, or Madness, G. Ireland: Leicester, 1782.

Ashe, Isaac. 'Some Observations on General Paralysis'. *JMS*, vol. 22, no. 97, April 1976, pp. 82–91.

Atkin, I. Classification of Psychological Disorders'. *BMJ*, November 2nd, 1946, p. 666.

Batty Tuke, John. 'A Pathological Classification of Mental Disease'. *JMS*, July, 1870, vol. 16, no. 74, pp. 195–210.

Baugh, L.D.H. 'Some Observations on Confusional Insanity'. *BMJ*, vol. 2, no. 2337, October 14th 1905, pp. 949–951.

Blandford, G. Fielding. 'The Lumleian Lectures on the Diagnosis, Prognosis and Prophylaxis of Insanity: Lecture I'. *BMJ*, April 6th, 1895, pp. 741–747.

Blandford, G. Fielding. 'The Lumleian Lectures on the Diagnosis, Prognosis and Prophylaxis of Insanity: Lecture II'. *BMJ*, April 13th, 1895, pp. 797–800.

Boyd, R. 'Statistics of Pauper Insanity'. *JMS*, vol. 17, 1871, pp. 221–225.

Brend, William A. 'Correspondence: War Neurosis'. *BMJ*, March 21st, 1942, p. 395.

Browne, J.C. 'Skae's Classification of Mental Diseases: A Critique'. *JMS*, vol. 21, no. 95, October 1875, pp. 339–365.

Bruce, A. Ninian. 'The Out-patient Treatment of Early Medical Disorder. The Neurological Clinic and Some of Its Function' Recorded in 'Minutes from The Medico-Psychological Association of Great Britain and Ireland: Eightieth Annual General Meeting of the Association'. *JMS*, vol. 67, no. 279, October 1921 pp. 511–556.

Bucknill, J.C. *The Care of the Insane and their Legal Control*, London: Macmillan, 1880.

Bucknill, J.C. 'The Diagnosis of Insanity'. *The Asylum Journal of Mental Science*, vol. 3, no. 20, May 1857, pp. 141–185.

Bucknill, J.C. and Tuke, Daniel H. *A Manual of Psychological Medicine*, Blanchard and Lea, 1858.

Bury, Judson S. 'Prognosis in Relation to Disease of the Nervous System'. *BMJ*, November 9th, 1901, pp. 1389–1396.

Church, William S., Living, E., et al., *The Nomenclature of Diseases: Drawn up by a Joint Committee Appointed by the Royal College of Physicians of London*, fourth edition, HMSO, 1906.

Clouston, Thomas. Annual Report of the Royal Edinburgh Asylum for the Insane, 1877, Royal Edinburgh Asylum, 1878.

Clouston, Thomas. 'Facts for the Teetotallers'. *JMS*, July 1870, vol. 16, no. 74 pp. 261–262.

Clouston, Thomas. *Lectures on Mental Diseases*, 2nd edition, J & A Churchill, 1892.

Clouston, Thomas. *Lectures on Mental Diseases*, 4th edition, J & A Churchill, 1904.

Clouston, Thomas. 'Skae's Classification of Mental Disorder'. *JMS*, January, 1876, vol. 21, no. 96, pp. 500–532.

Craig, Maurice. 'Delusional Insanity'. *Hospital*, vol. 22, no. 549, April 3rd, 1897, pp. 9–10.

Crichton, Alexander. *An inquiry into the nature and origin of mental derangement: comprehending a concise system of the physiology and pathology of the human mind and a history of the passions and their effects*, Cadell Jr. & Davies, 1798, p. 5.

Crichton Miller, Hugh. 'Anxiety and Hysteria'. *BMJ*, November 27th, 1943, pp. 687–688.

Crichton-Miller, Hugh. *The New Psychology and the Parent*, Jarrolds, 1922.

Cullen, William. *Synopsis Nosologiae Methodicae*, trans. William Jackson, W. Jackson, 1827, pp. 11–12.

Deas, P. Maury. 'Five Years of Statistics' *JMS*, vol. 25, no. 109, April 1879, pp. 8–19.

Dillon, F. 'Classification of Psychological Disorders'. *BMJ*, October 19th, 1946, p. 588.

Drapes, T. 'On the Maniacal-Depressive Insanity of Kraepelin'. *JMS*, vol. 55, no. 228, January 1909, pp. 58–64.

Fahet, M., '"On Some of the Latent Causes of Insanity", excerpts (translated) from *Leçons Cliniques de Médicine Mentale*, Paris, 1854'. *Journal of Psychological Medicine and Mental Pathology*, vol. 7, 1854.

Freeman, Walter and James W. Watts. 'Psychosurgery: An Evaluation of Two Hundred Cases Over Seven Years'. *JMS*, vol. 90, no. 379, pp. 532–537.

Freud, S. The *Standard Edition of the Complete Psychological Works, vol. 1 (1886–1899)*, trans. James Strachey and Anna Freud, Hogarth Press, 1966.

Glover, Edward. 'A Psycho-Analytic Approach to the Classification of Mental Disorders'. *JMS*, vol. 78, no. 323, October 1932, pp. 819–842.

Gowers, William R. 'A Lecture on the Prognosis and Treatment of Syphilitic Disease of the Nervous System'. *JMS*, April, 1903, pp. 773–778.

Gowers, William R. 'The Lettsomian Lectures on Syphilis and the Nervous System'. *BMJ*, February 9th 1889, pp. 283–285.

Green, George. 'The Prognosis in Dementia Paralytica'. *JMS*, vol. 52, no. 217, 1906, pp. 84–305.

Griesinger, Wilhelm. *Mental Pathology and Therapeutics*, trans. C. Lockhart Robinson and James Rutherford, The New Sydenham Society, 1867.

Hack-Tuke, Daniel. *A Dictionary of Insanity*, P. Blakiston, 1892.

Hack-Tuke, Daniel. 'On the Best Mode of Tabulating Recoveries from Insanity in Asylums Reports'. *JMS*, Vol 26, no. 115, October 1880, pp. 375–382.

Hadfield, J.A. 'War Neurosis: A Year in a Neuropathic Hospital'. *BMJ*, February 28th, 1942, pp. 281–285.

Havelock, John G. 'A Case of Recurrent Mania'. *JMS*, vol. 4, no. 179, October 1896, pp. 817–81.

Hart, Bernard. 'A Philosophy of Psychiatry'. *JMS*, vol. 54, no. 226, July 1906, pp. 473–490.

Henderson, D.K. and Gillespie, R.D. *A Textbook of Psychiatry for Students and Practitioners*, 3rd edition, OUP, 1932.

Henry, Eustace M. 'A Case of "Dementia Praecox"'. *JMS*, vol. 50, no. 210, July 1904, pp. 516–521.

Hitchman, John. "The Pathology of Insanity: A Lecture, Delivered May 25th, 1850, in the Middlesex County Asylum, Hanwell'. *Journal of Psychological Medicine and Mental Pathology*, vol. 3, 1850, pp. 501–521.

Hughlings Jackson, John. 'Remarks on the Diagnosis and Treatment of Diseases of the Brain'. *BMJ*, vol. 2, no. 1438, July 1st, 1888, pp. 111–117.

Humphreys, Noel A. 'Statistics of Insanity in England, with Special Reference to Its Alleged Increasing Prevalence'. *Journal of the Royal Statistical Society*, vol. 53, no. 2, June 1890, pp. 201–252.

Hutchison, Robert, et al., *The Nomenclature of Diseases: Drawn up by a Joint Committee Appointed by the Royal College of Physicians of London*, 6th edition, Her Majesty's Stationary Office, 1931.

Kraepelin, Emil. *Dementia Praecox and Paraphrenia*, trans. R. Mary Barclay, ed. George Robertson, Chicago Medical Book Co., 1916.

Kraepelin, Emil. 'On the Question of Degeneration' republished in *History of Psychiatry*, vol. 18, no. 3, 2007, pp. 399–404.

Lane, Edward B. 'Some Cases of Alternating Insanity with One Case of Recovery'. *Boston Medical and Surgical Journal*, vol. 116, January 20th, 1887, pp. 52–56.

Laycock, Thomas. *The Principles and Methods of Medical Observation and Research*, Edinburgh University, 1863.

Lord, J.R. 'The Clinical Study of Mental Disorders: The Presidential Address at the 85th Meeting of the Royal Medico-Psychological Association'. *JMS*, vol. 72, no. (S)298, August 1926, pp. 1–79.

Lord, J.R. and Fleming, G.W.T.H. 'The Revision of the Classification of Mental Disorders: Report by the Clinical Psychiatry Sub-Committee of the Research and Clinical Committee'. *JMS*, vol. 78, no. 320, January 1932, pp. 177–201.

Maclay, W.S., and Whitby, J. 'In-patient Treatment of Civilian Neurotic Casualties'. *BMJ*, October 1942, p. 449–451.

Major, Herbert C. 'Dr Major on Statistical Tables of the Causes of Insanity'. *JMS*, vol. 23, no. 104, January 1878, pp. 573–575.

Major, Herbert C. 'Remarks on the Results of the Collective Record of the Causation of Insanity'. *JMS*, vol. 30, no. 129, pp. 1–7.

Mapother, Henry. 'Emil Kraepelin'. *JMS*, vol. 73, no. 303, 1927, pp. 509–515.

Maudsley, Henry. 'On Some of the Causes of Insanity'. *JMS*, January 1867, vol. 1, no. 60.

Maudsley, Henry. *Responsibility in Mental Disease*, D. Appleton & Company, 1895.

Mercier, Charles. *A Text-Book of Insanity*, Macmillan, 1902.

Mercier, Charles. 'Kinds of Insanity', delivered to the British Medical Association: Swansea 1903: Section of Psychological Medicine'. *JMS*, Volume 49, no. 207, October 1903, pp. 776–780. (p. 776).

Mercier, Charles. 'The Data of Alienism'. *JMS* vol. 28, no. 123, October 1882, pp. 333-343; vol. 28, no. 124, January 1883, pp. 496–510; vol. 9, no. 125, April 1883, pp. 31–41; vol. 30, no. 131, October 1884, pp. 369–377, pp. 369–377.

Mercier, Charles. 'The Nature of Insanity'. *JMS*, vol. 27, no. 120, January 1882, pp. 512–527.

Mercier, Charles. 'The Statistical Tables'. *JMS*, vol. 50, no. 211, October 1904, pp. 672–697.

Mercier, Charles. 'The Study of Insanity'. *JMS*, vol. 27, no. 118, July 1881, pp. 166–177.

Mercier, Charles. 'The Study of Insanity'. *JMS*, vol. 27, no. 118, October 1882, pp. 166–177.

Mercier, Charles. 'What Insanity Is'. *Sanity and Insanity*, Scott, 1890, pp. 97–139.

Meyer-Gross, William, Slater, Eliot, and Roth, Martin. *Clinical Psychiatry*, Cassell, 1954.

Monroe, Henry. 'One Nomenclature of the Various Forms of Insanity'. *The Asylum Journal of Mental Science*, vol. 2, no. 17, April 1856, pp. 286–305.

Mott, Frederick W. 'The Genetic Origin of Dementia Praecox'. *JMS*, vol. 68, no. 283, October 1922, pp. 333–347.

Nicolson, David. Reports Upon Broadmoor Criminal Lunatic Asylum with Statistical Tables for the Year 1889, HMSO, 1890.

Pearson, Karl. 'On the Inheritance of Insanity'. *BMJ*, May 7th, 1905, pp. 1175–1176.

Penrose Lionel, S. 'Correspondence', 25th September 1953. MH 99/34 held by the National Archives, Kew Gardens.

Penrose, Lionel, S. Correspondence to R. Tomsett, the Board of Control. Mr Corbett's proposals for revising the Index Cards. Diagnostic Lists, Carlos Paton Blacker, Collected Papers.

Penrose, Lionel, S. 'Social Aspects of Psychiatry: The Importance of Statistics'. *JMS*, vol. 9, no. 389, October 1946, pp. 713–718.

Pilkington, Francis. 'Review: W.H.O. and Mental Health 1949–1961. W.H.O. Geneva 1962'. *JMS*, vol. 109, no. 458, January 1963, p. 154.

Pinel, Phillippe. *Nosographie philosophique ou La méthode de l'analyse appliquée à la médecine*, Paris, 1797.

Pinel, Phillipe. *Traité médico-philosophique sur l'aliénation mentale*, Chez J. Ant. Brosson, 1800.

Prichard, J.C. *A Treatise on Insanity and Other Disorders Affecting the Mind*, Sherwood, Gilbert, and Piper, 1835.

Rayner, Henry. 'Classification of Insanity'. *JMS*, vol. 32, no. 138, July 1886.

Rayner, Henry. 'The Classification of Insane States in Revised Statistical Tables'. *JMS*, vol. 51, no. 212, January 1905, pp. 140–143.

Rees, John Rawlings. *The Shaping of Psychiatry by War*. Chapman and Hall, 1945.

Reeve, Henry. 'Phillippe Pinel, "Traité Medico-Philosophique sur l'Aliénation Mentale ou la Manie"'. *The Edinburgh Review*, vol. 2, April–July 1803, pp. 160–172.

Reich, Wilhelm. *The Mass Psychology of Fascism: Translated from the German Manuscript*, trans. Mary Boyd Higgins, Orgone Institute Press, 1946.

Revington, G.T. 'The Neuropathic Diathesis, or the Diathesis of the Degenerate'. *JMS*, vol. 34, no. 146, July 1888, pp. 167–176.

Richard Robert Leeper, 'Some Reflections on the Progress of Psychiatry: The Presidential Address at the Ninetieth Annual Meeting of the Royal Medico-Psychological Association Held in Dublin'. *JMS*, vol. 77, no. 319, October 1931, pp. 683–691.

Robertson, George. 'Obituary: Alexander Reid Urquhart'. *JMS*, vol. 63, no. 263, October 1917, pp. 629–631.

Robertson, William Ford. 'Chronic Bacterial Infections in Dementia Praecox'. Lecture and responses recorded in Minutes from The Medico-Psychological Association of Great Britain and Ireland: Eightieth Annual General Meeting of the Association. *JMS*, vol. 67, no. 279, October 1921 pp. 511–556 (pp. 543–546)

Robinson, Lockhart C. 'Suggestions Towards an Uniform System of Asylum Statistics (with Tabular Forms)'. *JMS*, vol. 7, no. 36, January 1861, pp. 195–211.

Rowson, Lionel A. 'Classification of Psychological Disorders'. *BMJ*, November 9th, 1946, p. 709.

Sands, Dalton, E. 'Classification of Psychological Disorders'. *BMJ*, November 23rd, 1946, pp. 793–794.

Sands, Dalton, E. 'Electro-convulsion Therapy in 301 Patients in a General Hospital: With Reference to Selection of Cases and Response to Treatment'. *BMJ*, August 31st, 1946, pp. 289–293.

Sands, Dalton, E. 'Treatment of Psychiatric Patients in General Hospitals: A Social Experiment'. *BMJ*, May 22nd, pp. 628–630.

Sargant, W. 'Physical Treatment of Acute War Neurosis: Some Clinical Observations'. *BMJ*, November 14th, 1942, p. 574–576.

Skae, David. 'A Rational and Practical Classification of Insanity'. *JMS*, vol. 9, no. 47, October 1863, pp. 309–319.

Skae, David. Of the classification of the various forms of insanity on a rational and practical basis: being an address delivered at the Royal College of Physicians, London, at the annual meeting of the Association of Medical Officers of Asylums on 9th July, 1863, Royal College of Physicians, 1863.

Skae, David, et al. 'Report of the Committee Appointed at a Meeting of Member of the Medico-Psychological Association, Held at the College of Physicians, Edinburgh, on 25th November, 1869, for the Purpose of Taking Certain Questions Relating to the Uniform Recording of Cases of Insanity and to Medical Treatment of Insanity into Consideration'. *JMS*, vol. 16, no. 74, July 1870, pp. 223–232.

Smith, Percy. 'Adjourned Annual Meeting of 1904'. *JMS*, vol. 51, no. 215, October 1905, pp. 733–772.

Smith, Percy. 'The International Committee for the Study of the Causes and Prophylaxis of Mental Disease'. *JMS*, vol. 56, no. 234, 1910, pp. 389–405.

Sutton, S.W. 'Letters, Notes, Etc.: Coined Medical Words'. *BMJ*, July 5th, 1941, p. 38.

Sykes, Lieut.-Col. 'Statistics of the Metropolitan Commission in Lunacy'. *Journal of the Statistical Society of London*, vol. 3, no. 2, July, 1840, pp. 143–160.

Symonds, C.P. 'Correspondence: Classification of Psychological Disorders'. *BMJ*, September, 1946, p. 436.

Symonds, C.P. 'The Human Response to Flying Stress'. *BMJ*, December 4th, 1943, pp. 703–706.

Thompson, D.G. 'The Prognosis in Insanity'. *JMS*, vol. 29, no. 126, July 1883, pp. 188–205.

Thomson, Courtauld. 'Correspondence: A National Council for Mental Hygiene'. *BMJ*, April 1st 1922, 1(3196): 538

Thurnam, John. *Observations and Essays in the Statistics of Insanity: Including an Inquiry into the Causes Influencing the Results of Treatment in Establishments for the Insane; To Which are Added the Statistics of the Retreat*, Near York, Simpkin Marshall, 1845, pp. 39–40.

Turner, John. 'The Classification of Insanity'. *JMS*, vol. 58, no. 40, January 1912, pp. 9–25.

Urquhart, A.R. 'Nomenclature of Mental Diseases'. *JMS*, vol. 49, no. 205, April 1903, pp. 236–245.

Webster, John. 'Statistics of Bethlem Hospital with Remarks on Insanity'. *Medico-chirurgical Transactions*, vol. 26, 1843, pp. 374–416.

West, Ranyard. 'Correspondence: War Neurosis: The "Awareness" of Fear'. *BMJ*, March 21st, 1942, p. 395.

Wood, T. Outterson. 'The Early History of the Medico-Psychological Association'. *JMS*, vol. 42, no. 177, 1896. pp. 241–260.

Addresses and Lectures

Armstrong Jones, Robert. 'Medico-Psychological Association of Great Britain and Ireland: Presidential Address on the Evolution of Insanity, delivered July 26th, 1906'. *JMS*, vol. 51, no. 215, October 1905, pp. 629–661.

Leeper, Richard Robert. 'Some Reflections on the Progress of Psychiatry: The Presidential Address at the Ninetieth Annual Meeting of the Royal Medico-Psychological Association Held in Dublin'. *JMS*, vol. 77, no. 319, October 1931, pp. 683–691.

Urquhart, A.R. 'The Morison Lectures on Insanity, with Special Reference to Heredity and Prognosis. *JMS*, vol. 52, no. 217, April 1907, pp. 233–321.

Urquhart, A.R. 'The Presidential Address delivered at the Fifty-Seventh Annual Meeting of the Medico-Psychological Association, held at the Royal College of Physicians, Edinburgh, on the 21st July, 1898'. *JMS*, vol. 44, no. 187, October 1898, pp. 673–693.

Worth, R., 1935. 'Four Decades of Psychiatry: The Presidential Address at the Ninety-Fourth Annual Meeting of the Royal Medico-Psychological Association, held in the Middlesex Guildhall, Westminster, July 3, 1935'. *JMS*, vol. 81, no. 335, pp. 755–765.

Laws and Acts of Parliament

1845 County Asylums Act

1845 Lunacy Act

1866 Idiots Act

1890 Lunacy Act

1913 Mental Deficiency Act

1930 Mental Treatment Act

1948 National Health Service Act

Obituaries

'Obituary: Henry Sutherland'. JMS, vol. 48, no. 200, January 1902, pp. 208–209.

'Obituary: Herbert Francis Hayes Newington'. *JMS*, vol. 63, no. 263, October 1917, pp. 461–467.

'Obituary: John Sibbald'. JMS, July 1905, vol. 51, no. 214, pp. 636–637.

'Obituary: William Chapman Begley'. *JMS*, vol. 33, no. 142, July 1887, pp. 337–339.

'Obituary: William Henry Parsey'. JMS, vol. 30, no. 129, April 1884, pp. 166–167.

'The Late C.A. Mercier'. JMS, vol. 67, no. 276, January 1921, p. 146.

Donkin, H. Bryan. 'Obituary: Charles Arthur Mercier'. *JMS*, vol. 66, no. 272, January 1920, pp. 1–10.

SECONDARY SOURCES

Ackerknecht, Erwin. 'Anticontagionism Between 1821 and 1867'. *Bulletin for the History of Medicine*, vol. 22, 1948, pp. 562–593.

Andrew Scull, *Madhouse: A Tragic Tale of Megalomania and Modern Medicine*, Yale University Press, 2005.

Andrews, J., and Digby, A., eds. *Perspectives on Class and Gender in the History of British and Irish Psychiatry*, Rodopoi, 2004, pp. 149–171.

Angel, Katherine, Edgar Jones, and Neve, M. *European Psychiatry on the Eve of War : Aubrey Lewis, the Maudsley Hospital, and the Rockefeller Foundation in the 1930s*. Wellcome Centre for the History of Medicine, 2003.

Ankeny, R.A. 'The Overlooked Role of asses in Causal Attribution in Medicine'. *Philosophy of Science*, vol. 81, no. 5, December 2014, pp. 999–1001.

Augstein, H.F. 'James Cowles Prichard's Anthropology: Remaking the Science of Man in Early Nineteenth Century Britain'. *Clio Medica*, vol. 52, 2016.

Augstein, H.F. 'JC Prichard's Concept of Moral Insanity—A Medical Theory of the Corruption of Human Nature'. *Medical History*, vol. 40, 1996, pp. 311–343.

Barfoot, M. 'David Skae: Resident Asylum Physician; Scientific General Practitioner of Insanity'. *Medical History*, no. 53, 2009, pp. 469–488.

Barfoot, M. '"To Ask the Suffrages of the Patrons": Thomas Laycock and the Edinburgh Chair of Medicine'. *Medical History*, Supplement no. 15, pp. 1–226.

Bartlett, Peter. The Poor Law of Lunacy: The Administration of Pauper Lunatics in Mid-Nineteenth Century England (with special Emphasis on Leicestershire and Rutland), PhD Thesis, UCL, 1993.

Bartlett, Peter, and David, Wright, eds. *Outside the Walls of the Asylum: The History of Care in the Community 1750–2000*, Athlone Press, 1999.

Bashford, Allison. 'Global Biopolitics and the History of World Health'. *History of the Human Sciences* vol. 19, no. 1, 2006, 67–88.

Bashford, Alison. *Global Population: History, Geopolitics, and Life on Earth*, Columbia University Press, 2014.

Beer, D., and Berrios, G. 'The Notion of Unitary Psychosis: A Conceptual History'. *History of Psychiatry*, vol. 5, 1994, pp. 13–36.

Bentall, Richard P. *Madness Explained: Psychosis and Human Nature*, Penguin, 2003.

Berrios, German. '19th Century Melancholia and Depression'. *British Journal of Psychiatry*, vol. 153, no. 3, pp. 298–304.

Berrios, German. 'Alzheimer's Disease: A Conceptual History'. *International Journal of Geriatric Psychiatry*, vol. 5, no. 6, 1990, pp. 355–365. Web.

Berrios, German. 'Dementia During the Seventeenth and Eighteenth Century'. *Psychological Medicine*, vol. 7, no. 4, November 1987, pp. 829–837.

Berrios, German. 'Early Electroconvulsive Therapy in Britain, France and Germany: A Conceptual History'. Berrios and Freeman eds., *150 years of British psychiatry. vol. 2, The Aftermath*, Athlone, 1996, pp. 3–15.

Berrios, German. 'Introduction to J.C. Prichard and the Concept of 'Moral Insanity''. *History of Psychiatry*, no. 10, 1999, pp. 111–126.

Berrios, German. *The History of Mental Symptoms: Descriptive Psychopathology Since the Nineteenth Century*, Cambridge University Press, 1996.

Berrios, German, and Freeman, H., eds. *150 Years of British Psychiatry: 1841–1991*, Gaskell, 1991.

Berrios, German, and Porter, Roy. *A History of Clinical Psychiatry: The Origin and History of Psychiatric Disorders*. Athlone, 1995.

Beveridge, Allan. 'Thomas Clouston and the Edinburgh School of Psychiatry'. G.E. Berrios and Hugh Freeman eds., *150 Years of British Psychiatry 1841–1991*, Gaskell, 1991, pp. 359–388.

Beveridge A.W., and Renvoize, E.B. 'Electricity: A History of Its Use in the Treatment of Mental Illness in Britain During the Second Half of the 19th Century'. *British Journal of Psychiatry*, vol. 153, January 1988, pp. 157–162.

Bewley, Thomas. *From Madness to Mental Disorder: A History of the Royal College of Psychiatrists*, RCPsych Publications, 2008.

Black, K. 'Psychiatry and the Medical Model'. E. Rubin and C. Zorumski eds., *Adult Psychiatry*, 2nd edition, Blackwell, 2005, pp. 3–15.

Blashfield, Roger K. *The Classification of Psychopathology*. Springer US, 1984.

Bolton, Derek, and Hill. J. *Mind, Meaning and Mental Disorder*. Oxford University Press, 2004.

Boorse, Christopher. 'Health as a Theoretical Concept'. *Philosophy of Science*, vol. 44, no. 4, 1977, pp. 542–573. Web. 15 July 2016.

Borowry, Iris. *Coming to Terms with World Health: The League of Nations Health Organisation 1921–1946*, Peter Lang, 2009.

Bowden, P., and Chetwynd, R.V. 'Pioneers in Forensic Psychiatry. Charles Arthur Mercier (1852–1919): Wit Without Understanding'. *Journal of Forensic Psychiatry*, vol. 5, no. 2, 1994, pp. 321–353.

Broughton, Trev Lynn. 'Henry Reeve (1813–1895), Translator and Magazine Editor'. *Oxford Dictionary of National Biography*, January 3rd, 2008.

Burnham, John C. 'Transnational History of Medicine after 1950: Framing and Interrogation from Psychiatric Journals'. *Medical History*, vol. 55, no. 1, pp. 3–26.

Busfield, J. *Men, Women and Madness: Understanding Gender and Mental Disorder*. Macmillan, 1996.

Busfield, J. 'The Female Malady? Men, Women and Madness in Nineteenth Century Britain'. *Medical Sociology*, vol. 28, no. 1, February 1994, pp. 259–277.

Bynum, W.F. 'Nosology'. W.F. Bynum and R. Porter eds., *Companion Encyclopedia of the History of Medicine*, pp. 335–355.

Bynum, W.F. 'Rationales for Therapy in British psychiatry 1780–1835'. *Medical History*, vol. 18, 1974, pp. 317–334.

Bynum, W.F. 'Tuke's *Dictionary* and Psychiatry at the Turn of the Century'. Berrios and Freeman eds., *150 Years of British Psychiatry: 1841–1991*, Gaskell, 1991, pp. 163–179.

Bynum, W.F., Porter, R., and Shepherd, M. *The Anatomy of Madness: Essays in the History of Psychiatry, vol. III: The Asylum and Its Psychiatry*, Routledge, 1988.

Canguilhem, George. *The Normal and the Pathological*, trans. Carolyn R. Fawcett, MIT Press, 1991.

Carpenter, Peter K. 'Thomas Arnold: A Provincial Psychiatrist in Georgian Britain'. *Medical History*, vol. 33, 1989, pp. 199–216.

Casper, Stephen T. *The Neurologists: A History of a Medical Speciality in Modern Britain*, c. 1789–2000. Manchester University Press, 2014.

Casper, Stephen T., and Jacyna, L. Stephen, eds. *The Neurological Patient in History*. University of Rochester Press, 2012.

Chamberlin, E., and Gilman, S., eds. *Degeneration: The Dark Side of Progress*. Columbia University Press, 1985.

Chaney, S. 'The Action of the Imagination: Daniel Hack-Tuke and Late Victorian Psycho-Therapeutics'. *History of the Human Sciences*, vol. 30, no. 2, pp. 17–33.

Cherry, Steven. *Mental Health Care in Modern England: The Norfolk Lunatic Asylum, St Andrew's Hospital, 1810–1998*. Boydell P., 2003.

Clark, M.J. '"Morbid Introspection", Unsoundness of Mind, and British Psychological Medicine c.1830–1900'. Bynum, Porter and Shepherd eds., *The Anatomy of Madness: Essays in the History of Psychiatry: vol. 3, The Asylum and its Psychiatry*, Tavistock, 1988, pp. 71–101.

Clarke, M.J. 'The Rejection of Psychological Approaches to Mental Disorder in Late Nineteenth Century British Psychiatry'. Andrew Scull ed., *Mad Houses, Mad Doctors and Madmen: The Social History of Psychiatry in the Victorian Era*, Athlone, 1981.

Clifford Rose, F. 'William Cullen'. *History of British Neurology*, Imperial College Press, 2011,

Compton, Wilson M., and Guze, Samual B. 'The Neo-Kraepelinian Revolution in Psychiatric Diagnosis'. *European Archives of Psychiatry and Clinical Neuroscience*, vol. 245, no. 4–5, 1995, pp. 196–201.

Conrad, Peter. *The Medicalization of Society : On the Transformation of Human Conditions into Treatable Disorders*, Johns Hopkins University Press, 2007.

Cooper, Rachel. *Classifying Madness: A Philosophical Examination of the Diagnostic and Statistical Manual of Mental Disorders*, Springer, 2005.

Cooper, Rachel. 'Disease.' Studies in History and Philosophy of Science Part C: Studies in *History and Philosophy of Biological and Biomedical Sciences* vol. 33, no. 2, 2002, pp. 263–282.

Cooper, Rachel. 'Understanding the DSM-5: Stasis and Change'. *History of Psychiatry*, vol. 29, no. 1, pp. 49–65.

Cooper, Rachel. 'What Is Wrong with the DSM?'. *History of Psychiatry*, vol. 15, no. 1, February 2004, pp. 5–25.

Cooper, Rachel. 'Why Hacking Is Wrong About Human Kinds'. *The British Journal for the Philosophy of Science* vol. 55, no. 1, 2004, 73–85.

Cooter, Roger. 'Phrenology and British Alienists c.1825–1845: Part II: Doctrine and Practice'. *Medical History*, vol. 20 no. 2, April 1976, pp. 135–151

Cooter, Roger, and Stein, Claudia. *Writing History in the Age of Biomedicine*. New Haven: Yale University Press, 2013.

Copeland, J.R.M. 'Classification and the British Glossary of Mental Disorders'. *British Journal of Psychiatry*, vol. 119, no. 551, October 1971, pp. 413–418.

Croft, Hazel. 'Rethinking Civilian Neurosis in the Second World War'. Peter Leese and Jason Couthamel eds., *Traumatic Memories of the Second World* War, pp. 95–117

Crossley, D. 'The Introduction of Leucotomy: A British Case History'. *History of Psychiatry*, vol. 4, 1993, pp. 553–564.

Crowther, M. 'From Workhouse to NHS Hospital in Britain 1929–1948.' Hillam and Bone eds., *The Poor Law and After*, Liverpool: Liverpool Medical History Society, 1999, pp. 38–49.

Crowther, M. *Social Policy in Britain 1914–1939*. Macmillan Education, 1988.

Crowther, M.A. *The Workhouse System 1834–1929: The History of an English Social Institution*, Methuen, 1983.

Cunningham, Andrew. 'Identifying Disease in the Past: Cutting the Gordian Knot'. *Asclepio*, vol. 54, 2002 pp. 13–34.

Daston, Lorraine. *The Empire of Chance: How Probability Changed Science and Everyday Life*, Cambridge University Press, 1989.

Daston, Lorraine, and Galison, Peter. *Objectivity*. Zone Books, 2007.

Dawson, W.R. 'Notes on Two Cases illustrating the Difference Between Katatonia and Melancholia Attonita'. *JMS*, vol. 49 no. 207, 1903, pp. 686–689.

Decker, H.S. 'How Kraepelinian Was Kraepelin? How Kraepelinian Are the Neo-Kraepelinians? From Emil Kraepelin to DSM-III.' *History of Psychiatry* vol. 18, no. 3, 2007, pp. 337–360.

Demazeux, Steeves. 'The Ideal of Scientific Progress and the DSM'. Steeves Demazeux and Patrick Singy eds., *The DSM-5 in Perspective: Philosophical Reflections on the Psychiatric Babel*, Springer, 2015, pp. 3–24.

Desrosières, Alain. *The Politics of Large Numbers: A History of Statistical Reasoning*, Harvard University Press, 1998.

Dicks, H.V. *Fifty Years of the Tavistock Clinic*. Routledge & Kegan Paul, 1970.

Digby, Anne. *Madness, Morality, and Medicine: A Study of the York Retreat, 1796–1914*, Cambridge University Press, 1985.
Digby, Anne. 'The Changing Profile of a Nineteenth-Century Asylum: The York Retreat'. *Psychological Medicine*, vol. 14, no. 4, 1984, pp. 739–748.
Dixon, Thomas. *From Passions to Emotions: The Creation of a Secular Physiological Category*, Cambridge University Press, 2003.
Dixon, Thomas. 'Patients and Passions: Languages of Medicine and Emotion, 1789–1850'. Fay Bound Alberti ed., *Medicine, Emotion, and Disease, 1700–1950*, Palgrave Macmillan, 2006.
Doroslow, D.B. 'Performing a Cure for Schizophrenia: Insulin Coma Therapy on the Wards'. *Journal of the History of Medicine and Allied Sciences*, vol. 62, 2007, pp. 213–243.
Dowbiggin, 'Delusional Diagnosis? The History of Paranoia as a Disease Concept in the Modern Era'. *History of Psychiatry*, vol. 9, 2000, pp. 37–69.
Dyde, Sean. 'Cullen, a Cautionary Tale'. *Medical History*, vol. 59, no. 2, 2015, pp. 222–240.
Eghigian, G. 'A Drifting Concept for an Unruly Menace: A History of Psychopathy in Germany'. *ISIS*, vol. 106, no. 2, 2015, pp. 283–309.
Eghigian, G., ed. *The Routledge History of Madness and Mental Health*, Routledge, 2017.
Eldergill, Anselm. *Mental Health Review Tribunals: Law and Practice*. London: Sweet and Maxwell, 1998.
Ellis, Robert. 'The Asylum, the Poor law, and a Reassessment of the Four-Shilling Grant: Admissions to the County Asylums of Yorkshire in the Nineteenth Century'. *Social History of Medicine*, vol. 19, no. 1, 2006, pp. 55–71.
Engstrom, Eric J. *Clinical Psychiatry in Imperial Germany*, Cornell University Press, 2003.
Engstrom, Eric J. 'Emil Kraepelin: Psychiatry and Public Affairs in Wilhelmine Germany'. *History of Psychiatry* vol. 2, no. 6, 1991, pp. 111–32.
Engstrom, Eric J. '"On the Question of Degeneration" by Emil Kraepelin (1908)'. *History of Psychiatry*, vol. 18, no. 3, 2007, pp. 389–98.
Ewan, John H. *A Handbook of Psychiatry*. William Wood and Company, 1934.
Fink, Max, and Taylor, Michael A. *Endocrine Psychiatry: Solving the Riddle of Melancholia*, Oxford University Press, 2010.
Finn, Michael Anthony. The West Riding Lunatic Asylum and the Making of the Modern Brain Sciences in the Nineteenth Century, PhD Thesis, University of Leeds, 2012.
Fleck, Ludwik. *Genesis and Development of a Scientific Fact*, trans. Fred Bradley, Robert K. Merton and Thaddeaus J. Trenn, University of Chicago Press, 2008.
Foucault, Michel. *Discipline and Punish: The Birth of the Prison*, Penguin, 1991.

Foucault, Michel. *Madness and Civilisation: A History of Insanity in the Age of Reason*, trans. Richard Howard, Routledge, 1989.
Foucault, Michel. The *Birth of the Clinic: An Archaeology of Medical Perception*, trans. A.M. Sheridan, Routledge, 1989.
Foucault, Michel. *The Order of Things: An Archaeology of the Human Sciences*, trans. Alan Sheridan, Routledge, 2002.
Freis, David. *Psycho-Politics Between the World Wars: Psychiatry and Society in Germany, Austria, and Switzerland*, Palgrave, 2019.
Gadamer, Hans-Georg. *Truth and Method*, trans. Joel Weinshamer and Donald G. Marshall, London: Bloomsbury, 2013.
Gaukroger, Stephen. *The Collapse of Mechanism and the Rise of Sensibility: Science and the Shaping of Modernity, 1680–1760*, Oxford University Press, 2010.
Gaukroger, Stephen. *The Natural and the Human: Science and the Shaping of Modernity, 1739–1841*, Oxford University Press, 2016.
Goffman, Erving. *Asylums: Essays on the Social Situation of Mental Patients and Other Inmates*, Penguin, 1991.
Goldstein, Jan. *Console and Classify: The French Psychiatric Profession in the nineteenth Century*, Cambridge University Press, 1988.
Graham Richards. 'Psychology and the Churches in Britain 1919–39: Symptoms of Conversion'. *History of the Human Sciences* vol. 13, no. 2, 2000, pp. 57–84.
Greenberg, Gary. *The Book of Woe: The DSM and the Unmaking of Psychiatry*, Scribe, 2013.
Grob, Gerald N. 'Review: Madness to Mental Illness: A History of the Royal College of Psychiatrists'. *Journal of the History of Medicine and Allied Sciences*, vol. 67, no. 3, July 2012, pp. 509–510.
Guthrie, Douglas. *The Medical School of Edinburgh*, Oliver and Boyd, 1964.
Hacking, Ian. *Historical Ontology*. Harvard University Press, 2002.
Hacking, Ian. 'Lost in the Forest: A Review of the DSM-5'. *LRB*, vol. 35 no. 15, August 8th, 2013, pp. 7–8.
Hacking, Ian. *Mad Travelers: Reflections on the Reality of Transient Mental Illnesses*, Harvard University Press, 2002.
Hacking, Ian. *Rewriting the Soul: Multiple Personality and the Sciences of Memory*, Harvard University Press, 1998.
Hacking, Ian. *The Taming of Chance*, Palgrave, 1990.
Hare, E. 'Was Insanity on the Increase?'. *BJP*, vol. 142, no. 5, May 1983, pp. 439–455.
Hayward, Rhodri. 'Germany and the Making of 'English' Psychiatry: The Maudsley Hospital 1908–1939'. Volker Roelcke, Paul J. Weindling and Louise Westwood eds., *International Relations in Psychiatry: Britain, Germany and the United States to World War II*, University of Rochester Press, 2013, pp. 67–90.

Hayward, Rhodri. *The Transformation of the Psyche in British Primary Care 1880–1970*, Bloomsbury, 2014.

Healy, David. *Mania: A Short History of Bipolar Disorder*, John Hopkins University Press, 2008.

Hecker, E. cited in Kendler, K., and Engstrom, E. 'Kahlbaum, Hecker, and Kraepelin and the Transition from Psychiatry Symptom Complexes to Empirical Disease Forms'. *American Journal of Psychiatry*, vol. 174, no. 2, February 1st, 2017, pp. 102–109.

Heidberger, Michael. 'Naturphilosophie'. *The Routledge Dictionary of Philosophy*, Taylor and Francis, 1998.

Henderson, David Kennedy. *The Evolution of Psychiatry in Scotland*, E. & S. Livingstone, 1964.

Hess, Volker, and Mendelsohn, Andrew J. 'Case and Series: Medical Knowledge and Paper Technology, 1600–1900'. *History of Science*, vol. 48, no. 3, 2010, pp. 287–314.

Hide, Louise. 'In Plain Sight: Open Doors, Mixed-sex Wards and Sexual Abuse in English Psychiatric Hospitals, 1950s–Early 1990s'. *Social History of Medicine*, vol. 31, no. 4, November 2018, pp. 732–753.

Hill, S.A. 'Mania, Dementia and Melancholia in the 1870s: Admissions to a Cornwall Asylum'. *Journal of the Royal Society of Medicine*, vol. 96, no. 7, July 2003, pp. 361–363.

Hirschmüller, Albrecht. 'The Development of Psychiatry and Neurology in the Nineteenth Century', trans. Magda Whitrow. *History of Psychiatry*, vol. 10, 1999, pp. 395–423.

Hoenig, J. 'Schizophrenia'. Berrios and Porter eds., *A History of Clinical Psychiatry: The Origin and History of Psychiatric Disorders*, Routledge, 1995, pp. 336–348.

Hoff, P. 'Kraepelin'. Berrios and Porter eds., *A History of Clinical Psychiatry: The Origin and History of Psychiatric Disorders*, Routledge, 1995, pp. 261–279.

Honigsbaum, Frank. *Health, Happiness and Security*, London: Routledge, 1989.

Huertas, R. 'Esquirol: Between Doctrine and Clinical Practice'. *History of Psychiatry*, vol. 19, no. 2, 2008, pp. 123–140.

Hunter, Richard, and McAlpine, Ida. *Three Hundred Years of Psychiatry 1535–1860: A History Presented in Selected English Texts*, LLC, 2013.

Irving, Allen. *Brock Chisholm: Doctor to the World*, Fitzhenry & Whiteside, 1998.

Jablensky, Assen. 'Living in a Kraepelinian World: Kraepelin's Impact on Modern Psychiatry'. *History of Psychiatry*, vol. 18, no. 3, 2007, pp. 381 –88.

Jackson, Mark. *The Borderland of Imbecility: Medicine, Society and the Fabrication of the Feeble Mind in Late Victorian England*, Manchester University Press, 2000.

Jacyna, L.S. Scientific Naturalism in Victorian Britain: an Essay in the Social History of Ideas, Unpublished Ph.D. Thesis, University of Edinburgh, 1980.

Jacyna, L.S. 'Somatic Theories of Mind and the Interests of Medicine in Britain, 1850–1879'. *Medical History*, vol. 26, no. 233–258.

Jacyna, L.S. 'The Physiology of Mind, the Unity of Nature, and the Moral Order in Victorian Thought'. *British Journal for the History of Science*, vol. 14, 1981, pp. 109-132.

Jansson, Åsa. 'From Statistics to Diagnostics: Medical Certificates, Melancholia, and 'Suicidal Propensities'. Victorian Psychiatry'. *Journal of Social History*, vol. 46, no. 3, Spring 2013, pp. 716–731.

Jansson, Åsa. 'Mood Disorders and the Brain: Depression, Melancholia, and the Historiography of Psychiatry'. *Medical History*, vol. 55, no. 3, July 2011, pp. 393–399

Jenner, F.A. 'Erwin Stengel: A Personal Memoir'. G. Berrios and H. Freeman eds., *150 Years of British Psychiatry: 1841–1991*, Gaskell, 1991.

Jones, David. *Disordered Personalities and Crime: An Analysis of the History of Moral Insanity*, Routledge, 2016.

Jones, Edgar. 'An Atmosphere of Cure: Frederick Mott, Shell Shock and the Maudsley'. *History of Psychology*, vol. 25, 2014, pp. 412–421 (p. 415)

Jones, Edgar. '"The Gut War": Functional Somatic Disorders in the UK During the Second World War'. *History of the Human Sciences*, vol. 25, no. 5, 2012, pp. 30–48.

Jones, Kathleen. *Asylums and After: A Revised History of the Mental Health Services: From the Early 18th Century to the 1990s*, Athlone Press, 1993.

Jones, Kathleen. 'Law and Mental Health: Sticks or Carrots'. Berrios and Freeman eds., *150 Years of British Psychiatry*, Gaskell, 1991, pp. 89–102.

Jones, Kathleen. *Mental Health and Social Policy, 1845–1959*, Routledge, 1960.

Jones, Kevin Matthew. 'The Disappearance of "Medical Psychology" and the Controversy over the Medical Section During the Early 1950s'. *History and Philosophy of Psychology*, vol. 19, no. 1, 2018.

Kaufmann, Doris. 'Science as Cultural Practice: Psychiatry in the First World War and Weimar Germany'. *Journal of Contemporary History* vol. 34, no. 1, 1999, pp. 125–44.

Kendell, R.E., et al., 'Diagnostic Criteria of American and British Psychiatrists'. *Archives of General Psychiatry*, vol. 5, 1971, pp. 123–130.

Kendig, Catherine, ed. *Natural Kinds and Classification in Scientific Practice*, Routledge, 2016.

Kendler, K. 'David Skae and His Nineteenth Century Etiologic Psychiatric Diagnostic System: Looking Forward by Looking Back'. *Molecular Psychiatry*, vol. 22, pp. 802–807.

Kevles, David. *In the Name of Eugenics: Genetics and the Uses of Human Heredity*, University of California Press, 1995.

Klein, R. *The New Politics of the NHS: From Creation to Reinvention*, 3rd edition, Longman, 1995.

Koselleck, Reinhart. *The Practice of Conceptual History: Timing History, Spacing Concepts*, trans. Todd Samuel Presner et al., Stanford University, 2002.

Kuhn, Thomas S. *The Structure of Scientific Revolutions: 50th Anniversary Edition*, The University of Chicago Press, 2012.

Kutchins, Herb, and Kirk, Stuart A. *Making Us Crazy: DSM: The Psychiatric Bible and the Creation of Mental Disorders*, Free Press, 1997.

Laing, R.D., and Easterton A. *Sanity, Madness and the Family: Families of Schizophrenics*, Penguin, 1964.

Lawlor, Clark. *From Melancholia to Prozac: A History of Depression*, Oxford University Press, 2012.

Leff, Alex. 'Clean Round the Bend—The Etymology of Jargon and Slang Terms for Madness'. *History of Psychiatry*, vol. 9, 2000, pp. 155–162.

Leigh, Denis. 'James Cowles Prichard'. Proceedings of the Royal Society of Medicine: Section of Psychiatry with Section of the History of Medicine, 1955, pp. 586–590.

Leonhard, Perris C. 'Cycloid Psychosis: Clinical Section'. Berrios and Porter eds., *A History of Clinical Psychiatry: The Origin and History of Psychiatric Disorders*, Routledge, 1995, pp. 421–430.

Lewis, Aubrey. 'British Psychiatry in the First Half of the Nineteenth Century: Philippe Pinel and the English'. *Proceedings of the Royal Society of Medicine*, vol. 48, February 1955, pp. 581– 586 (p. 582).

Linden, S. and Jones, E. 'German Battle Casualties: The Treatment of Functional Somatic Disorders During World War 1'. *Journal of the History of Medicine*, vol. 68, no. 4, October 2013, pp. 627–58.

Lock, Margaret. 'DSM III as a Culture-Bound Construct: Commentary on Culture-Bound Syndromes and International Disease Classifications'. *Culture, Medicine and Society*, vol. 11, 1987, pp. 35–42.

Lovie, A.D. 'Three Steps to Heaven: How the British Psychological Society Found its Place in the Sun'. G.C. Bunn, A.D. Lovie, and G.D. Richards eds., *Psychology in Britain: Historical Essays and Personal Reflections*, BPS Books, 2004.

Löwy, Ilana. 'Labelled Bodies: Classification of Disease and the Medical Way of Knowing'. *History of Science*, vol. 49, no. 3, 2011, pp. 299–315.

Lum, G. 'Making Sense of Knowing-How and Knowing-That'. Christopher Winch and Mark Addis eds., *Education and Expertise*, Wiley, 2008, pp. 117–137.

Mack, A.H., et al. 'A Brief History of Psychiatric Classification: From the Ancients to DSM-IV'. *Psychiatric Clinics of North America*, vol. 17, no. 3, September 1994, pp. 515–523.

Mackenzie, C. A Family Asylum: A History of the Private Madhouse at Ticehurst in Sussex, 1792–1917, PhD thesis, UCL, 1986.

Magnello, Eileen and Hardy, Ann, eds. *The Road to Medical Statistics*, Rodopi, 2002.

Marland, Hilary. *Dangerous Motherhood: Insanity and Childbirth in Victorian Britain*, Palgrave, 2004.

Marland, Hilary. '"Destined to Be a Perfect Recovery": The Confinement of Puerperal Insanity in the Nineteenth Century'. Melling and Forsythe eds., *Insanity, Institutions and Society, 1800–1914: A Social History of Madness in Comparative Perspective*, Routledge, 1999, pp. 137–156.

Marx, Otto. 'What Is the History of Psychiatry?' *History of Psychiatry*, vol. 3, 1992, pp. 279–292.

McCandless, P. 'Liberty and Lunacy: The Victorians and Wrongful Confinement'. Andrew Scull ed., *Madhouses, Mad-doctors, and Madmen*, 339–362.

Mellettt, D.J. 'Bureaucracy and Mental Illness: The Commissioners in Lunacy 1845–1890'. *Medical History*, vol. 21, pp. 221–250.

Melling, Joseph, and Forsythe, Bill. *The Politics of Madness: the State, Insanity and Society in England, 1845–1914*, Routledge, 2006.

Micale, Mark S. 'Hysteria and Its Historiography: the Future Perspective'. *History of Psychiatry*, vol. 1, 1990, pp. 33–124.

Micale, Mark S. 'On the 'Disappearance' of Hysteria: A Study in the Clinical Deconstruction of a Diagnosis'. *Isis*, vol. 84, no. 3, 1993, pp. 496–526.

Micale, Mark S. 'The Ten Most Important Changes in Psychiatry Since World War II'. *History of Psychiatry*, vol. 25, no. 4, 2014, pp. 485–491.

Micale, Mark S., and Paul Lerner, eds. *Traumatic Pasts: History, Psychiatry, and Trauma in the Modern Age, 1870–1930*. Cambridge University Press, 2001.

Michael, P. *Care and Treatment of the Mentally Ill in North Wales, 1800–2000*. University of Wales Press, 2003.

Millard, Chris. 'Concepts, Diagnosis and the History of Medicine: Historicising Ian Hacking and Munchausen Syndrome'. *Social History of Medicine*, vol. 30, no. 3, August 2017, pp. 567–589.

Misbach, J., and Stam, Henderikus J. 'Medicalizing Melancholia: Exploring Profiles of Psychiatric Professionalization'. *Journal of the History of the Human Sciences*, vol. 42, no. 1, pp. 41–59.

Mol, Annmarie. *The Body Multiple: Ontology in Medical Practice*, Duke University Press, 2002.

Moncrieff, Joanna. *The Myth of the Chemical Cure: A Critique of Psychiatric Drug Treatment*, Palgrave Macmillan, 2007.

Murphy, Elaine. 'The Administration of Insanity in England 1800 to 1870'. Roy Porter and David Wright eds., *The Confinement of the Insane: International Perspectives, 1800–1965*. Cambridge University Press, 2003.

Murphy, Terrence D. 'Medical Knowledge and Statistical Methods in Early Nineteenth-Century France'. *Medical History*, vol. 25, 1981, 301–319.

Noll, Richard. *American Madness: The Rise and Fall of Dementia Praecox*, Harvard University Press, 2011.

O'Neal, John C. 'Understanding and Interpreting Confusion: Philippe Pinel and the Invention of Psychiatry'. *Lumen*, no. 26, 2007, pp. 243–258.

Pichot, Pierre. 'Nosological Models in Psychiatry'. *British Journal of Psychiatry*, vol. 164, no. 2, February 1994, pp. 232–240.

Pick, Daniel. *Faces of Degeneration: A European Disorder c.1848–1918*, Cambridge University Press, 1993.

Pickersgill, Martyn. 'Debating DSM-5: Diagnosis and the Sociology of Critique'. *Journal of Medical Ethics*, 2014, no. 40, pp. 521–525.

Pickersgill, Martyn. 'From Psyche to Soma? Changing Accounts of Antisocial Personality Disorders in the *American Journal of Psychiatry*'. *History of Psychiatry*, vol. 21, no. 3, pp. 294–311.

Pickren, W., and Fowler, R. 'Professional Organisations'. Freidheim and Weiner, eds. *Handbook of Psychiatry, Volume 1: History of Psychiatry*, Hoboken: John Wiley & Sons, 2003, pp. 535–554.

Pomata, G. 'The Medical Case Narrative: Distant Reading of an Epistemic Genre'. *Literature and Medicine*, vol. 32, no. 1, 2014, pp. 1–23.

Pons, J.H., and Berrios G. 'J.H. Pons on "Sympathetic Insanity": With an Introduction by G.E. Berrios'. *History of Psychiatry*, vol. 25, no. 3, September 2014, pp. 364–76.

Porter, D. 'Public Health and Centralisation: the Victorian British State'. *Health, Civilisation and the State: A History of Public Health from Ancient to Modern Times*, pp. 117–127.

Porter, R. *Mind-forg'd manacles : A History of Madness in England from the Restoration to the Regency*, Penguin, 1990.

Porter, R. 'Psychiatry'. *The Greatest Benefit to Mankind*, Harper Collins, 1997.

Porter, R. *The Greatest Benefit to Mankind: A Medical History of Humanity from Antiquity to the Present*, Fontana Press, 1999.

Porter, R. 'The Patient's View: Doing Medical History from Below'. *Theory and Society*, vol. 14, no. 2, 1985, pp. 175–98.

Porter, R. and Jones C., eds. *Reassessing Foucault: Power Medicine and the Body*, Routledge, 1994.

Porter, T. *Genetics in the Madhouse: The Unknown History of Human Heredity*, Princeton University Press, 2018.

Porter, T. *Trust in Numbers: The Pursuit of Objectivity in Science and Public Life*, Princeton University Press, 1995.

Price, Elfed Huw. 'Do Brains Think? Comparative Anatomy and the End of the Great Chain of Being in 19th-Century Britain'. *History of the Human Sciences*, vol. 25, no. 3, pp. 32–50.

Quirk, Vivian, and Gaudillière, Jean-Paul. 'The Era of Biomedicine: Science, Medicine, and Public Health in Britain and France after the Second World War'. *Medical History*, vol. 52, pp. 441–452.

Renwick, C. *Bread for All*, Palgrave, 2017.

Richard Foulkes, 'William Terriss'. *Oxford Dictionary of National Biography*, Oxford University Press.

Roelcke, Volker. 'Biologizing Social Facts: An Early 20th Century Debate on Kraepelin's Concepts of Culture, Neurasthenia, and Degeneration'. *Culture, Medicine, and Psychiatry*, vol. 21, no. 4, 1997, pp. 383–403.

Rogers, A., and Pilgrim, D. *Mental health policy in Britain*, Basingstoke: Palgrave, 2001.

Rose, Clifford F. 'William Cullen'. *History of British Neurology*, Imperial College Press, 2011, pp. 67–68.

Rose, N. *Governing the Soul: Shaping of the Private Self*, Free Association Books, 1999.

Rosenberg, Charles E. 'Contested Boundaries: Psychiatry, Disease, and Diagnosis'. *Perspectives in Biology and Medicine*, vol. 49, no. 3, 2006, pp. 407–424.

Rosenberg, Charles E. *Explaining Epidemics and Other Studies in the History of Medicine*, Cambridge University Press, 1992.

Rosenberg, Charles E. 'The Tyranny of Diagnosis: Specific Entities and Individual Experience'. *The Milbank Quarterly*, vol. 80, no. 2, June 2002, pp. 237–260.

Rousseau, George S. 'Depression's Forgotten Genealogy: Notes Towards a History of Depression'. *History of Psychiatry*, vol. 11, 2000, pp. 71–106.

Sapolsky, Robert. *Behave: The Biology of Humans at Our Best and Worst*, Penguin, 2017.

Saunders, J. 'Quarantining the Weak-Minded: Psychiatric Definitions of Degeneracy and the Late-Victorian Asylum'. W.F. Bynum, R. Porter and M. Shepherd eds., *The Anatomy of Madness: Essays in the History of Psychiatry: vol. 3, The Asylum and Its Psychiatry*, Tavistock, 1988, pp. 273–296.

Scull, A. *Decarceration: Community Treatment and the Deviant: A Radical View*, Polity, 1984.

Scull, A. 'The Rise of the Asylum'. *The Most Solitary of Afflictions: Madness and Society in Britain 1700–1900*, Yale University Press, 1993, pp. 3–45.

Scull, A. 'The Social History of Psychiatry in the Victorian Era'. Andrew Scull ed., *Mad Houses, Mad Doctors and Madmen: The Social History of Psychiatry in the Victorian Era*, Athlone, 1981, pp. 5–33.

Scull, A. 'Was Insanity Increasing? A Response to Edward Hare'. *BJP*, vol. 144, no. 4, April 1984, pp. 432–436.

Sellers, Laura Mary. Managing Convicts, Understanding Criminals: Medicine and the Development of English Convict Prisons, c.1837–1886, PhD thesis, University of Leeds, July 2017.

Shepherd, Ben. *A War of Nerves: Soldiers and Psychiatrists in the Twentieth Century: 1914–1994*, Harvard University Press, 2000.

Shepherd, Ben. "Pitiless Psychology': The Role of Prevention in British Military Psychiatry in the Second World War'. *History of Psychiatry*, vol. 10, October 1999, pp. 491–524.

Shepherd, Michael. 'Psychiatric Journals and the Evolution of Psychological Medicine'. *Psychological Medicine*, vol. 22, 1992, pp. 15–25.

Shorter, Edward. *A History of Psychiatry: From the Age of the Asylum to the Age of Prozac*, Wiley and Sons, 1997.

Shorter, Edward. 'The History of Nosology and the Rise of the *Diagnostic and Statistical Manual of Mental Disorder*'. *Dialogues in Clinical Neuroscience*, vol. 17, no. 1, pp. 59–67.

Showalter, E. *The Female Malady: Women, Madness and English Culture, 1830–1980*, Virago, 1987.

Smith, Roger. *Between Mind and Nature: A History of Psychology*, Reaktion Books, 2013.

Smith, Roger. 'Legal Frameworks for Psychiatry'. Berrios and Freeman eds., *150 Years of British Psychiatry*, Gaskell, 1991, pp. 137–151.

Smith, Roger. 'The Boundary Between Insanity and Criminal Responsibility in Nineteenth-Century England'. Andrew Scull ed., *Mad Houses, Mad Doctors and Madmen: The Social History of Psychiatry in the Victorian Era*, Athlone, 1981, pp. 363–377.

Smith, Roger. 'The History of Psychological Categories'. *Studies in History and Philosophy of Biological and Biomedical Sciences*, vol. 36, 2004, p. 55–95.

Star, S.L. *Regions of the Mind: Brain Research and the Quest for Scientific Certainty*, Stanford University Press, 1989.

Stein, Dan J., Phillips, Katharine A., Bolton, Derek, Fulford, K.W.M., Sadler, John Z., and Kendler, K. 'What Is a Mental/Psychiatric Disorder? From DSM-IV to DSM-V'. *Psychological Medicine*, vol. 40, no. 11, November 2010, pp. 1759–1765.

Steinberg, H. 'The Sin in the Aetiological Concept of Johnann Christian Heinroth'. *History of Psychiatry*, vol. 5, no. 4, December 2004, pp. 299–344.

Suzuki, Akihito, 'Framing Psychiatric Subjectivity: Doctor, Patient and Record-Keeping at Bethlem in the Nineteenth Century'. Joseph Melling and Bill Forsythe eds., *Insanity, Institutions and Society, 1800–1914: A Social History of Madness in Comparative Perspective*, Routledge, 1999.

Szaz, T. 'The Myth of Mental Illness'. *American Psychologist*, vol. 15, no. 2, pp. 113–118.

Szasz, T. *The Myth of Mental Illness: Foundations of a Theory of Personal Conduct*, Harper, 2010.

Szreter, Simon. *Fertility, Class and Gender in Britain, 1860–1940*, Cambridge, 1996.

Takabayashi, A. 'Surviving the Lunacy Act of 1890: English Psychiatrists and Professional Development During the Early Twentieth Century'. *Medical History*, vol. 61, no. 2, pp. 246–269.

Taylor, Barbara. *The Last Asylum*, Penguin, 2014.

Thomson, M. 'Mental Hygiene in Britain During the First Half of the Twentieth Century: The Limits of International Influence'. Volker Roelcke, Paul Weindling, and Louise Westwood eds., *International Relations in Psychiatry: Britain, Germany, and the United States to World War II*. University of Rochester Press, 2010, pp. 134–55.

Timms, Noel. *Psychiatric social work in Great Britain, 1939–1962*, Humanities Press, 1964.

Tomes, Nancy. 'The Great Restraint Controversy: A Comparative Perspective on Anglo-American Psychiatry in the Nineteenth Century'. *Anatomy of Madness*, vol. III, pp. 190–225.

Toms, Jonathan. *Mental Hygiene and Psychiatry in Modern Britain*, Palgrave, 2013.

Toms, Jonathan. 'Political Dimensions of "the Psychosocial": The 1948 International Congress on Mental Health and the Mental Hygiene Movement'. *History of the Human Sciences*, vol. 25, no. 5, 2012, pp. 91–106.

Topham, Jonathan. 'Science, Print, and Crossing Borders: Importing French Science Books into Britain, 1789–1815'. D.N. Livingstone and C.W.J. Withers eds., *Geographies of Nineteenth-Century Science*, University of Chicago Press, 2011, pp. 311–344.

Turner, Trevor. *A Diagnostic Analysis of the Casebooks of Ticehurst House Asylum, 1845–1890*, Cambridge University Press, 1992.

Turner, Trevor. 'Henry Maudsley: Psychiatrist, Philosopher and Entrepreneur'. *Psychological Medicine*, vol. 18, no. 3, August 1988, pp. 551–574.

Turner, Trevor. 'Not Worth Power and Shot: The Public Profile of the Medico-Psychological Association c.1851–1914'. Berrios and Freeman eds., *150 Years of British Psychiatry*, Gaskell, 1991, pp. 3–18.

Wakefield, Jerome C. 'The Concept of Mental Disorder: Diagnostic Implications of the Harmful Dysfunction Analysis'. *World Psychiatry*, vol. 36, no. 3, October 2007, pp. 149–156.

Wallace, Edwin R., and Gach, John, eds., *History of Psychiatry and Medical Psychology: with an Epilogue on Psychiatry and the Mind-Body Relation*, Springer, 2008.

Wallis, Jennifer. *Investigating the Body in the Victorian Asylum Doctors, Patients, and Practices*, Palgrave Macmillan, 2017.

Wallis, Jennifer. 'The Bones of the Insane'. *History of Psychiatry*, vol. 24, no. 2, 2013, 196–211.

Webster, C. 'Psychiatry and the early National Health Service: the role of the Mental Health Standing Advisory Committee'. Berrios and Freeman eds., *150 Years of British Psychiatry*, Gaskell, 1991, pp. 103–106.

Webster, C. *The Health Services Since the War vol. 1*, HMSO, 1996.

Weiner, D.B. 'Betrayal! The 1806 Translation of Pinel's *Traité' medico-philosophique sur l'aliénation mentale, ou la manie*'. *Generus*, vol. 57, 2000, pp. 42–50.

Weiner, D.B. 'The Madman in the Light of Reason. Enlightenment Psychiatry: Part II. Alienists, Treatises, and the Psychologic Approach in the Era of Pinel'. Edwin R. Wallace and John Gach eds., *History of Psychiatry and Medical Psychology: With an Epilogue on Psychiatry and the Mind-Body Relation*, pp. 281–304.

Werlinder, H. 'Psychopathy: A History of Concepts'. *Series Acta Universitatis Upsaliensis*, no. 6, Almqvist & Wiksell, 1978, pp. 218–249.

Wilson, A. 'On the History of Disease Concepts: The Case of Pleurisy'. *History of Science*, vol. 38, no. 3, 2000, pp. 271–319.

Wilson, A. 'Viewpoint: Science's Imagined Pasts'. *ISIS*, vol. 108, no. 4, December 2017, pp. 814–826.

Woods, Angela. *The Sublime Object of Psychiatry: Schizophrenia in Clinical and Cultural Theory*, Oxford, 2011.

Woods, Evelyn A. and Carlson, Eric T. 'The Psychiatry of Philippe Pinel'. *Bulletin of the History of Medicine*, vol. 35, no. 14, 1961, pp. 14–25.

Wright, David. 'Delusions of Gender?: Lay Identifications and Clinical Diagnosis of Insanity in Victorian England'. *Sex and Seclusion, Class and Custody*, Clio Medica, 2003, pp. 149–176.

Wright, David. 'The Certification of Insanity in Nineteenth-Century England and Wales'. *History of Psychiatry*, vol. 9, no. 35, 1998, pp. 267–290.

Zilboorg, Gregory. *A History of Medical Psychology*, W.W. Norton, 1967.

Index

K. M. Jones, *Psychological Classification and Diagnosis in Asylum Statistics, 1800–1948*, Mental Health in Historical Perspective,
https://doi.org/10.1007/978-3-031-46154-5

FSC
www.fsc.org
MIX
Papier | Fördert
gute Waldnutzung
FSC® C083411

Kolibri 360 GmbH
Ferdinand-Jühlke-Straße 7
99095 Erfurt, Deutschland
produktsicherheit@kolibri360.de